NATURE DOCTORS

Pioneers in Naturopathic Medicine

Second Edition

Friedhelm Kirchfeld
&
Wade Boyle

NCNM Press • Portland, Oregon

Managing Editor: Nora J. Sande
Production and typography: Bergner Communications
Editing: Ronald L. Johnson and Howard Asinoff, ND
Indexing: Eileen Ridge
Cover Photograph: Father Kneipp, Archdukes Joseph and Francis Ferdinand of Austria. Taken from *Universal Naturopathic Encyclopedia Directory and Buyer' Guide: Year Book of Drugless Therapy for 1918-19, Volume 1.* Edited by Benedict Lust, ND, DO, DC, MD. 1918

First Edition 1994
Second Edition 2005—Second printing 2008

Published by NCNM Press
National College of Natural Medicine
049 SW Porter Street
Portland, Oregon 97201 USA
www.ncnm.edu

Printed in the United States of America
with recycled paper and soy ink.

International Standard Book Number (ISBN): 978-0-9771435-0-4
Library of Congress Control Number (LCCN): 2005931021

Dedicated to nature doctors everywhere
past, present and future

In Memoriam

Wade Francis Boyle, N.D.

(1945-1993)

Wade Boyle was born February 6, 1945 in Pittsburgh. He received a bachelor's degree in English from College of Wooster and a master of divinity from Hartford Seminary Foundation, Hartford, Connecticut. While working as a minister at a church in Hartford, he learned about a vegetarian diet, alternative medicine, and heard naturopathic medicine discussed on a radio talk show by Dr. S. G. Soderstrom. He sought treatment from Dr. Soderstrom and sent for a catalog from National College of Naturopathic Medicine in Portland. He then had a dream that he was with his family when his father had a heart attack and he did not know what to do. He awoke very upset about the helplessness he felt. He resolved to study naturopathy so he could take care of his family as well as his larger family—humanity.

Wade Boyle never thought that becoming a naturopathic physician would be a way of earning a living, but would simply provide him a means of learning about health and healing. He graduated from National College in 1983. For eight years, Wade served at the Mantell Clinic in Cranberry, Pennsylvania, outside Pittsburgh, using herbs, hydrotherapy and nutrition to treat thousands of chronically ill patients, many of them with cancer, the disease which eventually took his own life. Most recently he set up a practice in his hometown of East Palestine, Ohio. He taught at the Canadian College of Naturopathic Medicine and the Chautaqua Institution. He was a popular teacher in botanical medicine at conventions of the American Association of Naturopathic Physicians (AANP). At the 1993 AANP convention he received the President's Award for his contributions to naturopathic medicine.

Wade Boyle wrote a column on the history of naturopathic medicine for the Naturopathic Physician, and was an associate editor of Medical Herbalism. He founded Buckeye Naturopathic Press, which publishes books on herbal medicine and other naturopathic topics. He authored Lectures in Naturopathic Hydrotherapy with Dr. André Saine, which is used as a modern textbook in naturopathic colleges, Herb Doctors, short biographies of pioneers in nineteenth-century American botanical medicine, and Official Herbs, a book tracing the inclusion or exclusion of medicinal herbs in the various editions of the *U.S. Pharmacopoeia* between its first publication and

1990. He also edited and published Reading the Eye, Pulse and Tongue for the Indicated Remedy, a collection of articles by Eli Jones, MD, (1850-1933).

Wade Boyle has also contributed to the clinical practice of naturopathic botanical medicine, which he defined as "botanical medicine in support of nature cure" as opposed to "expecting the herb to do the work." He also developed a botanically-oriented physical examination, using various palpation techniques to find the indicated herbal remedy. He was the first to admit negative clinical results and because of this has introduced new insights about indications, contraindications, and adverse effects into the herbal materia medica.

> Those who knew Wade will remember his humility, his kindness, his wry sense of humor, his careful attention to both scholarly and clinical details, his passionate love of both nature cure and medicinal plants, and his desire to preserve these for humanity in an era dominated by reductionist medical science.
> (Bergner 1993, 11 & Traub 1993, 23).

Acknowledgments

Acknowledgments may be of little interest to the general reader, but they offer great satisfaction to the authors who wish to express their gratitude to those people who helped them on their journey. Our first thanks go to two authors whose books were excellent examples of naturopathic history and provided valuable information about the German nature doctors. They are Alfred Brauchle, who wrote *Die Geschichte der Naturheilkunde in Lebensbildern (History of Nature Cure in Biographies),* and Karl E. Rothschuh (1908-1985), author of *Naturheilbewegung, Reformbewegung, Alternativbewegung (Nature Cure Movement, Reform Movement, Alternative Movement).* Brauchle himself was a noted nature doctor and Rothschuh, who founded the Institute for History of Medicine at the University of Münster, was a medical historian with a critical, yet fair analysis of the nature cure movement in Germany. Without Professor Rothschuh's kind personal guidance we would never have known the Archive of the Eden Foundation in Bad Soden, which houses the best collection of German nature cure literature. Since we had only a few hours to admire the treasures of this library, we were completely dependent on the librarian, Frau Marianne Venzke, for patiently supplying us with photocopies of journal articles. We also wish to thank Peter Fenton, Hon. Secretary and Treasurer of the Incorporated Society of Registered Naturopaths (Great Britain), who sent us valuable information about the "Scottish Lindlahr," James C. Thomson. Seeking information about Stanley Lief, the "British Benedict Lust," we contacted Jean Edwards, a childhood friend living near London, whose energetic research at the library of the British College of Naturopathy and Osteopathy provided us vital information.

On this side of the Atlantic our first acknowledgment goes to John B. Lust, N.D., who succeeded his uncle, Benedict Lust, as editor of *Nature's Path* magazine, and who was a noted naturopathic author in his own right. He left the Benedict Lust Collection to the National College of Naturopathic Medicine in Portland, Oregon upon his death in 1985. Among the many valuable books was an almost complete set of Benedict Lust's *Naturopath,* documenting the struggles and achievements of American naturopathy in the first half of this century. We also wish to thank Laura Lust Proctor for graciously providing us with information about Benedict and Louisa Lust as well as rare photographs of her uncle. We received valuable support from Jared Zeff, N.D., L.Ac., Academic Dean of the National College of Naturopathic Medicine, and Linda McNaughton Simpson, who transferred several handwritten chapters onto a disk with her magical computer skills. We thank Emily A. Kane for taking time from her naturopathic medical studies at Bastyr College in Seattle to give us invaluable photographic assistance. We are grateful to George A. Freibott, N.D., President of the American Naturopathic Association, for offering a different viewpoint of events in the history of American naturopathy. Thanks also goes to Joseph C. Keating, Jr., PhD, an eminent chiropractic historian, who sent us many articles illuminating the close but not always friendly relationship between the chiropractic and naturopathic profession in the past. Dr. John Bender, his successor in Waterloo, Ontario, graciously provided us with Dr. Arno R. Koegler's biography.

Wade Boyle died on October 3, 1993 - a deep shock for all of us who have known him as a unique friend, doctor, researcher, lecturer and writer. This book, which would have fewer flaws if he had lived to complete it, is a tribute to him. It was his wish that the book would be dedicated "to nature doctors everywhere, past, present and future." He embodied the best of all of them in an exemplary fashion.

We also feel the deepest sympathy for his wife Karen Boyle who supported her husband's work with great love. She told us that the hope of completing the book was an important factor in her husband's struggle with his final illness. In accordance with her husband's wishes she read the manuscript before it was published and improved it with many valuable suggestions.

After Wade's death I engaged Ron Johnson, a Portland poet and teacher of creative writing, for editing and improving the manuscript. I also thank Howard Asinoff, N.D., who, as an experienced editor and proofreader, provided further improvements to the text. They did a superb job.

Finally we thank Jill Stansbury, N.D., for her graceful cover design. We admire her for this rare combination of being not only a Professor of Botanical Medicine at the National College of Naturopathic Medicine but also an accomplished artist.

As the co-author I was handicapped by my inadequate command of the English language, but it was my advantage as a native of Germany to have access to the German sources used in *Nature Doctors.* I consider my contribution to the book an expression of my gratitude to the staff and students of the National College of Naturopathic Medicine in Portland. They hired me as a librarian in 1978 and offered me the exciting opportunity to build up the first naturopathic library. I was never happier in any other job than I was being among these high-minded and dedicated present and future "nature doctors" who had such a strong belief in the value of their concept of health and healing.

Table of Contents

Photographs and Illustrations

PREFACE

The modern American public is just now being reintroduced to naturopathy, the medical art which originated in Germany using natural agents such as air, light, water, food and herbs to stimulate the body's own natural healing powers. To understand the naturopathic medicine of the present, one must understand its origins. Unfortunately, even doctors of naturopathic medicine who are experts in its practice often have a limited knowledge of their historical tradition. In 1987, Jonathan Wright, M.D., then Chairman of the Board of the John Bastyr College of Naturopathic Medicine, sent a questionnaire to the staff, students and alumni of the college, asking, "What is a Naturopathic Physician?" The responses were noteworthy for their lack of agreement and the absence of any clear, unifying principles. Naturopathic physicians have long been noted for being mavericks who go their own ways. This characteristic of rugged individualism may be required to survive in a persecuted profession, but a sense of belonging may be created by a better knowledge of the profession's historical origins and the guiding principles from which it evolved.

Physicians and students of naturopathy may have an unclear picture of their roots as insufficient information has been readily available to them. Our book is an attempt to correct this. There have been several well-researched histories of other schools of unorthodox medicine. They include Kaufman (1971), Coulter (1977, 1973) and Winston (1993) on homeopathy; Griggs (1981), Boyle (1988) and Wood (1992) on eclectic and herbal medicine; Weiss & Kemble (1967), Donegan (1986) and Cayleff (1987) on water cure; Shelton (1968), Whorton (1982) and Griggs (1986) on the health reform and natural hygiene movement; Gevitz (1982) on osteopathy and Wardwell (1992) and Moore (1993) on the chiropractic profession which can even boast its own *Journal of Chiropractic History*. But the history of naturopathy has remained neglected. *Other Healers*, edited by Norman Gevitz (1988), includes essays on botanical medicine, the water cure movement, homeopathy, osteopathic medicine, chiropractic, Christian Science, etc., but naturopathy is omitted, and such important "other healers" as Benedict Lust and Henry Lindlahr are not even listed in the index.

Bits and pieces of historical information on naturopathy can be found in the older journals, especially in Benedict Lust's *Naturopath*. George Cody's chapter on the history of naturopathic medicine in *A Textbook of Natural Medicine* (Pizzorno 1987) was a laudable attempt to compile a historical account from them. More recently the medical anthropologist Hans A. Baer gave a concise overview of the history of American naturopathy in his article "The Potential Rejuvenation of American Naturopathy as a Consequence of the Holistic Health Movement" (Baer 1992). However, the only significant works about the history of nature cure were published in German. This is not surprising since the nature cure movement originated and still enjoys its greatest popularity in German-speaking countries. Among these works Alfred Brauchle's *Naturheilkunde in Lebensbildern (Nature Cure in Biographies)*, first published in 1937, still provides the most thorough account of the history of nature cure, despite some ideological and scholarly flaws. Brauchle was perhaps too far-reaching in what he claims as the territory of nature cure. He included such early water-doctors as Siegmund and Johann Siegmund Hahn; the great propagandist of vegetarianism and Life Reform in Germany, Eduard Baltzer; the inventors of Swedish massage, Per Henrik Ling and Major Thure Brandt; food and fasting doctors such as Edward Hooker Dewey, Alexander Haig, Max Bircher-Benner, Ragnar Berg and Mikkel Hindhede; and such representatives of the "psychotherapeutic nature cure" as Franz Anton Mesmer and Emile Coué.

We are more selective and focus only on those personalities who fell indisputably within the naturopathic camp and who had no allegiances outside it. We also strive more for depth than completeness and concentrate on the doctors most crucial for the development of nature cure and naturopathy. This, of course, lead to a few painful but necessary exclusions.

We do not claim to necessarily present the definitive work on the history of naturopathic medicine as we are not medical historians and worked with limited means. Our factual errors and errors of interpretation will hopefully be corrected by future historians with access to better sources. A case in point is Benedict Lust. We were informed that his family is in possession of an autobiography but we were unable to obtain it. In 1946, *Nature's Path* featured an article about Dr. Jesse Mercer Gehmann, who became Lust's successor as the President of the American Naturopathic Association. In listing his achievements, this article praised him as the well-known author of several books, including "the only authorized biography of Dr. Benedict Lust, written during the past six years . . . to be released at the Golden Jubilee Celebration of the Founding of Naturopathy" (611-12). One can only wonder what happened to this biography because no other reference to it could be found.

Despite its shortcomings we hope that this work will inspire students of naturopathic medicine to return to the wisdom of Kneipp, Lindlahr, Lust and the other pioneers, which still offers valuable guidance for the practice of modern medicine, naturopathic or otherwise.

The Predecessors

Introduction

Nature cure was a system for treating diseases with natural agents such as water, air, diet, herbs and sunshine which developed in nineteenth-century Europe. Naturopathy was the combination of nature cure and homeopathy, spinal manipulation and other natural therapies which were developed in early twentieth-century America. Naturopathic medicine is the application of the principles of naturopathy within the context of modern scientific knowledge that has evolved throughout the last half of this century. The term nature doctor has been used to describe the practitioners of all three of these permutations of nature-based medicine.

Natural therapies have been used to treat disease since ancient times. Indeed, the earliest doctors had little to work with other than herbs, foods, water, fasting and tissue manipulation. These gentle treatments did not obscure the body's own healing power, and the *vis medicatrix naturae* or "healing power of nature" became a basic tenet of the Hippocratic school and remains one of the central themes of naturopathic philosophy. Belief in the "healing power of nature" has never been the exclusive province of naturopathic medicine, as the medical historian, Max Neuburger, elaborated in his work, *The Doctrine of the Healing Power of Nature throughout the Course of Time*:

> The problem of the healing power of nature is a great, perhaps the greatest of all problems, which has occupied the physician for thousands of years. Indeed . . . the aims and limits of therapeutics are determined by its solution (Neuburger 1932, 864).

Neuburger examined how this doctrine is woven through the fabric of medical history like a red thread and how every important medical author has had to take a position for or against it. Nature doctors have been the greatest champions of this doctrine, but it has also been the cornerstone of the medical theories of Paracelsus, Jan Baptista Van Helmont, Thomas Sydenham, Georg Ernst Stahl, Christoph Wilhelm Hufeland and others.

A number of these physicians are philosophical antecedents to the nature cure movement of the nineteenth century, but since they are already prominent in the history of medicine they will be touched on only briefly here.

Hippocrates (460-377) is often considered the earliest predecessor of naturopathic physicians. Brauchle began his *Nature Cure in Biographies* with him. But not everyone agreed that the "father of medicine" could be claimed as a forerunner of naturopathic medicine. The most extreme position was taken by Herbert Shelton:

> Hippocrates inclusion in the list of nature doctors seems to rest on the fact that he stressed the effort of the body to heal itself. He said: 'nature is healer of all diseases,' and 'let foods be your medicine and your medicines your foods . . . ' If such statements entitle him to a place in naturopathy, why not include Morris Fishbein, who is guilty of uttering numerous such statements? . . . Hippocrates was the originator of the bleeding practice that resulted in the spilling of more blood than war and wild beasts caused. He was the author of the anti-phlogistic and depleting plans of practice that sent millions of earth's inhabitants to untimely graves (Shelton 1949, 89).

The *Corpus Hippocraticum*, the collection of Hippocratic writings, was actually the work of different authors belonging to two different schools, which symbolized the eternal polarity of medicine. The school of Cos represented the vitalistic, empirical approach to health, while the school of Cnidos promoted the rationalistic, analytical approach. As Dubos stated so well:

> The Hippocratic writings are multifaceted and occupy a place in medicine corresponding to that of the Bible in the literature and ethics of Western peoples. As in the Bible, everyone can find in them something relevant to his preoccupations which has never been stated better and more succinctly (Dubos 1959, 117).

Focusing primarily on the vitalistic teachings of Cos, naturopathy is indebted to Hippocrates for formulating its fundamental credo of the *vis medicatrix naturae,* which the physician can support but never replace. Hippocrates also realized that treating a disease meant treating the patient as a whole:

> The very word 'physician'- from the Greek root meaning nature - was used by Hippocrates to denote that every practitioner of medicine 'was to be skilled in Nature and must strive to know

> what man is in relation to food, drink, occupation, and what effect these have on him.' Moreover, the physician should never forget that disturbances in any organ correspond to a disturbance of the whole person and that 'to heal even an eye, one must heal the head and even the whole body ' (Dubos 1959, 120).

Between Hippocrates and Paracelsus there was a physician who has received too little recognition as a "predecessor." This was the great Jewish philosopher, scholar and physician, Maimonides (1135-1204). A lonely figure in the medieval wilderness of polypharmacy, Maimonides zealously kept abreast of the latest medical discoveries and critically examined the great medical texts of the past. Centuries before the evolution of holistic medicine he prescribed holistic practices.

> The physician must keep in mind that the heart of every sick person is narrow and that every healthy person has an expanded soul. Therefore, the physician must remove emotional experiences that cause shrinking of the soul (Hoffman 1986, 28).
>
> And in order to strengthen the vital powers, one should employ musical instruments and tell patients gay stories which make the heart swell and narratives that will distract the mind and cause them and their friends to laugh. One should select as attendants and caretakers those who can cheer up the patient. This is a must in every illness (Maimonides 1958, 47).

In direct contrast to many of his medical colleagues, Maimonides downplayed the importance of drugs and surgery and argued that diet, exercise, and mental outlook were the key elements for attaining health. The success of his natural healing methods attracted the attention of the royal family in Cairo. In 1185 he became court physician to the Grand Vizier and later to the Sultan Saladin. The basic recommendations of his fascinating work, *The Preservation of Youth*, are pure nature cure. He wrote it for a dissolute young prince who suffered from a host of disorders from depression to indigestion and warned him that "overeating is like a deadly poison to any constitution and the principal cause of all diseases" (Hoffmann 1986, 29). Addressing the prince's sedentary lifestyle, he advocated daily, vigorous exercise. Against the prince's hypochondriac tendencies he warned:

> In spite of your caution and carefulness, you will not be able to prevent minor things from developing in the human body. For example: Now the stool will be soft and now hard, one day you may find a change in your digestion or experience a slight head-

> ache or an ache in another part of your body, and many similar things. And be very careful not to begin treating it medically, rushing to take a medication that is supposed to remove this minor ailment . . . Because if you undertake to medicate these minor conditions, there are two possibilities: Either your act will be erroneous, the opposite of what nature intends, and you will lose and suffer injury, or your action will be correct and you will restore to nature its natural function, but at the same time train your body to lag behind and to do the normal only with outside help (Maimonides 1958, 72).

The writings of Paracelsus (1493-1541) are as multifaceted and as open to multiple interpretations as the Hippocratic writings. Living at a crucial turning point in the history of Western civilization, when the medieval heaven-centered concept of the world was giving way to the Renaissance view of nature and man as the center of interest, Paracelsus was one of the most fascinating figures in the history of medicine.

His real name was Theophrastus, but he defiantly adopted the pen-name Paracelsus which meant "better than Celsus," the great Roman encyclopedist, who had ruled medical science for centuries. In 1527, at the height of his career, Paracelsus publicly cast the famous textbook of medieval medicine, the Canon of Avicenna, into a bonfire which his students made in the marketplace. It became a symbol of rebellion against unthinking acceptance of ancient doctrines. The medical students of that period, who rarely saw a patient before they graduated, were aroused by Paracelsus' battle cry: "The patients are your textbook, the sickbed is your study" (Pachter 1951, 16). They were inspired by his refusal to believe that patients were doomed just because the books did not provide a treatment. It was Galen and Avicenna, Paracelsus argued, who were bankrupt, not medicine.

Paracelsus, a restless pilgrim for truth, studied at the universities of Germany, Italy and France, crisscrossed Europe several times:

> And wherever I went I eagerly and diligently investigated and sought after the tested and reliable arts of medicine. I went not only to the doctors, but also to the barbers, bathkeepers, learned physicians, women, and magicians who pursued the art of healing; I went to alchemists, to monasteries, to nobles and common folk, to the experts and the simple . . . (Paracelsus 1958, 4).

Paracelsus was the first physician of his era to take up Hippocrates' neglected concept of the healing power of nature, and he never tired of repeating that "mumia cures all wounds, protect them from external enemies and they will be healed" (Pachter 1951, 213). The "mumia" was the inner balsam or life power inherent in the flesh. Paracelsus spoke out against the atrocious medieval practices of dressing surgical wounds with concoctions of cow dung, viper fat, feathers and moss. He insisted that wounds be kept clean. "If you prevent infection, Nature will heal the wound all by herself." He appealed to the doctors to turn to nature as the only true physician: "Nature is the physician, not you. From her you must learn, not from yourself; she compounds the remedies, not you" (Paracelsus 1958, 91).

It should be noted that Paracelsus had a more realistic view of nature than many of the later nature doctors who equated nature with paradise, who saw only its idyllic, healing qualities and ignored its darker, destructive powers.

> Even while still in the womb, unborn, man is burdened with the potentialities of every disease, and is subject to them. And because all diseases are inherent in his nature, he could not be born alive and healthy if an inner physician were not hidden in him. But wherever diseases are, there are also physicians and medicine! Each natural disease bears its own remedy within itself. Man has received from nature both the destroyer of health and the preserver of health. And just as the destroyer strives continuously to destroy and to kill man, so the preserver works with equal vigor and zeal to preserve him . . . (Paracelsus 1958, 76).

However, all his praise of nature's healing power did not make Paracelsus a nature doctor. As Rothschuh pointed out, it was Paracelsus who introduced such chemical drugs as antimonial and arsenical compounds, lead nitrates, chlorides of iron and gold, copper sulphates and bismuth and tin compounds. "It was the exaggerated use of such drugs in the medical practice of the early nineteenth century which was one of the main reasons for the 'nature doctors' to condemn the scientific medicine of their times as 'poison medicine' and turn away from it" (Rothschuh 1983, 50).

But Paracelsus remains one of the most quotable physicians, and his expressions remain apt for physicians of any persuasion:

> The art of medicine is rooted in the heart. If your heart is false, you will also be a false physician; if your heart is just you will also be a true physician (Paracelsus 1958, 72).

Unlike Hippocrates or Paracelsus, Christoph Wilhelm Hufeland (1762-1836), is never mentioned as a predecessor in the American naturopathic literature, though in Germany medical doctors who specialize in natural therapeutics celebrate him as a shining example of a truly holistic physician in the best Hippocratic tradition. He had an open mind toward such different schools of healing as homeopathy, Mesmerism and water cure. Each year the professional organization of these specialists in natural therapies awards the Hufeland Medal to one of its outstanding members.

Hufeland was closely associated with famous poets and philosophers of the Weimar classical period. Schiller, Wieland, Herder and Fichte became his patients. It was Goethe who procured him a position as a professor at Jena, where his lectures on the art of prolonging life drew large audiences. He became one of the most respected physicians of his time. His special concern for public health matters led him to have the first morgue built in Germany, to prevent people from being mistakenly buried alive. He also insisted upon the quarantine of smallpox patients to fight the spread of that disease.

In 1780 he accepted an appointment as royal physician to the King of Prussia. When Napoleon's army threatened to invade Berlin, he left his family in Berlin and followed the royal couple to Eastern Prussia because the queen needed his special care. Grateful for his services, she gave him the financial support needed for the establishment of an outpatient clinic where the poor of Berlin could be treated free of charge.

Hufeland was eminently successful as a practitioner, teacher and a leader of the medical profession. He wrote several well-known books, among them the *Enchiridion Medicum* or *The Practice of Medicine: The Result of Fifty Years' Experience* (1836). He was one of the pioneers of medical journalism in the nineteenth century, editing four journals. Hufeland's Journal was the most respected journal of its time. In his writings Hufeland was an ardent advocate of the concept of the healing power of nature. The first chapter of his *Enchiridion Medicum* is entitled "Physiatric" and started with the sentence "All cures of diseases are caused by Nature; the medical art is only Nature's servant and cures through her." One of his favorite sayings was, "Do little, leave everything to Nature." He wrote:

> Every patient is a temple of Nature. Approach him with reverence and respect, free yourself from all frivolity, selfishness and unscrupulousness and then Nature will look favorably upon you and reveal her mysteries to you (cited in Brauchle 1951, 40).

Hufeland was a great friend of water cure and mineral springs, and he often prescribed them in his own practice. He knew most of the springs himself visited them before writing his treatise on mineral springs in Germany. His greatest success was his book *The Art of Prolonging Human Life*, first published in 1796, which became one of the most widely read books on the subject of preventive medicine, and can be considered the first natural health best-seller. It was reprinted numerous times and translated into many languages, even Chinese. Only Kneipp's *My Water Cure* a century later had comparable success.

Hufeland coined the seemingly twentieth-century term, "macrobiotics," to describe the art of prolonging life. Later editions of his book were entitled *Macrobiotic: The Art of Prolonging Life*. George Oshawa, an admirer of Hufeland, who started the modern macrobiotic movement, borrowed this term from him. For Hufeland, macrobiotic was different from medical art:

> The object of the medical art is health; that of the macrobiotic, long life . . . The medical art must consider every disease as an evil, which cannot be too soon expelled; the macrobiotic, on the other hand, shows that many diseases may be the means of prolonging life (Hufeland 1870, ix).

He spoke about the curative powers of fever, inflammation and suppuration and how their suppression can cause disease. Most of the basic concepts of the later nature doctors can be found in *Macrobiotic*. Concerning feverish diseases he wrote:

> As soon as one perceives these symptoms, nothing is so necessary as to lessen one's nourishment, which strengthens the disease, and to follow the beneficent instinct of Nature, which every animal, to its great advantage obeys on such occasions. Let the patient abstain from eating, for Nature, by rejecting food, shows that she is incapable of digesting it; and let him drink a little more than usual, but only water, or some other light beverage. One ought also to be kept quiet; to lie in the best position, for the lassitude sufficiently shows that Nature requires her strength for modifying the disease . . . These simple means, prescribed to us so clearly by Nature herself, are capable, would we only listen to her voice, of checking an infinite number of diseases in their very birth (Hufeland 1870, 281).

The following paragraph, written by Hufeland, could have been written by the "sun doctor," Arnold Rikli, some seventy years later:

> But there are agents . . . which have a friendship for, and an affinity to, the vital power; and which are capable of exciting, invigorating, and, in great probability, of affording it a subtle nourishment. These, in particular, are light, heat, and air, or rather oxygen; three celestial gifts, which, with great propriety, may be called the friends and guardian spirits of life . . . . Light is, without

> doubt, the most intimate friend and relation of life . . . . The life of every created being is the more perfect the more it enjoys the influence of light. Let a plant or an animal be deprived of light, notwithstanding every nourishment, care, and cultivation, it will first lose its color, then its strength, and at last, entirely decay (Hufeland 1870, 41).

Hufeland was deeply influenced by the philosopher Jean-Jacques Rousseau (1712-1778), and Rousseau's ideal of a simple, healthy life in the country pervades every line of his *Macrobiotic*:

> All the melancholy consequences of a sedentary life and overstraining the mental faculties would disappear, if people, some hours every day, or a few months in the year, would take hold of a spade or a mattock and cultivate their field or their garden . . . . Such rustication will again restore the equilibrium between the mind and the body, which the writing-desk so often destroys (Hufeland 1870, 244-245).
>
> A day spent in the country, under a serene sky, amidst a circle of agreeable friends, is certainly a more positive means of prolonging life than all the vital elixirs in the world. Laughter, that external expression of joy, must not here be omitted. It is the most salutary of all the bodily movement; for it agitates both the body and the soul at the same time; promotes digestion, circulation, and respiration; and enlivens the vital power in every organ (Hufeland 1870, 267).

With his call "Return to Nature!" Rousseau must be considered the true spiritual father of the nature cure movement. If anything struck the Age of Reason like a thunderbolt, it was the famous first lines of Emile: *"Tout est bien sortant des mains de l'auteur des choses, tout degenere entre les mains de l'homme:"*

> Everything is good as it leaves the hands of the Author of things; everything degenerates in the hands of man. He forces one soil to nourish the products of another, one tree to bear the fruit of another. He mixes and confuses the climates, the elements, the seasons. He mutilates his dog, his horse, his slave. He turns everything upside down; he disfigures everything; he loves deformity, monsters. He wants nothing as nature made it, not even man (Rousseau 1979, 33).

Rousseau regarded medicine as "an art more pernicious to men than all the ills it claims to cure" (1979, 54). He wrote:

> Do you want to find men of true courage? Look for them in places where there are no doctors, where they are ignorant of the consequences of illnesses, where they hardly think of death .... The only useful part of medicine is hygiene. And hygiene is itself less a science than a virtue. Temperance and work are the two true doctors of man. Works sharpens his appetite, and temperance prevents him from abusing it (Rousseau 1979, 55).

By substituting Nature for God, Rousseau glorified her in a way which might sound naive and sentimental but which expresses the modern longing for an inviolate nature:

> I looked for some wild spot in the woods, a deserted little place where no trace of a human hand could be detected, where no intruder could push himself between me and Nature. What magnificence Nature unfolded before my eyes in ever new variations? The gold of the broom and the purple of the heather filled me with astonishment, deeply moving my heart with their beauty. The majesty of the trees which covered me with their shadows filled me with awe. Without stopping and warning she includes us in the whirl of her dance and carries us away with her until we are exhausted and slip out of her arms (cited in Rothschuh 1983, 74).

With his "naturism" Rousseau supplied the ideological basis for nature cure. Rothschuh distinguished between three essential elements which characterized the nature cure movement:

> 1) A strongly emotional attitude towards nature which can be defined as "naturism."
>
> 2) A theory of health, disease, treatment and cure which we know as nature cure or naturopathy.
>
> 3) A preference for certain treatment methods which are considered natural (physiotherapy) such as the application of water, light, air, movement, diet, etc. (1983,19).

The leitmotif of naturism was "Return to Nature" and you will live a happy, healthy life. The French word "naturisme" means faith in the divine power of Nature. Naturism was not only concerned with healing but also strove for the salvation of humankind. Vegetarianism, hydropathy, nudism and the absolute condemnation of "poisonous" drugs were all expressions of this attempt to save humankind from the ills of civilization. Rousseau tapped such a deep vein of cultural sentiment that his precepts not only provided the nature cure movement of 100 years ago with a philosophical foundation, but they also continue to ring with meaning for millions today who may never have read Rousseau nor heard of naturopathy.

Most nature doctors of the nineteenth century were deeply influenced by Rousseau, most directly J.H.Rausse,Theodor Hahn and Adolf Just, who entitled his famous nature cure book *Return to Nature!* Vincent Priessnitz, the first nature doctor, was even called the "Rousseau of Water Cure" (vom Walde 1898, 221). Priessnitz, a Silesian peasant, may never have heard of Rousseau, but his homespun philosophy of health evolved in a cultural atmosphere pervaded by Rousseau's naturism. Certainly many of his patients considered their pilgrimage to Priessnitz' Gräfenberg a literal "return to nature" which they hoped would result in a return to health.

Part 1

The European Nature Cure Pioneers

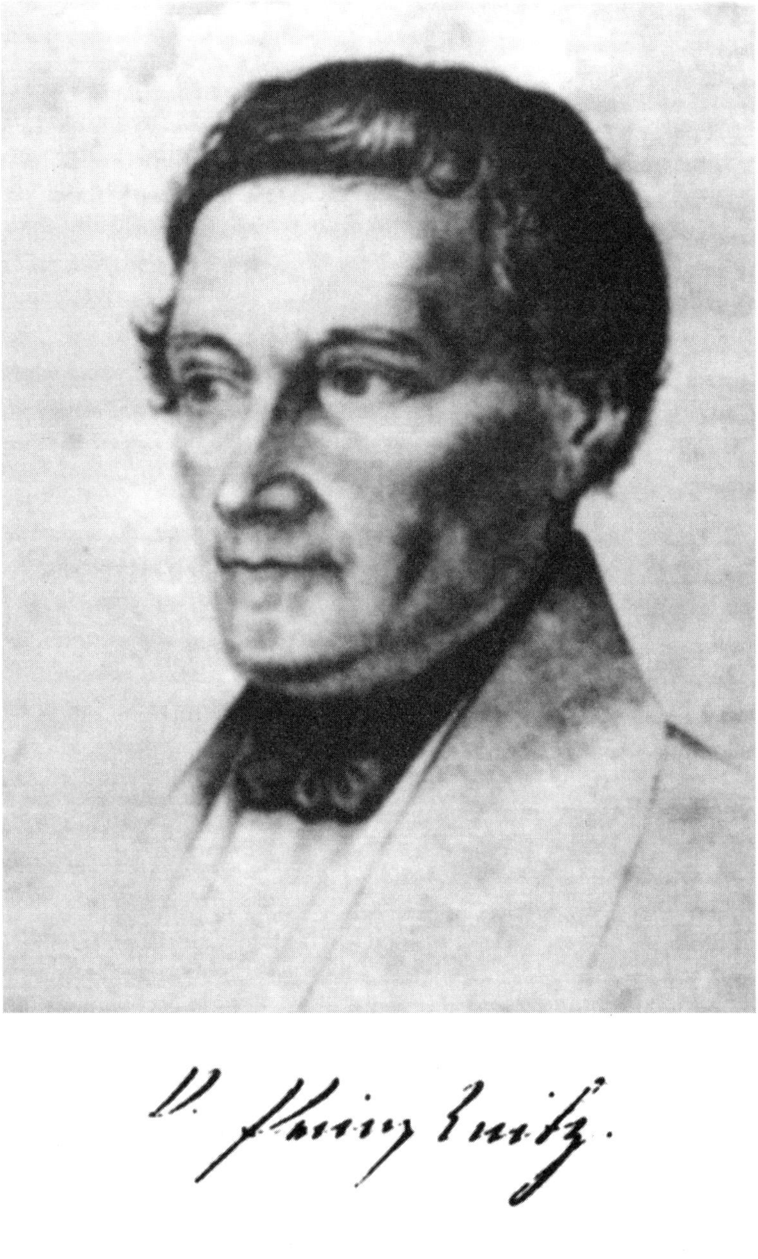

Vincent Priessnitz
(Shelton 1968, 93)

Foundations of Nature Cure

Vincent Priessnitz

(1799 - 1852)

Vincent Priessnitz was born a peasant and never went to medical school, yet he became one of the most famous healers of the nineteenth century. Besides curing thousands of patients of stubborn conditions, he set in motion the forces which would lead to the establishment of hydrotherapy as a legitimate medical entity, which allowed the simple methods of natural healing at his time to evolve into naturopathic medicine of today.

Priessnitz was born October 4, 1799 at Gräfenberg, a small village in the Sudetes Mountains of southern Silesia, now Czech Republic. He was the youngest of five children. As a boy Priessnitz received a rudimentary education at a Catholic school in the neighboring village of Freiwaldau, but had to quit school to manage the family farm after an older brother, who was to take over the farm, died of brain fever, and his father went blind in grief.

His village was in the same region where the early water doctors Sigmund Hahn (1664-1742) and his son Johann Sigmund Hahn (1696-1773) had made extensive use of cold water in their medical practices. An old man in the neighborhood is said to have shown the young lad how to treat cattle with water, and the boy Priessnitz was credited with curing his father's hide-bound, feverish cow by cold water application.

Once Priessnitz was tending his father's cattle in a mountain pasture. He observed a stag, wounded in the thigh by hunters, hobble into a mountain spring and situate itself with the injured limb submerged in the cold flowing water. Each day the stag returned to treat itself. "Great was his [Priessnitz'] joy to observe the animal improve day to day, till it finally got well" (Metcalfe 1898, 12). Interestingly, Gräfenberg mountain was part of the Hirschbad Kamm or Stag's Bath Ridge of the Sudetes. These pine-forested mountains abounded in fresh water springs, one of which had carried Priessnitz' family name for 200 years since an ancestor was killed there trying to rescue his "lovely daughter" from Swedish soldiers during the Thirty Years War.

Overworked on the farm to the point of carelessness, Priessnitz experienced a number of accidental injuries which gave him the opportunity to

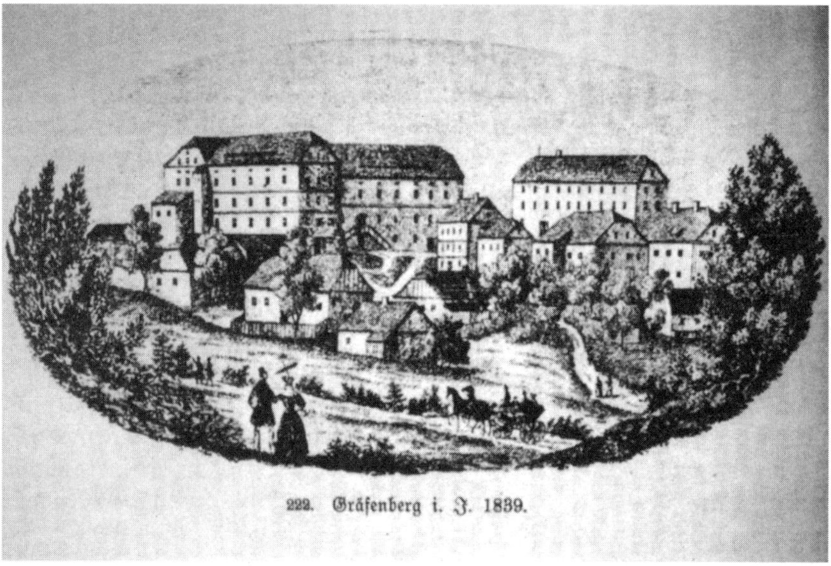

Gräfenberg in the year 1839
(vom Walde 1898)

practice on himself the healing powers of cold water. At only thirteen he sprained his wrist, and found it felt much better under the cold stream of a water pump. Since he couldn't keep his wrist under the pump and attend to his chores, he wrapped it in a wet bandage which he renewed quickly as it dried. Thus was born the "Priessnitz compress," eventually adopted into regular medical practice and which remains to this day an entry in medical dictionaries.

At seventeen, Priessnitz was run over by a horse-drawn wagon carrying a heavy load of wood. The local surgeon pronounced the critical injuries incurable and left the teenager to his fate. But Priessnitz, who had already become "a kind of medical advisor to his neighbors," set the broken ribs himself by pressing his abdomen against the edge of an arm chair, and bound himself with a bandage wrung out in cold water. He took to his bed, moistening the bandage whenever it was dry, and drinking large amounts of cold water. In 10 days he was up attending to his chores. He wore the bandage for the next year after which he pronounced himself fully recovered.

Because of this and other similar experiences, he felt dutybound to share his discoveries with others. Whenever he heard of anyone having a sprain, bruise, or other external injuries, he recommended cold water treatments, which he often applied himself. So successful was he that at the age of nineteen he was invited to Bohemia and Moravia to give treatments. Throughout this time he used only sponge ablutions, and he came to be known as the Schwamm or sponge doctor.

At first, Priessnitz did not charge for his services and made numerous house calls. Eventually experience showed him that people who came to his home and paid for treatment were cured the most quickly, so he changed his practice accordingly.

Three doctors from Freiwaldau incited the authorities against Priessnitz, since his success was diminishing their practices. "Even in Priessnitz' day," according to Lust, "there was a jealous medical profession" (1918, 223). In the early years he was frequently arrested and tried for illegal practice of medicine, but he was always acquitted because he used only water, not medicine. During one trial a patient was called as a witness, and the judge asked him who had cured him. "They all have helped me," the patient answered "The doctors, the apothecaries, and Priessnitz. The former helped me get rid of my money, and Priessnitz to get rid of my illness" (Metcalfe 1898, 21). One physician sent by the state to investigate Priessnitz frequently referred patients to Gräfenberg thereafter.

At one point, in frustration, the authorities, who were convinced Priessnitz must be employing drugs or sorcery, "raided his place and wrecked it in search of his secret. They cut up all his sponges . . . but the mystery was not revealed" (Lust 1918, 224). In 1829, when the magistrate in Freiwaldau prohibited him from using his "bewitched" sponge, Priessnitz' replied: "This is even better; then I use only my hands. Thus life comes to life" (Schönenberger 1931, 47). After this Priessnitz never employed sponges but used only the flat hand for applying water which he found to be even more effective.

These persecutions didn't embitter Priessnitz, who accepted them with equanimity and silence, but rather they spread his fame throughout the region, bringing him ever more patients. Soon he was forced to graduate from caring for external injuries to also treating many forms of internal disease. By trial, error, and astute observation he invented new ways to use cold water against disease. Others, such as the Hahns and the great water cure propagandist Eucharius Ferdinand Christian Oertel (1765-1850), had recognized the value of cold water for health, but they had not really understood its many possibilities. Philo vom Walde listed 56 different cold water applications in his Priessnitz book. Chief among them was the wet sheet pack. In the words of James C. Jackson, "If Vincent Priessnitz had never done anything else for mankind but to have discovered and brought into use this form of hydrotherapy, he would have done enough to make him immortal" (1874, 2).

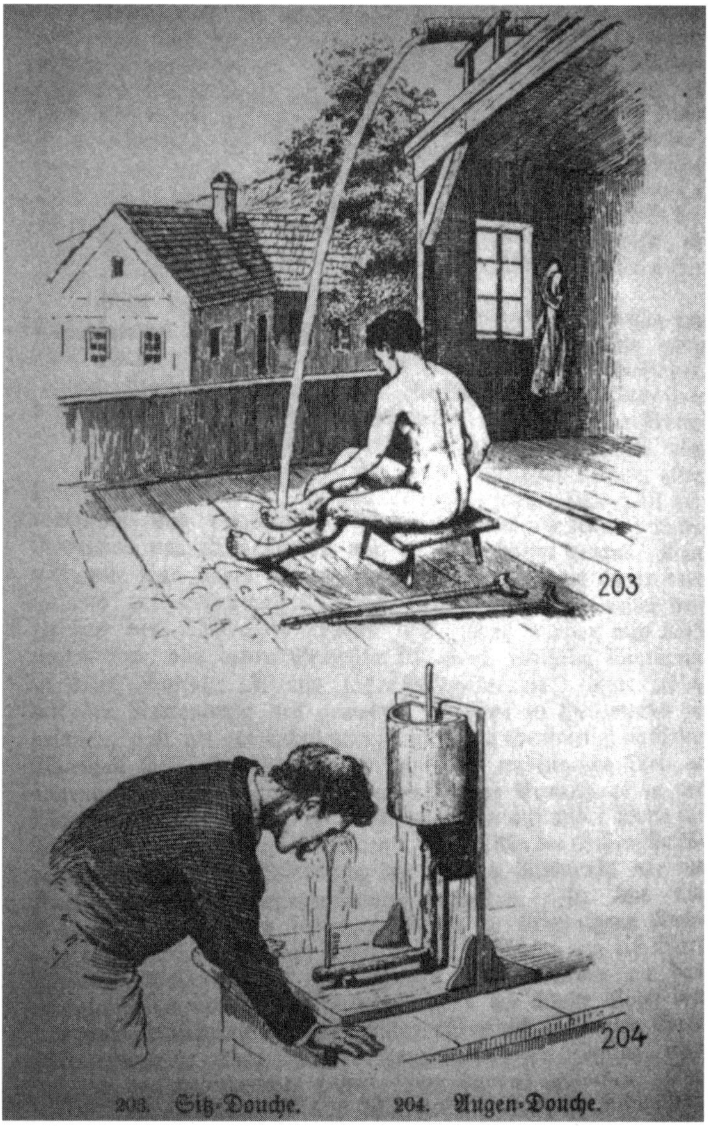

Sitz douche and eye douche
(vom Walde 1898)

By 1826 he had opened his own hydrotherapeutic institution, and in 1829, the first year records were kept, he had forty-five patients in residence. By 1833 this number grew to 200, increasing to 800 in 1838 and 1600 in 1840. Besides members of royalty and clerical dignitaries Priessnitz eventually counted such luminaries as Chopin, Gogol and Napoleon III among his patients.

During this period of phenomenal growth and clinical success, complaints against Priessnitz from the medical profession escalated proportionately. By 1838 the pressure was so great that the Austrian government created a special commission to investigate Priessnitz. The commission, headed by Baron Turkheim, traveled to Gräfenberg and made an in-depth investigation to settle the matter once-and-for-all, which it did. Turkheim's report to the Imperial Cabinet at Vienna is worth quoting:

> That Priessnitz is no ordinary man even his enemies must admit. He is no imposter, but is filled with the purest zeal to help others whenever he is asked to do so; and he is particularly fitted to do this. The number of those, who call Priessnitz a quack and a man of selfish motives, only constitute a small minority, and are mostly doctors and surgeons from the surrounding districts whose incomes are reduced by his practice, and who therefore get up complaints against him.
>
> Unassuming, modest, ever ready to give his patients help, untiring by day and night, obliging, firm and consistent in his actions, Priessnitz possesses qualities which are inadmissible in an imposter. Notwithstanding the most careful investigations, I have been unable to trace a single instance wherein he was activated by selfish motives . . .
>
> The Imperial Commission has pronounced unanimously against closing the Gräfenberg establishment, as it has proved itself efficient in many cases . . . (Metcalfe 1898, 28-30).

After this stunning endorsement of his practice, the Austrian government decreed that Priessnitz should enjoy the same privileges as medical doctors, and that henceforward no one should ever harass him. The government even went so far as to build new roads to facilitate access to his establishments. Ultimately, the Emperor of Austria bestowed upon Priessnitz a large gold medal for civic merit, the highest mark of distinction in Austria. Thus ended almost two decades of prosecution and harassment, and Priessnitz was finally free to practice healing as he saw fit.

Physically Priessnitz was a little above middle size, and it was his habit to go about dressed in a plain frock coat. His complexion was fair, although pitted slightly by smallpox. His light hair was cut short. He spoke so little that when he did say something, it was treated like truth from the Delphic Oracle. He was unfailingly humble—quite innocent of self-promotion or puff. As one royal fan put it, "We do not know which to admire more, his rare genius, his perseverance, or his modesty" (Metcalfe 1898, 35).

A no-nonsense person, Priessnitz had a wry sense of humor. A count came to Gräfenberg for treatment and one day remarked to Priessnitz, "My dear sir, in your place I would make short work of all hypochondriacs." Smiling, Priessnitz replied, "In that case I should be obliged to begin with your Excellency" (Metcalfe 1898, 55-56). About a lady who did not show the slightest inclination to privations and restrictions, Priessnitz said: "There we have another one who would like the entire water cure in a cup of coffee" (Schönenberger 1931, 46).

Priessnitz could read, but his writing skills were limited, and his busy practice gave him little time for literary pursuits. His only book, *Familien-Wasserbuch (Family Water Book)*, was sketchy. To learn his method of healing, other physicians had to travel to Gräfenberg to observe, which they did in large numbers. In 1839 alone, 120 doctors came to study the cure. Given Priessnitz' laconic manner and his poor teaching ability, his students had to follow close by his side and observe for weeks at a time. It is only through their writings and those of some of his patients that we have any record of Priessnitz' methods.

From the start Priessnitz preferred soft water over mineral water because of its ability to dissolve impurities, and he never used hot water because he thought it was debilitating. His techniques for employing cold water evolved over the years. By the 1840s, a typical day for a patient would be the following: Awaken at 4 a.m. to be wrapped in numerous blankets to sweat for up to several hours, then plunged briefly into a cold tub. This would be followed immediately by a brisk walk, after which a simple breakfast of bread, cold milk, and fruit was served. At 10 a.m. a cold douche (shower) was taken followed by simultaneous sitz and foot baths. A "plentiful but coarse" dinner would be served at 1 p.m. The douche was repeated at 4 p.m., and the sitz and foot baths taken again at 7 p.m. A supper similar to the breakfast was then served, and the patient retired at 9:30 p.m. During free time, patients walked the Gräfenberg mountain trails, as much as 1,000 miles in three months, or about 10 miles per day, and drank copiously of cold water from the mountain springs. Indeed, patients would often "amuse themselves" by wagering who could drink the most (Claridge 1843, 11).

They were required to walk considerably just to take their daily douches. The six available douches were springs of water running out of the mountain, conveyed by pipes into huts where they fell about 15 feet in a stream the thickness of one's wrist. They were scattered throughout the Gräfenberg forest.

This formed the general pattern of therapy, but Priessnitz was famous for treating no two patients alike. He was "a genius in the art of individual treatment" (Detmar 1951, 101). He rejected all rule-of-thumb therapy. "Our task," he was fond of saying, "is not to treat the disease, but the patient" (65). He individualized his treatments according to his own system of diagnosis based on close observation of the patient and the reaction of the skin to cold water treatment, which he often timed with a watch. Priessnitz told one patient who was hesitant about taking his first cold-water plunge in the dead of night, "Get into the big bath, for only then can I prescribe treatment for you." The patient, relaying the story, said "I jumped in and out again in the flash of an eye. He then looked me all over by the light of the lantern and congratulated me on the good cure ahead. 'Why?' I asked. 'Because your body after the very first bath is red all over. If it remains white, a cure may take years. You will have an easy cure'" (63).

In Priessnitz' own words, "When I examine a patient's appearance, especially his eyes and his skin, I see before me a picture, so to say, of his diseased state; I see what is the matter with him, and at the same time the exact means to overcome the disease which causes his sufferings. I then prescribe accordingly" (Metcalfe 1898, 78). He would immediately tell a patient whether or not he could cure him, and frequently rejected applicants for treatment. Priessnitz declined to accept as many as twenty percent of the patients who came to him. But after accepting a patient, he could often predict the course of disease and cure. The precision with which Priessnitz diagnosed his patients often surprised them, and they regarded him "almost as one endowed with supernatural power" (Metcalfe 1898, 10).

A complete cure would take from four weeks up to two years, and averaged six months or more. From his earliest experiments on himself and his neighbors Priessnitz noticed that a skin rash would sometimes develop over the areas of the body treated with cold water, and he assumed that this was morbific matter being drawn out of the body. He subsequently based his therapy on the body-fluid theory (humoral pathology), and he set the goal of expelling bad fluids by violent means. The best method in his view was the healing crisis, generating an acute disease in the patient, manifested by fever and boils, which would throw off the toxic material and leave the patient free of both acute and chronic disease. The suggestion that the skin eruptions were the "result of infections introduced by unsterile and perhaps unclean linen" (Donegan 1986, 186) is unsupported by any evidence. Much of Priessnitz' success was based on understanding of the benefits of this process, his courage to put patients through it and his consummate skill in managing such a crisis. He always changed treatment during a crisis, switching from dry packs to wet sheet packs and suspending douches.

Priessnitz inspired his patients with confidence and courage, and his look and touch had a powerful influence on them. Such was the unbounded confidence of the patients in him, "that everyone ardently desires to pass through this ordeal (healing crisis), being the sure road to health." A stranger to Gräfenberg would have been "struck by the novelty of hearing people compliment one another, on being informed that they have passed a feverish night, or that rash or boils have broken out on some part of the body" (Claridge 1843, 28). Most physicians, then and now, would run the other way when confronted with a healing crisis, but Priessnitz "possessed an imperturbable self-reliance" (Houghton 1851, 70). His years of practice convinced him, as he said, that "anything brought forth by water, the water will cure" (Metcalfe 1898, 99).

Priessnitz also attached great importance to the value of fresh air. As "an absolute air fanatic" he laid the groundwork for the development of the air bath of the later back-to-nature movement, and the windows in his sickrooms had to stand open at all times. After being locked out of his clinic during persecution, he said, "If I had no water, I could cure with air!" (Schönenberger 1931, 138). He used air as a thermal and as a mechanical stimulant. In his "air-water bath" the patient was not allowed to dry himself with towels but had to create a draft by beating his wet body with a sheet to activate his inactive skin. He felt people should warm themselves by exercise and not heavy clothes, even in winter, and he would not let his patients wear wool or flannel next to the skin. In fact, Priessnitz considered heat from external sources a bad thing not only in water and clothing but also in food. Meals were served more or less cold. Priessnitz presided at every meal at the central table in the great common dining hall and answered patients' questions. He never restricted the amount of food his patients ate, but liked to see them eat heartily to keep up their strength for his rigorous treatments. Mealtime visitors were surprised to see the patients eating more like field hands than invalids.

Priessnitz' critics ridiculed the severity of his treatments. After describing Colonel Claridge's treatment under Priessnitz, which Claridge himself found so satisfactory that he wrote a book about it, Weiss and Kembel stated, "Such irksome treatment . . . was inflicted for varying periods on patients" (1967, 7). They quoted a contemporary critic of Priessnitz who said that to endure the treatments at Gräfenberg "required the courage of the lion, the strength of the bull, and the stomach of the hog" (12). Another modern historian described the wet sheet pack as "wrapping the patient like a bale of goods" (Turner 1967, 1967).

Priessnitz was the first to admit the rigor of his treatments. "It is true my patients have a hard time of it," he said, "but one cannot do too much for one's health." And he had little patience with the faint-hearted. "To use the water cure, a person must have force of will," he said. "Those who have a weak character or show no inclination to strengthen it, had better remain away from the water cure" (Metcalfe 1898, 86). There is evidence that in the last years of his practice Priessnitz made his treatments gentler, favoring the wet sheet pack over other sweating packs, moderating the cold-water temperatures and limiting the water drinking and exercise.

How successful was Priessnitz in his practice? We know that of the over 40,000 patients he treated, only 45 died under his care. "In truth," one writer said, "a figure to put us modern doctors to shame" (Detmar 1951, 64). Detractors asserted that these deaths occurred from the severe treatments, but supporters of Priessnitz claimed that most of the deaths were of patients who were already moribund and whom Priessnitz consented to treat out of pity. His critics claimed that Priessnitz cured only 1 in 20 patients (Weiss 1967, 13), but this is not consistent with the fact that thousands of people came from all over the world, including Peru, Egypt, Brazil, and Lapland to seek treatment. And Gräfenberg was a remote location in an age of difficult transportation, 260 miles from Berlin, 200 miles from Dresden, and 175 miles from Vienna. It took from 10-14 days to get to Gräfenberg from England via steamboat, railway, and carriage (Claridge 1843, 48). It is unlikely that thousands of patients over dozens of years would endure such hardships for a five-percent chance of getting better, and it is inconsistent with the testimony of numerous patients and visitors.

We know from Claridge's own words of the satisfactory results of his treatment, and he quotes numerous others who witnessed the effectiveness of Priessnitz' therapy. A Dr. Behrend admitted to being skeptical at first but then stated: "'I have seen asthmas and pleurisies completely cured in three to four days by cold water only" (7). He also mentioned observing routine cures of smallpox, measles, ringworm, syphilis, gout, and tic douloureux. "The efficacy of water," he concluded, "is so clearly manifested that doubt is impossible" (8). Such testimony from medical doctors is all the more convincing, considering Priessnitz distrusted MDs, at whose hands he had suffered so much. He never went out of his way to cultivate their favor.

Priessnitz was not vengeful toward those who had harmed him, however. A story circulated about how Priessnitz saved the child of Syndie, who had led the persecution against him.

> The Syndie's five children all took scarlet fever and were treated by an ordinary doctor. Three died. The father then begged the aid of Priessnitz, who said he would help only if the doctors were dismissed. To this the father could not agree and a fourth child died. The father then put the last child wholly in the hands of Priessnitz, who plunged it into ice-water for a minute or so, felt the body carefully all over, repeated the plunge four or five times, then allowed the child to fall asleep. When it woke, the fever was gone (Turner 1967, 158-159).

Although Priessnitz was known to say, "Nothing is impossible to nature, diet and cold water" (Claridge 1843, 42), he was often more circumspect. He readily admitted that his treatments were not a panacea, but he firmly believed he could "cure all curable disease" (10). He was apparently successful with syphilis and smallpox, infectious diseases which were quite prevalent in his day. One witness observed, "At Gräfenberg, M. Priessnitz, by the sweating process, made a certain, speedy and safe cure of all cases of syphilis" (38). Syphilis was discovered to be curable by fever therapy later when doctors in malarial regions observed that syphilitics who contracted malaria were often saved from their original disease. Priessnitz, himself a victim of smallpox, was very confident of his ability to cure that disease. "Smallpox is only dangerous and disfiguring because people are wrongly treated" (Metcalfe 1898, 90), he said. He claimed to have cured each of the many smallpox cases which came to Gräfenberg with never a death nor a disfigurement. He relied on the wet sheet pack, changed as frequently as every half hour. So sure of this treatment was Priessnitz that he chose not to have his own son vaccinated against smallpox. He believed, as many doctors after him, that vaccinations predisposed the patient to other diseases such as scrofula.

The following case from Joel Shew, one of Priessnitz' most notable American students, is typical of the cases he recorded at Gräfenberg:

> A medical man from Sweden came to Gräfenberg, supported by two crutches, and by a servant. At one time, during treatment, a feverishness came upon him. Priessnitz applied successively, eighteen sheets in the day, and then a bath. In a week he went about with only a stick, and in ten days more, he walked as well as anyone (Shew 1849, 22).

Priessnitz' water treatments were effective. One medical doctor who visited Gräfenberg said, "I witnessed cures of such an extraordinary nature as to lead me to believe that Priessnitz must be acting under divine inspiration" (Claridge 1843, 33). Regardless of whether or not Priessnitz' nature treatments were enhanced by supernatural guidance, we must conclude, along with Dr. Detmar that "his enormous successes, even among serious invalids, are historically established and irrefutable" (1951, 101). If Claridge is reliable, the following passage well illustrates the success Priessnitz achieved. In describing the annual Gräfenberg ball commemorating Priessnitz' birthday, Claridge wrote:

> I do not know a more touching scene than seeing invalids, who, by his (Priessnitz') means, had regained the use of their limbs approach him, throw their crutches at his feet, and join in the maze of the waltz. Monarchs might have envied him his feelings on such occasions (35).

Priessnitz, a devoted family man, married in 1828 his beloved Sophie, the daughter of a wealthy magistrate whose wife he had cured of gout. Sophie was fair and good-looking, clever, and "a natural in manners." She managed the domestic economy of the large Priessnitz household with great skill, and was a source of strength and comfort to her husband during the persecutions he endured. "A rare treasure was this amiable and superior woman" (Metcalfe 1898, 25).

She and Priessnitz had eight children. When first married she had "no great faith" in Priessnitz' system of health and insisted their children be treated in the orthodox way, to which Priessnitz agreed. But when one of the children contracted measles and died under the regular doctor's care, she turned their medical care over to her husband. After that time she never had a moment's apprehension about them, and adopted the water treatment even for her own health. She was accustomed "during the six weeks previous to her accouchement to take a cold bath every day. To this she owes the happiness of a prompt and easy accouchement, and her speedy establishment in health" (Claridge 1843, 39). But after one birth she had "a severe attack of child-bed fever induced by the excitement of being visited, for several days after her confinement, by a number of ladies of rank." Her husband cured her in two days by a series of wet sheet packs and tepid baths (Shew 1849, 22).

Priessnitz loved his children intensely and valued their company, but this was rarely possible due to the heavy demands of his clinic work. Some of his children showed a predilection for the cold water treatments. His only son, "when sick, acted as his own physician and would tell the nurse: 'I want a dripping sheet. I must have another compress. That does me good'" (Metcalfe, 1898, 65). Priessnitz hired a teacher, whom he had successfully treated, as governess for his beloved children. When she fell seriously ill on a trip with the children, she was promptly cured by Priessnitz' eldest daughter who was skillful in the water treatments.

Priessnitz was also deeply religious, a devout Roman Catholic without prejudice against other denominations, who considered religion an indispensable part of healthy human life. He was civic-minded and participated actively in the communal life of Gräfenberg. Though thrifty by nature, Priessnitz was incredibly generous in his charity. At the height of the severe famine which struck Europe in 1846, as many as 300 people received food daily at Priessnitz' house.

In 1847 Priessnitz, weakened by overwork, collapsed with scarlet fever. His recovery under self-prescribed water treatments was complicated by the loss of his favorite daughter to marriage. Then the Revolution of 1848, which swept Europe the next year, profoundly upset the conservative Priessnitz. The breakdown of authority had a "crushing effect" on him and renewed his decline. "Truth and confidence are no more," he said (Metcalfe 1898, 67).

This took a toll on Priessnitz that showed in his face. At the age of fifty "his complexion was yellowish and weather-beaten, and his face deeply wrinkled" (Weiss 1967, 14). At about this time he said, "I believe that the end is approaching. I do not think that my complaint can be cured" (Metcalfe 1898, 67). Yet he still continued a full schedule of professional duties. Finally, in July, 1851 Priessnitz announced that he would no longer go to Freiwaldau to give treatments. He deteriorated so quickly that his wife sent for all of their children. Buoyed by the return of his family, Priessnitz felt better temporarily and made plans to erect a new building for his practice. "I am going to treat myself thoroughly," he said. "If eruptions of the skin show themselves, I can get well; if not, there will be no new building." (70) But the call to his patients was strong and Priessnitz continued to overwork himself. His wife watched him closely, ready to call for medical help, but Priessnitz refused a doctor to the end. He died at Gräfenberg of failure of the left lung, liver, and kidneys—all probably the direct or indirect result of the accidental injuries he had suffered as a teenager which helped set him on his course as a healer.

The suggestion that Priessnitz' "premature" death at age 52 "potentially discredited" his system (Cayleff 1987, 27) ignores the fact that he probably would not have survived into adulthood without the water treatments he administered to himself after the serious crush injuries to his chest. Also, the autopsy report suggests that decades of impingement on the vital organs by the improperly corrected chest injuries had prematurely shortened his life. This could be interpreted to say that the water treatments gave Priessnitz 35 extra years of life and enabled him to accomplish all that makes him worthy of our attention today.

The death of Vincent Priessnitz, the Genius of Cold-water, was reported "in newspapers over the civilized world" (Weiss 1967, 3) and "mourned by hundreds of thousands." His funeral procession was headed by 30 priests and extended the entire three miles from Gräfenberg to Freiwaldau. During the solemn procession:

> No sound was audible save the rushing of water from the springs which seemed to send their last farewell to him who had drawn them forth from their quiet to minister to the health of Europe (Metcalfe 1898, 74-75).

Priessnitz' wife, Sophie, who had been born in 1805, survived her husband by three years, dying in August of 1854.

Weiss and Kemble asserted that following Priessnitz' death "his patients dispersed and his water cure came to an end. There was no one to carry on his work" (1967, 14). But this is untrue. After Priessnitz' death, Josef Schindler, M.D. (1814-1891), succeeded Priessnitz' in Gräfenberg at the request of his family and "continued the methods of his teacher in exemplary fashion for another forty years" (Detmar 1951, 66). During the cholera epidemics of 1855 and 1866 Schindler treated 190 cholera patients with Priessnitz' methods and only one patient died. It was Schindler who introduced hydrotherapy to Wilhelm Winternitz (1834-1912), a professor from the University of Vienna, who established a scientific basis for it and taught it to Simon Baruch (1840-1921) and John Harvey Kellogg (1852-1943), American medical doctors who successfully brought these methods to the United States.

In 1898, Metcalfe gave detailed travel tips to his British countrymen who might wish to journey to Gräfenberg. As late as the 1920s Lust noted that Gräfenberg was the site of two large water cure institutions carrying on Priessnitz' work (1927, 270-271). Even today monuments erected by grateful patients in honor of Priessnitz, and remnants of the former grandeur of the spa can be found in the town of Jeseník (Freiwaldau) and Láznè Jeseník (Bad Gräfenberg), two kilometers above Freiwaldau. Modern travel guides to Czechoslovakia give the following description:

> Most of the surviving buildings, including the main spa building, are of the early years of the century. The cold water cure is still recommended for those suffering from nervous complaints, respiratory diseases and metabolic disorders, but the spa today has the faded character of a place past its heyday (Jacobs 1992,

> 309). There is a wonderful Art Nouveau monument to the spa's founder in the Kurpark, presiding god-like over the skinny sick on his right and on the "cured" (or at least plump) on his left (Humphreys, 1991, 251)

But Priessnitz' legacy went far beyond the remains of Gräfenberg. Not only did he make natural treatments so well known that his name was literally a household word throughout Europe, but also hundreds of water cure institutions had been established throughout the continent, America, and the British Isles based on the water cure principles he had laid down. His American patients and students returned from Gräfenberg afire with the new gospel of natural treatment and helped set in motion a health reform movement which swept America and paved the way for the transplantation of the Nature Cure movement from Europe to America some 50 years later.

How did "an illiterate hind of the Silesian mountains" (Shew 1850, ix), have such a tremendous impact? Although he was not "illiterate," his education was limited, and this ironically may have helped him discover the healing power of natural treatments. Claridge quoted a friend's doctor as saying:

> I fancy he (Priessnitz) is so completely ignorant of human anatomy, that if asked where the liver was situated, he would be at a loss to say, but that he can cure the liver complaint there is not the slightest doubt (1843, 33).

Despite his lack of scientific training Priessnitz became an amazingly successful doctor. A friend with access to science books offered to bring medical texts to Priessnitz, but Priessnitz rejected the offer, saying he was afraid they would warp his mind. "Doctors have learned too much," he used to say. "If they want to be good water doctors, they would have to forget a lot!" (Metcalfe 1898, 98) Priessnitz found not only doctors but also their teachers to be problems. "It is always professors of medicine who are my worst pupils," he complained (vom Walde 1899, 153). During his 25 years of practice he was visited by at least 1200 physicians, some who studied with him for several months. Since quite a few tried to influence the patients in various ways, Priessnitz was forced to include the following paragraph in his house rules: "If any physicians are present, I request that they abstain from any judgment towards the patients; if unable to do so, to leave the premises as soon as possible" (Schönenberger 1931, 48).

His keen, inquiring mind, unprejudiced by the scientific world-view of his age, "pierced the hidden secrets of nature!" By untiring observation and diligent experimentation he, in the words of one of his many royal fans, "brought to light facts which the science of centuries had been unable to discover" (Metcalfe 1898, 34).

Turner, in his book, *Taking the Cure*, a condescending put-down of the water cure movement, ridiculed Priessnitz as the "Demon of Gräfenberg" (145). Weiss and Kemble suggested Priessnitz owned a brewery and distillery in addition to his water cure establishment, and that in private he indulged in wine, coffee and brandy, which he forbade his patients. They also suggested he may have paid a bribe to suppress a favorable report about a health-care competitor, Johann Schroth, and substituted a favorable report about himself (1967, 11-12).

These charges are probably not true, but if they are, they would do little to detract from the accomplishments of Priessnitz whom other writers deemed "one of the most astounding geniuses of modern times" (Metcalfe 1898, v), "a second Columbus" (Rausse 1858, x) and "the benefactor of mankind "(Claridge). Schieferdecker compared him favorably to Luther as a reformer (1844, 20), and four countries (Czechoslovakia, Poland, Hungary and France) erected permanent national memorials in gratitude for the healthful services rendered their citizens by Priessnitz (Turner 1967, 162).

Belittlers of Priessnitz also liked to point out that he became very wealthy and suggested it was because of greed and high fees, which reflected some defect of character. It is true that Priessnitz was rich, but it was not from his fees, which were quite modest , but rather by gifts from grateful patients. Polish counts, cured at Gräfenberg, would dedicate a prize riding horse or even an entire team to show their gratitude. As Lust stated, Priessnitz lived in luxury in the midst of "worldly goods showered upon him not only from emperors, kings and princes . . . but also from the common people given to him in thankfulness and appreciation for the cure" (1927, 270).

Even historians favorably disposed toward the water cure movement he generated seem reluctant to give Priessnitz' methods their due. A recent study, which granted that Priessnitz probably did heal people, speculated that it was because of his skillful touch and refusal to use heroic medicines:

> His success stemmed from removing patients from the stresses and excesses that often induced their illnesses, providing a pleasant communal setting, implementing diet and exercise regimens that strengthened the body, ceasing heroic therapeutics, letting nature help right what was reversible, involving patients in their own cure through habit reformation, and applying the mystical healing powers attributed to Priessnitz personally (Cayleff 1987, 21).

While all these factors probably did contribute to his success, there seems to be an unwillingness to admit that the skillful use of so ordinary a substance as water could also have played a role.

Criticisms of Priessnitz were undercut by his fame and popularity. During his day, his name was literally a household word throughout Europe. A letter to him from the United States addressed "Herr Priessnitz, Europe" was delivered with no problem, and by his death, over 200 books had been written about him (vom Walde 1899, 31 & 34). Herman Melville refers to him in his 1857 novel *The Confidence Man* as the "well-meaning Preisnitz" (sic) (Melville, 1857, 110).

Priessnitz has always been granted the status of "father of hydrotherapy" but rarely is acknowledged as the progenitor of naturopathic medicine. Priessnitz is important to the history of naturopathic medicine as the first person to whom the term "Naturarzt" (nature doctor) can be applied. He was the first to systematize and promote a natural method of healing which was comprised "externally of pure water, of fresh air, of skin friction and kneadings, of clothing, and internally of simple diet, of pure-water drinking, all used in judicious conjunction with open air exercise (preferably hillside walking), and open air rest" (Metcalf 1898, 102). As one writer mildly put it, "He evidently cares to stick as close to nature as he can" (Houghton 1851, 147). This has proven a solid foundation for naturopathic medicine.

Priessnitz also understood, utilized and articulated in rudimentary form many principles of naturopathic medicine often attributed to Henry Lindlahr, who codified them over a half century after Priessnitz in his important work, *Nature Cure*. These include toxicity as a basis of disease, the idea of chronic disease as a result of suppressive treatments of acute disease, and the concept of the healing crisis as the basis for radical cure.

Finally, Priessnitz paved the way for Kneipp, Lust, Lindlahr and all future nature doctors by popularizing natural treatments throughout the western world, and by testing, perfecting and proving their efficacy in tens of thousands of cases. He also demonstrated the passionate devotion to his patients and the dogged determination in the face of persecution from established medicine which has been required of naturopathic physicians to this very day.

Perhaps the soundest assessment of Priessnitz came from Simon Baruch, a medical doctor, a generation removed from Priessnitz who, as an advocate of scientific hydrotherapy, despised the empirical tradition personified by Priessnitz but was grateful to Priessnitz for bringing water treatment to the attention of established medicine:

> His success was brilliant because he was a careful observer, a good judge of human nature, and his mechanical skill enabled

> him to invent various technical modifications of water treatment, many of which have been adopted by the profession and are still in use (Baruch 1892, 9).

Priessnitz was not only the simple, rustic character that has filtered down through history, but he was also a gifted healer and a man of great compassion, keen intellect and towering moral strength, a model for nature doctors of all times. Kneipp, Lindlahr, Lust, and other great innovators of natural therapy followed, but none of these can be judged of greater importance to the development of naturopathic medicine than the humble peasant, Vincent Priessnitz.

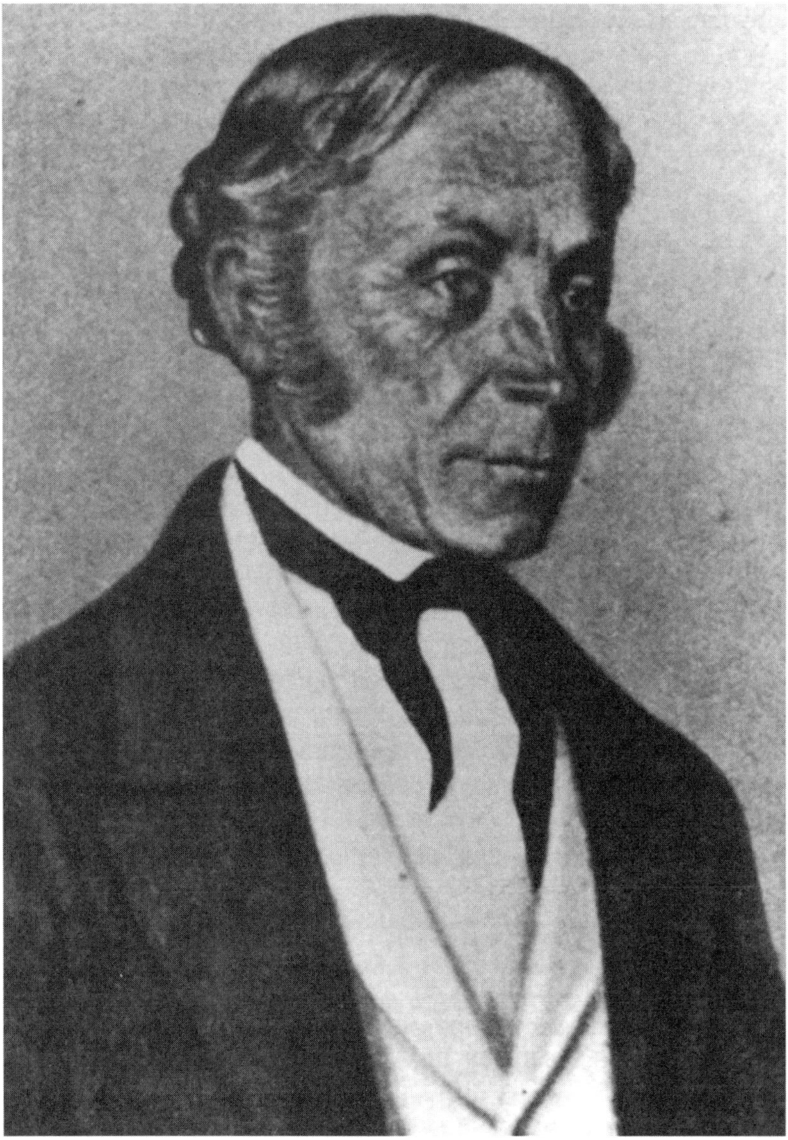

Johann Schroth
(Brauchle 1933, 36)

Priessnitz' Rival: Moist Heat, Thirst and Fasting Cure

Johann Schroth

(1798 - 1856)

Priessnitz' great rival and antagonist, not in numbers of patients but in the use of a different therapeutic system was Johann Schroth. Schroth was against Priessnitz' cold water applications or "frost regime," as Rausse called it, and prescribed long-lasting warm moist packs and even, if necessary, warm water bottles and hot baths. He prohibited drinking cold water, which played an important role at Gräfenberg, and he allowed his patients to drink a few glasses of warm wine in between "dry" days, when no fluid intake was permitted. Schroth advised his patients to rest in their packs for a long time and to move around only in moderation, while Priessnitz used vigorous exercise and work as a method to warm up the body before and after the cold water application.

Their dietary regimes were also diametrically opposed. Priessnitz recommended a hearty diet with lots of meat and milk to strengthen the body for the cold water treatment. Schroth subjected his patients to a salt- and fat-free dry diet without any meat or milk. It was his achievement to rediscover the age-old healing method of fasting and to employ it as a supplement to the water cure. It is, therefore, not surprising that some patients, who did not get the desired results from Priessnitz at the lofty heights of the Gräfenberg, fared better with Schroth in nearby Lindewiese, down in a picturesque river valley.

Johann Schroth was born in Lindewiese at the foot of the Gräfenberg on February 11, 1798, one and a half years before Vincent Priessnitz, who was a schoolmate in Freiwaldau and to whom he may have been distantly related. He was seven when his father, a farmer like Priessnitz' father, died. Schroth's mother married again after a short time, and young Johann was soon put to work on the family farm. He was such a good worker that his step-father decided to leave the farm to him instead of to his own sons. Besides his farm, Schroth established a livery stable and express business, and eventually became well-to-do.

Like Priessnitz, Schroth developed many of his important healing concepts from the close observation of nature and treating his own injuries. As a cavalry man and orderly to a veterinarian, Schroth also had contact with sick animals and showed a natural gift for treating them. When he returned home, he used his expertise in setting bones and treating fractures. In 1817, he was kicked by a horse, and his right knee-cap was broken. The medical treatment left considerable residual inflammation in the joint, and Schroth could no longer bend his knee. Unable to walk by the side of his loaded express cart, he used to climb up and ride on the top. One day a traveling monk, who thought Schroth was lazy, reproved him for riding in this way. After Schroth told him about his leg, the monk advised him to wash his knee with cold water several times a day. As this was inconvenient, Schroth fastened a wet bandage on the knee instead, renewing it at intervals. He found the effect to be wonderful. Inside the bandage there developed a very pleasant, moist warmth; the swelling disappeared, the hardened veins became soft, and after ten weeks, the former lame leg was as well as the other one.

Schroth sought to learn why these moist compresses brought about such remarkable results, so he looked for the answer in nature. While tilling the fields, he realized that seeds needed a warm humid soil for growth, much like a developing infant requires a warm, humid environment inside the mother's womb. He concluded that moist warmth is the most important condition for the development of plants and animals and that diseases were caused by its deficiency. Therefore, he reasoned, diseases could be cured by the application of wet heat. He also observed that horses, given much water, sweated more and tired out sooner than those kept without water, and that animals wounded by shooting recovered by fasting and refusing drink while keeping absolute rest.

His own cure, as well as Priessnitz' success, encouraged him to use wet bandages for injuries, sprains, dislocations, and swelling and stiffening of the joints. As Priessnitz, at the urging of his patients, advanced from the treatment of external injuries to internal ailments, so did Schroth begin to use warm wet packs combined with a dry diet for internal afflictions.

Brauchle wrote, "There can be no doubt that Schroth's career is inseparably linked to that of Priessnitz" (1951, 160). Schroth felt challenged by his former classmate and could not accept that Priessnitz alone should gain fame for healing the sick. The story goes that Schroth, at one point, courted Priessnitz' sister and was rejected. This may have challenged him as much as the patients who came down from the Gräfenberg without receiving much benefit from the cold water treatments and the copious water drinking.

Perhaps the wet heat and fasting were a more appropriate method of treatment for helping these "incurables."

Schroth never claimed that his method was a universal remedy and equally effective for all diseases. Like Priessnitz, however, he endured his share of persecutions and humiliations at the hands of the physicians. He was expelled from several communities where he went to treat the sick. He was accused of being a sorcerer, brought to court, charged with quackery and even thrown into jail.

By 1836, when Priessnitz was already a famous man, Schroth was still almost unknown. When his name was mentioned, he was scoffed at as an old cavalryman who was always drunk and deceived his patients with magnetism and hunger cure. Even Philo vom Walde wrote: "In the beginning, Schroth had his patients drink magnetized water, later brandy and finally wine in order to spur on the healing forces of the organism and as a stimulant of the weakened nerves," then added, "Alcohol must be considered more or less as a poisonous medicine, and its indulgence in excess by some patients in Lindewiese violates natural healing principles" (1898, 96-97). Mader defended the use of wine with the following reasons:

> "It is not easily practicable to eliminate alcohol or wine from the Schroth cure. Without the use of some alcohol most sufferers would not attempt these treatments at all, or they would not continue them with sufficient persistence. Whoever has observed dietary treatments, knows how difficult it is to make patients 'stick it out' without some alcohol. Strict diet, such as connected with the Schroth treatment, frequently brings about a morose and irritable patient, which reaches the point where the cranky sufferer becomes practically unbearable to all who come in contact with him. Therefore, the break in the monotony of the thirsting days offered by the patient's limited, periodic allowance of wine is very beneficial" (Mader 1927, 15-16).

According to modern Schroth-cure practitioners, unadulterated wine, sparingly used, has a stimulating effect on the heart and circulation and on the central nervous system. "The patient becomes more energetic in every respect" (Meyer-Camberg 1977, 263). Recently Schroth's use of wine received some posthumous vindication from the newest findings of epidemiologists who were puzzled about the low mortality rate from coronary heart disease in s France and attributed it in part to high wine consumption (Renaud 1992, 1523). However, the use of alcoholic beverages as therapy remains controversial within naturopathic circles.

Even after Schroth's fame grew, the number of his patients was never as overwhelming as Priessnitz'. Priessnitz treated 1304 patients in 1841 compared to Schroth's 77 patients. Even five years later in 1846 after Prince Bariatinsky had generated favorable publicity for Schroth, Lindewiese still had as few as 128 patients. Only in 1851, when Priessnitz could no longer visit his patients in Freiwaldau and Böhmischdorf, did the number of patients in Lindewiese increase considerably.

In 1840, Schroth was granted official permission to operate his establishment as his success with certain patients made an impression on the Austro-Hungarian authorities which had previously given Priessnitz the freedom to practice. The physician Baumbach, a former Priessnitz patient, said that Schroth was not so bad as he was portrayed on the Gräfenberg. His method proved that not only could the vigorous bathing and showering of Priessnitz be helpful, but also a strict diet and sweating could achieve excellent results. No doubt, Baumbach was one of the patients disappointed by Priessnitz who found the right treatment with Schroth. Also Dr. Lorenz Gleich, whose writings contributed much to the theory and terminology of Nature Cure, became an enthusiastic "Schrothian" after visiting Gräfenberg twice with less than spectacular results and then going to Schroth who helped him. He condemned Priessnitz' "old cold water pigtail" and sided more with Schroth (Rothschuh 1983, 75). Dr. W. Czybulka praised him in a publication which gave the first over-all picture of the Schroth cure. Schroth even won some powerful patrons from among royalty including the Russian Prince, Alexander von Bariatinsky, an adjutant to the Czar who made the long trip from St. Petersburg to Schroth as a last resort for an eye disease. He underwent a successful cure in 1846 and wrote a pamphlet which praised Schroth and condemned Priessnitz. Vom Walde, however, tells us that the prince's old ailment came back after his return home. For this reason, he asked a well-known Englishman, who was Schroth's patient at that time, to purchase and destroy all of his remaining pamphlets, as he felt regret to have written about Priessnitz in a derogatory way (98). Whether this story is credible is hard to say, since Philo vom Walde had an obvious bias in favor of Priessnitz.

Schroth's most spectacular cure was that of the Prince Wilhelm von Württemberg whose knee had been wounded by bullets in the battle of Novara. His condition was pitiful, and his physicians wanted to amputate his leg. "Finally someone called his attention to Schroth, and the Prince went to the peasant-physician, who within a few months brought about a cure of such thoroughness that the overjoyed Prince was able to dance a court ball and was as "happy as the happiest there" (Anonymous 1927, 338). In April 1850 he issued the following proclamation to "Messrs. Comrades in the

Army" in the Austrian *Soldiers' Friend* which drew many new patients to Lindewiese:

> The undersigned considers it his duty to draw the attention of his comrades with war injuries to a healing method which brings a safer recovery than all other methods known so far and applied by physicians. The farmer Johann Schroth in Niederlindewiese near Freiwaldau in Austria-Silesia has been treating fresh and old injuries in a very special way for many years with the best results. Unfortunately, they are too little known. His cure had been termed and derided by many as 'Semmelkur' (dry roll cure) because it was believed that he cured injuries with dry rolls. However, this is not true. Schroth's principle is to cut off, as much as possible, the injured parts from bad humors and he accomplishes this by subjecting his patients to the strictest diet. He does not permit water at all and reduces the food for the sick to wine and dry rolls in order to nourish and strengthen them simultaneously. At the same time he uses local wet packs which stay on for a longer or a shorter period depending on the condition of the injury. The cure cannot be called easy, but it is not excessively demanding either, and certainly not too much of a sacrifice for the safe restoration of health. To mention a few examples, I start with myself. A pointed bullet had penetrated my shin-bone directly under the knee; I had been bed-ridden for nine months, and there was no hope that I would keep my leg. At last, I turned to Schroth and he restored me completely in four months. At any time it will be my pleasure to give more information to my wounded comrades about the cure to which I owe my recovery and which will hopefully still help many others. Wilhelm, Duke of Württemberg, Captain at the Archduke Sigmund-Inf.Reg.No.45 (cited in Fenn 1982, 35-36).

People who knew and respected Schroth characterized him as a true healer with a warm, charming and confidence-inspiring personality. They emphasized his selflessness in treating many poor patients without charge and always being ready to help without pursuing his own advantage. They also said that he intuitively perceived the healing processes going on in his patients and knew how to support them at just the right moment. Like Priessnitz, Schroth never charged any consultation fee, but thanks to the gifts from rich patients he became quite wealthy later in life, although his wealth never reached the proportions of Priessnitz'.

Often in biographical works, too little recognition is given to the wives of famous men. Like Sophie Priessnitz, the good spirit of Gräfenberg who earned the respect of all patients as "Madame Priessnitz," Theresia Schroth was a great support to her husband. This is especially remarkable because these women, like their husbands, came from a peasant background and had no formal education. Yet they took responsibility for the care and accommodation of large numbers of patients besides keeping their own homes, raising children, and tending to farm duties.

According to Vom Walde, Priessnitz would not accept patients after they changed from him to Schroth. "I cannot do anything with somebody weakened by hunger and thirst," he supposedly said. "Come back in 6-12 months after you have recovered some strength at home again!" (98). Nonetheless, although Priessnitz and Schroth rejected each other's methods, they always spoke about each other with respect.

Schroth was a tall, gaunt man with a kind, benevolent face. However, the heavy burden of tending his farm while taking care of his patients, all while warding off persecutions, wore him down so much that he finally became extremely emaciated and exhausted. Brauchle dismisses as slander Vom Walde's contention that Schroth over-indulged in alcohol. Schroth died from an organic heart ailment at the age of fifty-eight on March 26, 1856, five years after Priessnitz. His son and successor, Emanuel Schroth, also died from a heart disease in the prime of life.

Like Priessnitz, Schroth was not a man of the pen, and he did not leave a written description of his method. However, numerous books and articles about the Schroth Cure were published by his successors in Lindewiese and by doctors who introduced the Schroth Cure in their own sanitariums. They developed and improved it while giving it a theoretical foundation. It is alive and practiced in Germany like the Kneipp Cure, though on a much smaller scale. Lindewiese, now located in the Czech Republic, lost its significance as the Schroth Cure Center after World War II when the Germans were driven out. According to a modern travel guide to Czechoslovakia, Lindewiese has not completely disappeared from the map as a spa: "Pleasant and old-fashioned is the tiny spa of Lipovà-Làznè (Lindewiese), 4 km due West of Jeseník (Freiwaldau) cozily set between trees and lush rolling meadows; founded in 1830 by a man called Schroth, its waters have been used since then for the treatment of obesity and rheumatism" (Jacobs 1992, 251). Dr. Hermann Brosig saved the cure, bringing it over to West Germany in 1949 and making Oberstaufen in the Bavarian Alpes the new "Lindewiese." Today, many thousands of patients visit Oberstaufen each year. A "Schroth Federation" with its own magazine keeps Schroth's memory alive and propagates his cure (Fenn 1982, 37).

Despite the early translation into English of Clemens Gehrke's enthusiastic book about the Schroth Cure applied to children's diseases (1881) and a series of articles about the Schroth Cure by Dr. Max Mader, one of Schroth's successors at Lindewiese, in the *Naturopath*, Schroth's methods never became popular in America. Every year over 2000 patients underwent the Schroth Cure in Lindewiese at that time (Mader 1926, 533).

One can only speculate about why the Schroth Cure never took hold in this country. Certainly the lack of a well-established tradition of health-spa attendance and lack of insurance coverage for such methods have played a role. In addition, fast-paced American life is not conducive to taking one or two months for a complete body overhaul. Schroth did not draw large numbers of American patients to Lindewiese who would transplant his ideas to this country as many Priessnitz enthusiasts had done.

The basic elements of the Schroth Cure are wet sheet packs, periodic alternation of dry and drinking days, and the Schroth diet. The three phases of the treatment are the preliminary, the main, and the supplementary. In the preliminary phase, the patient is gradually weaned from the usual diet to a more simplified fare of dry rolls, prunes, and water-based cereals. The Schroth diet, along with a strict regimen of alternate drinking and thirsting days, constitutes the main phase of treatment. The supplementary phase is a gradual return to the usual diet. Wet sheet packs are used to relieve thirst, equalize the body's temperature, and carry away toxins. The cure may take from one to three months according to the nature of the case. In prolonged treatments the patient may be given a "period of rest" of one to two weeks of normal diet before the strict program is resumed. The cure is complete when the patient's tongue is moist and perfectly clean, and the urine no longer contains sediments (Gray 1904, 185).

The effect on the body of alternating dry and drinking days is compared to the effect on a sponge which is cleansed by being filled with water, then squeezed out, filled with water and squeezed again until it is clean (Fenn 1982, 42). The overall process does not occur without the usual healing crises, which need close monitoring by the medical staff. One goal of the treatment is to induce a fever which helps the body burn off toxins. The treatment is considered especially useful for conditions arising from inertness of the skin as an excretory organ, from imperfect assimilation of food, and from poisons that have entered the body. The Schroth Cure requires extraordinary willpower and self-discipline. Schroth's own motto was: "Without battle no victory, without deprivation no enjoyment, without cleansing no healing" (Mader 1926, 532).

While Priessnitz focused his efforts on the generation of a skin crisis to detoxify the body of poisonous substances, the skin played a less important role in Schroth's program. Although he stimulated its activity with wet packs, Schroth regarded the skin crisis as merely a side crisis which only eliminated superficial morbid substances. His experiences convinced him that the urinary and intestinal crises played more important roles, and that true healing came only from a curative stimulation of the digestive system and the kidneys. But, as Brauchle stated, "If we take a closer look, both treatment methods do not contradict but complement each other, because the skin crises as well as the kidney and intestinal crises deserve our consideration" (Brauchle 1951, 162).

The complementary nature of the two systems is also emphasized by Gerhard Hildebrand and Benedict Lust. Hildebrand writes: "As strange as it may sound, only to such an extent that Schroth established himself as a competitor with Priessnitz, was progress made from the water cure to nature cure methods" (cited in Rothschuh 1983, 75). In a series of articles published in the *Naturopath* in 1926, Lust gave a report about his "Trip to the Fatherland" which included visits to the famous birthplaces of nature cure: Gräfenberg, Lindewiese, and Wörishofen. One of the highlights of this trip was when he brought the rival camps of Gräfenberg and Lindewiese together. His unique, vivid account deserves to be quoted at length:

> There was a keen rivalry for over 100 years between Johann Schroth School and Vincent Priessnitz School. Here you have two masters, they are using Nature's agents but each one uses it in a different way, and both arrive at the same end. Their principles constitute Basic Naturopathy.
>
> In visiting Wörishofen, Niederlindewiese and the Gräfenberg I was more than ever convinced that the Naturopathic idea including all that is rational and good in the healing art and adopting special methods for certain cases is the best. A naturopathic physician must stand above cults, he must above all be broad, never fanatical. He must have a full conception of what constitutes a real cure and he must know how to assist Nature with her own agents, with the congenial means of life, to purify, to cleanse, and to build up and so restore the normal state.
>
> Now to come back to our lecture at Niederlindewiese. In 150 years, it has never happened that the head physicians of Gräfenberg and Lindewiese sat at the same table. My coming brought about this wonderful reconciliation and understanding of the two leaders of the two meccas of the original Nature Cure. Dr. Ebelt was chairman and introduced us, and I was pleased to see so many Americans and English-speaking people at this large audience—intelligent and highly-cultured people practically

> from all parts of the world. We lectured in German and also in English. We told them about the advance of the Nature Cure Movement in the U.S.A. from the early days of Graham, Jennings, Thrall, and Dr. Gifford. We told them that in 1852 there were over 40 hydrotherapeutic establishments in the United States, established and conducted by doctors who were students of Vincent Priessnitz and Johann Schroth. I told them of the Naturopathic movement now, as it includes all methods of healing that are rational and sane, such as Chiropractic, Osteopathy, the Physical Culture Movement and also the Christian Science Movement, as well as the old Nature Cure, Eclecticism (sic) and Homeopathy. I was asked questions on these points.
>
> I started my lecture at 2:30 and finished at six o'clock, in the 'Gasthaus zur Sonne' in the big hall. Some drank good wine and some drank 'real' beer in the great old German style. Dr. Ebelt of the Gräfenberg and Dr. Max Mader of Lindewiese shook hands together and celebrated the feast of harmony and getting together for the benefit for all.
>
> The large number of patients that were present came from Gräfenberg and all the Schroth patients were there with their Doctors, headed by the great chief Max Mader.
>
> It was certainly a delightful time and Dr. Ebelt wrote me last week that those hours he will never forget. The grand-niece of V. Priessnitz, Dr. Mader, and Dr. Ebelt—all three were made honorary graduates of our school and honorary members of the American Naturopathic Association. All were very happy to receive this distinction from the parent school of Nature Cure in the U.S.
>
> This event is perpetuated by an inscription in gold lettering on the Gablenz Monument at Lindewiese and any reader of this magazine who ever visits over there will be pleased to see there our visit recorded in metal and stone (Lust 1927, 171-172).

After his return to New York Lust summed up what the trip to the two birthplaces of nature cure had meant to him: "I am now satisfied and happy that I visited Gräfenberg and Lindewiese, the two principle shrines of the Nature Cure. Priessnitz represents Hydrotherapy and all that goes with the old Nature Cure and Johann Schroth represented the fasting and the diet cure, the two mainstays of Naturotherapy" (Lust 1927, 272). If there is a dialectic in nature cure, then Johann Schroth represented a striking antithesis to Priessnitz' clearly-stated thesis. It was left to Benedict Lust and others to work out a suitable synthesis of these contrasting methods.

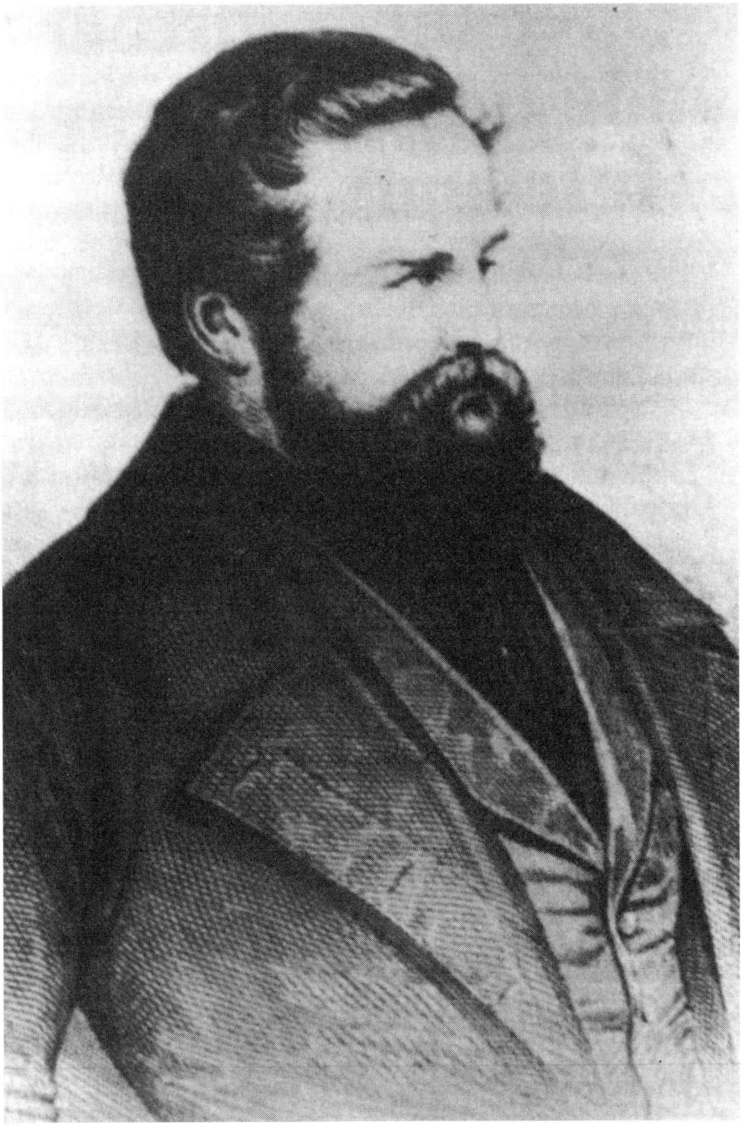

J. H. Rausse
(Rothschuh 1983, 20)

The Reformer of Water Cure

J. H. Rausse

(1805 -1848)

J. H. Rausse was the most important and influential of the many visitors to Gräfenberg to write about the taciturn Priessnitz and his methods. Ernst Kapp, a grateful patient Rausse cured of an eye disease, called him the "reformer of water cure" in an eulogistic biography written shortly after Rausse's death. Philo vom Walde, the Priessnitz advocate, acknowledged Rausse as a man of genius and the first to lay down the scientific principles of hydrotherapy (1898, 66). Richard Metcalfe, the great British hydrotherapist, called him "the most energetic in propagating the new method of healing in Germany."

He was born August 18, 1805 in Güstrow (Mecklenburg) where his father was employed as a superintendent of the Lutheran church. His real name was Heinrich F. Francke. His fellow university students gave him the nickname "Rausse," the French equivalent of the German word "Ross" meaning horse, due to his animal strength and wild temperament.

Rausse, who grew up with ten brothers and sisters, was a strong and healthy baby. The family physician predicted that he would become a Samson. When he was three years of age however, he was afflicted with diarrhea, which was treated with constipating drugs and a bland diet, and as a result he fell ill with constipation which was treated with strong doses of purgatives for the next two years. The physician himself was astonished that the young boy could tolerate such high doses which were normally given only to robust farmhands. These powerful overdoses made the boy so weak and frail that the physicians did not know what else to do but employ the strongest drug tonics. Incredibly, in his tenth year Rausse weighed no more than in his first year. When the doctors gave up on him and finally stopped medication altogether, he slowly, but never completely, recovered.

Rausse loved his mother dearly; he believed he inherited his pride, passion for the truth, and love of nature from her. However, he never forgave her for allowing him to be poisoned as a child. His sometimes unbearable suffering in the later years of his life reminded him of this. As Kapp wrote,

"Here we have the key to Rausse's enormous animosity against everything called medicine. Here is the key to the secret of his truly demonic desire to free himself and all similar victims of medical abuse from the evil enemy of medicinal substances" (1850, 16-17).

After a number of years as a student at the local gymnasium, a place he hated for its mind-killing pedantry, the rebellious Rausse was sent to the university to follow in his father's footsteps and study theology. However, he preferred carousing to studying and attended lectures on philosophy, science, and medicine irregularly and without any clear plan or goal. He was the center of attention wherever he went because of his quick-wittedness and originality, and well liked due to his abilities in drinking and fencing. A scar above his left eye from a duel in Berlin gave his already severe countenance an even more martial expression. He was removed from a number of universities because of his outspokenness and insubordination. Rausse said of this time:

> At the university I was a mixture of enthusiasm for nature, pleasure in physical exercise, and excessive debauchery. I lost not only self-respect, but also respect for humanity, for everything that is good and noble. I considered the theological writings as pure hypocrisy and since childhood I had never believed in the catechism or the Bible (cited in Kapp 1850, 30).

Concerning medicine he wrote, "From the first semester I regarded this science as a mindless repetition of an ancient system which had nothing to do with the true healing art" (30).

However, a great change occurred when he discovered the works of Jean-Jacques Rousseau, the Swiss-born political philosopher. They influenced his entire way of life from then on. He realized that he was more suited to an outdoor career than university studies, and he became a forest superintendent. He devoted himself entirely to the observation of nature and studied the plants and trees, the origins of springs and rivers, the formation of weather patterns, and the behavior of animals. "After living a dissolute and most unnatural life," wrote Kapp, "he went into the other extreme and wanted to become a complete man of Nature in the footsteps of Rousseau's Emile. Europe was the wrong place for this. He wanted to escape its corrupting civilization and find in America's virgin forests what he was looking for—Nature and true human freedom" (1850, 36).

Following Rousseau's call to return to nature, Rausse spent almost a year among the Osage Indians in North America living as a hunter, until he fell ill with yellow fever. Worn out and tired of life in America and of existence in general, he returned to Germany to die in his homeland. The sea journey however, had a beneficial effect on his health, and back in Europe he regained sufficient strength to resume working. To supplement his low salary as a forester he started a career as a writer and published *Travel Scenes from Two Worlds* about his adventure in the wilderness, and *The Star of Love*, a novel which reflected his own love story in a somewhat altered and eccentric way.

All these activities again aggravated his illness. Because of his deep aversion to any regular medical attention, he decided to try Priessnitz' water cure, which was becoming prominent. Rausse spent ten weeks in Gräfenberg during the fall of 1837 and was profoundly impressed by this completely new approach to healing. Its simplicity and closeness to nature reminded him of the truths he had discovered in Rousseau, and he began to ponder the principles underlying water cure which Priessnitz followed by intuition.

But Rausse's rebellious and inquiring nature brought him in conflict with Priessnitz' treatment plan. Once he discerned the physiological basis of the water cure, he was able to identify errors in its application in certain cases, including his own. He withdrew from Priessnitz' direct influence, continuing his cure according to his own judgment. Because of limited means, he had to interrupt his treatment before he was completely well. "I departed soon to return home after I was clear about the design of my cure," he wrote. "However, I would have never attained an understanding of the general as well as of my own water cure if Priessnitz' great and ingenious discoveries had not become the basis for my successive research and discoveries" (cited in Kapp 1850, 42).

Soon Rausse wrote down his observations on Gräfenberg in a small book entitled *The Spirit of the Graefenberg Water Cure* (1838), which caused a sensation and went through several editions. A year later he published his *Miscellanies to the Graefenberg Water Cure*, which was dedicated to Priessnitz and had as a motto, "Water Can Do It." In Kapp's opinion, nothing contributed more to Priessnitz' fame and recognition than this wonderfully written book — "neither the praise of the recovered patients nor the physicians who were converted to the new system nor all the other books which praised him" (1850, 51). The book opened with a hymn to the genius of Priessnitz which concluded: "Go up to those mountains; here, high above the nations stands the figure of that great man, embracing with one arm eternal, beneficent Nature and reaching forth the other to mankind, offering it restoration of health and happiness in a new era" (Rausse 1851, x).

The book made many friends, but also some enemies. Physicians who dared not attack the famous Priessnitz were only too grateful for the chance to tear apart an unknown author espousing Priessnitz' practices. "They slapped Rausse," wrote Kapp, "but meant Priessnitz" (1850, 51).

Rausse's arrogance and his biting polemics against their drug practice did little to endear him to the allopathic doctors. On the title page below his name Rausse had inscribed, "Truly Secret Magician and Medicus with the Tribe of Serpent Indians, Corresponding Member in all the Nations of Caraibes, and Hottentotts, Knight of Innumerable Orders from the States Lichtenhain, Ziegenhain and Passendorf." This was a parody of the physicians and their obsession with academic titles and honors. "These pages will probably not be without errors in minor details," he began immodestly, "but on the whole this book contains more truth than all the medical writings and systems since Galen to our present time—which of course does not mean much" (cited in Rothschuh 1983, 23).

Originally Rausse did not want to become a water doctor, but he was pressed into this new career by his enthusiastic readers and admirers. He was also influenced to enter the field professionally because of mistakes in water cure practices which he felt corrupted the true principles of hydrotherapy.

In 1844 he took over the water cure in Stuer (Mecklenburg). The influx of patients to his establishment was overwhelming and stirred great jealousy among the Mecklenburg allopaths. Their attacks upon him were savage but ill-advised, for the venomous wit of Rausse's counter-attacks devastated his adversaries. By 1847, when the Stuer establishment proved too small, he founded a larger water cure institution in Lehsen near Wittenberg. Kapp offers an interesting sketch of Rausse at this time.

> "Rausse was of medium size. His build was extraordinarily strong and muscular; his shoulders were broad, and his skull was enormous with a clearly arched forehead. He usually walked around with his head bent, reflecting, thinking, arms crossed behind the back, his hands playing with a stick. His gait was slow. His small, sonorous voice was in marked contrast to his strong stature. He did not put the slightest emphasis on outside appearance. In the avoidance of harmful food and drink he set an example for his patients; however, he often ate enormous portions and, perhaps sometimes more than was good for his stomach. He suffered quite often from vomiting which he considered a healing crisis." (Kapp 1850)

Despite his busy water cure practice, Rausse still found time to write inflammatory polemics, outstanding in their logic, wit, and astuteness. His last complete work, *Errors of Physicians and Others in the Practice of the Water*

Cure as Remedial Agent in the Prevention and Cure of Medicine, was published in 1847.

In this work he not only condemns the mistakes of physicians who were using the water in the wrong way or in combination with drugs, leeches, and bloodletting, but he also dared to criticize some of Priessnitz' excessively harsh methods. Philo vom Walde tried to refute him: "Priessnitz treated each of his patients in a special way. Therefore Rausse's generalizations don't do him justice. Only after a second longer stay on the Gräfenberg would Rausse have been entitled to write a 'Critic of Vincent Priessnitz' Water Cure Methods'" (1898, 89). Brauchle believed that some of Rausse's critical remarks about Priessnitz' were justified. However, considering the record Priessnitz established for success and safety, he concluded, "the significance of Rausse's objections seem to be exaggerated" (1951, 127).

When Rausse's water cure in Lehsen could no longer accommodate the ever-increasing number of patients, he moved to Alexandersbad near Wunsiedel in April of 1848. Here he began a book, *Instructions for the Use of the Water Cure Methods* (1850). Only the first part of this work came from his own pen. The second and third parts were written after Rausse's death by his cousin and disciple Theodor Hahn.

Rausse was not happy in Alexandersbad because of the excessive demands of the practice and the increasing deterioration of his health. He had received invitations to manage water cure establishments in the United States and in Switzerland and he soon reproached himself for not having accepted one of these offers. Rausse's last days of agonizing struggle are described by Theodor Hahn, who portrayed him as gloomy and ill-humored. In the first days of July, his vomiting and stomach pain worsened, he became very restless and thought seriously of shooting himself to be free from the unbearable pain. On July 12, 1848, death finally delivered him from his suffering at the age of 43. He died as lonely as he had lived. He had locked himself in his room and those who found him had to climb through a window to get in. His autopsy revealed pyloric stenosis and a hardened pancreas suggesting that he died either from stomach ulcer or stomach cancer (Kapp 1850, 70-82).

Rausse considered Priessnitz the discoverer of the water cure, but looked on himself as its master and perfecter. He rightly credited Priessnitz with discovering that cold water draws blood, strength, and warmth to the body parts it contacts; that cold water is curative only after the skin is warm, or even better, sweating; that, contrary to the prevailing medical opinion of his time, the sudden change from sweat pack to cold bath does no harm but rather increases the beneficial reaction of the entire organism; that chronic diseases must be transformed by cold water treatments into acute diseases before they can be cured. But Rausse felt that Priessnitz strayed from these truths when he lost touch with his extraordinary "instinct."

For Rausse instinct was everything. It represented the safest and most important guide for the preservation of health and the cure of disease. He wrote: "The inclinations and antipathies of instinct are the lead-strings by which Nature directs man and beast on the road to happiness and health. Man is not ordained for emancipation from the bonds of Nature; every digression from the voice of Nature is a revolt and outbreak, and the consequences are misery and afflictions" (1851, viii). Rausse was first drawn to Priessnitz because he felt he embodied the instinctual principles advocated by Rousseau. "Go into the woods and become humans," wrote Rousseau. This is exactly what Rausse believed Priessnitz had done at Gräfenberg. But, in Rausse's opinion, success spoiled Vincent Priessnitz. Fame and fortune distorted his instincts and led him into overly harsh treatments.

Despite his severe criticism of Priessnitz, Rausse respected him highly as a person and as a great pioneer in water therapy. While Rausse loved nothing better than to attack his allopathic enemies, it was agony for him to speak ill of the hero to whom he had been so devoted. He never forgot that Priessnitz had saved his life.

For his part, Priessnitz bore no grudge against Rausse for his unkind behavior and as late as 1845 recommended him to head a water cure establishment in Spain. "His praise of himself," Priessnitz said of Rausse, "will not give him any benefit, nor will it harm me" (cited in Rothschuh 1983, 24). Priessnitz appreciated their differences for what they were: disputes between a beloved father and a rebellious son wanting to make his own mark.

Rausse fought against what he considered wrong healing methods with passionate, polemical fervor. He felt allopathic medicine was harmful because it used strong drugs to force the body to give up its struggle for health. The result was not restoration of health but often a chronic condition and long-term debility. He understood that the power to heal was within the body and that curative treatments ought to stimulate that healing power rather than suppress it. He believed disease was caused by foreign material which had to be removed from the body for cure. Therefore, he was a strong advocate of the healing "crisis" as practiced by Priessnitz.

He also advocated treating the whole person rather than an isolated body part or organ because he recognized that all body functions are interrelated. He rejected any disease classification arguing that nature knew no genera or species but only individuals. Because no two patients were alike even if they had the same disease, his water cure concentrated on symptoms and emphasized the art of individualization. The nature cure movement would later take its battle cry, "Treat the patient, not the disease!" from this postulate. These and other essential concepts intuited by Priessnitz and articulated and developed by Rausse dominated nature cure philosophy thereafter. All of them can be found in the writings of their successors again and again (Rothschuh 1983, 22).

Nature cure historians agree that not only was Rausse an ingenious thinker and gifted writer, a "passionate fighter with quill and words," but also that he was possessed of a "demonic nature" full of inner tensions and subject to changing moods. With fervent eloquence he preached the importance of a life close to nature. Brauchle called him a Rousseau of the water cure because of Rausse's belief that the water cure had so much in common with Rousseau's dictum "Return to Nature" (1951, 123).

In Rothschuh's view:

> Rausse was a strange mixture of artist, apostle, and nature doctor—of ignorance and arrogance. He had a violent temperament and made as many enemies as friends. He was enormously inventive in finding insulting terms for allopathic physicians—the pill jesuits and poisoners. Indeed, the atmosphere between conventional medicine and nature cure has been seriously clouded ever since (Rothschuh 1983, 24).

Rausse was not a scientific thinker nor widely read in medicine. He was apparently unfamiliar with Hufeland, who had much in common with him philosophically and whose views could have been very useful to Rausse. One of his critics, Hirschel, because of Rausse's violent rantings against orthodox medicine, considered him mentally deranged and suffering from fixed delusion. This was exaggerated, especially in light of the medicine in his time, which offered sufficient reason for criticism. As Rothschuh noted, "One had only to look at the heroic bloodletting procedures and drugging abuses" (1983, 21). Even Philo vom Walde, who never forgave Rausse's criticism of Priessnitz, said: "Regardless of how many human foibles he had and how much he hurt Priessnitz' reputation, Rausse was a genius and a true water-Paulus who spread the message about the blessings of an unspoiled Nature to the world with fervent eloquence. His accomplishments for the development of the nature cure are immortal" (1898, 90).

Rausse is barely known and poorly appreciated in naturopathic circles today. This is unfortunate because his contributions to the understanding of the principles underlying nature cure which he articulated with such force and clarity still define the philosophy of naturopathic medicine. The radicalness of his doctrine is both refreshing and shocking.

The art of healing does not lie before us in the grey mysteries and doctrines of the future, but far behind us in the past of the green original life of nature. "Return" is the motto of the true healing art, not "forward" (cited in Rothschuh 1983, 23).

Water Cure and Vegetarianism

Theodor Hahn

(1824 - 1883)

Theodor Hahn is less known in the United States than in Germany, as none of his works have been translated into English. He is an important figure in the history of the nature cure movement because he carried on Rausse's clinical and theoretical work. On the cover of Benedict Lust's *Amerikanische Kneipp-Blätter* (1898-1901), a forerunner of *The Naturopath*, a bust of Hahn decorates the pedestal of a Kneipp monument beside busts of Schroth, Rausse, and Priessnitz.

Hahn was born on May 19, 1824, in Ludwigslust in Mecklenburg, the home province of Rausse. As a reaction to his first vaccination, he developed a rash which did not disappear until he was six years old, this despite continuous treatment with different lotions. At age four he began to suffer from serious asthma which could not be controlled by any drugs. Asthmatic attacks troubled him so much that it frequently interrupted his schooling. Despite the use of all the conventional drugs of his time (Belladonna once blinded him completely), nothing helped his condition. "Like so many nature doctors, Hahn's own suffering and disappointment with conventional medicine served as the starting point for his calling as a healer" (Brauchle 1951, 165).

> Originally Hahn wanted to become a physician himself, but he felt too weak to endure the long and strenuous education. Therefore he became an apprentice in a pharmacy where he proceeded to try the different medicines on himself—without any success. Disillusioned with the drug practice, he discovered Rausse's writings which inspired him to experiment with the water cure on himself. At about the same time, he was influenced by the story of the pharmacist Schreiber "who was cured at Gräfenberg after many futile attempts with drug therapies and who sold his pharmacy, his 'poison dump' as he called it, to become an advocate for the water cure" (Brauchle 1951, 165-166).

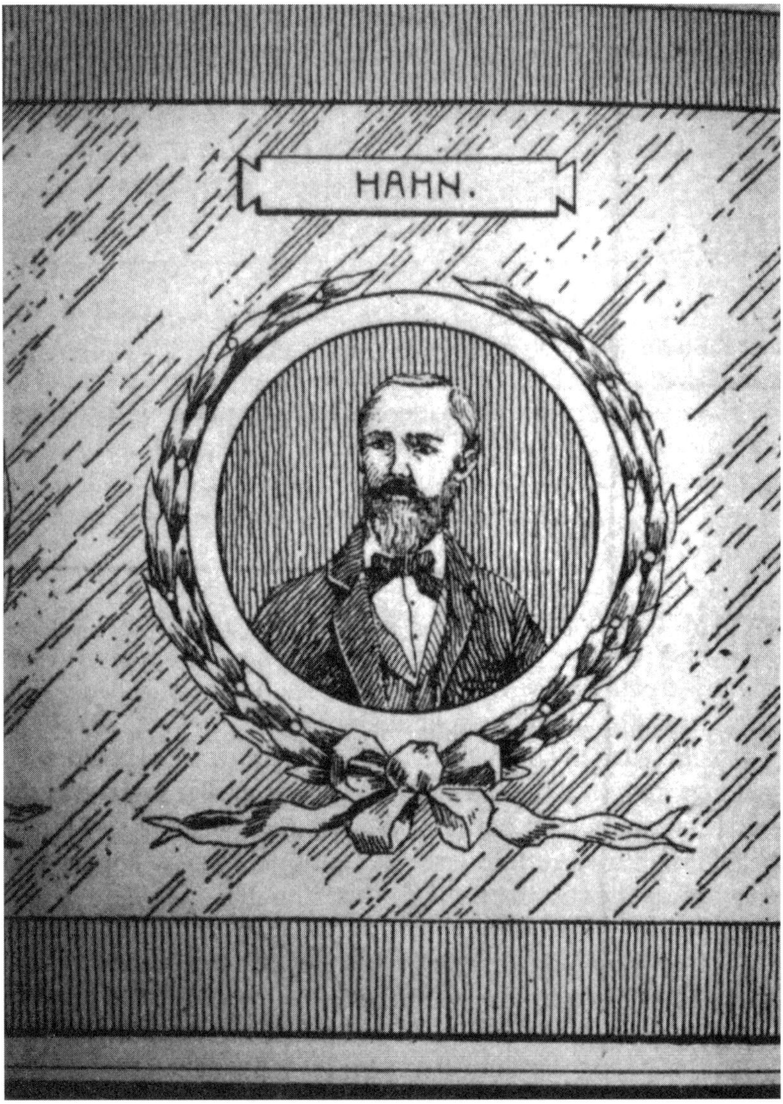

Theodor Hahn
(Amerikanische Kneipp-Blätter, March 1, 1898, title page)

Since Hahn was not completely comfortable with his own attempts at self-treatment—he wore a wet trunk compress night and day until it generated the expected strong rash—he decided to go to Lehsen to seek Rausse's advice. During this first consultation they discovered that they were cousins. Rausse recommended that Hahn come to him for treatments for six months in order to restore his health. Hahn started his water cure on October 1, 1847, and after a short experience became an enthusiastic follower and eloquent promoter. He accompanied Rausse when Rausse took over the larger water cure at Alexandersbad, and became both an assistant and friend. After Rausse's early death in 1848, Hahn took it upon himself to organize and publish the manuscripts which Rausse left. He completed the second part and third part of Rausse's last work, *Instructions for the Use of the Water Cure*, in 1851 and 1852.

It was here Hahn first used the term "Naturheilkunde" (Nature Cure). As Rothschuh pointed out, however, it was probably not Hahn but the Bavarian military physician, Lorenz Gleich (1798-1865), who coined the term in a lecture he gave in Munich on July 29, 1849 (1983, 25). Gleich, who had studied Priessnitz' and Schroth's methods in Gräfenberg and Lindewiese, deserves special recognition for the development of a new and coherent terminology in his *Physiatric Writings* (1860), a collection of his articles and lectures. He suggested dropping such old terms as "hydropath" and "water cure," which were no longer adequate to describe the increasing variety of methods and their practitioners, replacing them with such terms as "Naturheilkunde" (Nature cure), "Naturheilmethode" (nature cure methods), "Naturheilanstalt" (nature cure establishment), and "Naturheilarzt" (naturopathic physician) or "Naturarzt" (nature doctor). Today these terms are widely known and understood in Germany, but remain poorly recognized in America.

After Rausse's death, Hahn attended the University of Leipzig for a short time, married (his wife would have seven children) and settled down in the spring of 1849 as a lay practitioner in Schwerin. During this time he delved into many medical and dietetic writings and was especially drawn to Hufeland's *Macrobiotic:The Art of Prolonging Life* which convinced him of the bad effects of meat-eating. A year later he was put in charge of the Buchenthal water cure in the Canton St. Gallen, Switzerland, and then in 1852 he became the director of the Tiefenau water cure in the Canton Zuerich. There, he began prescribing a vegetarian diet for some of his patients. Later, all of his patients had to adhere to a strict vegetarian regime.

After several other changes, Hahn founded his own water cure, "Auf der Waid," in Oberwaid near St. Gallen in 1864. Here he treated his patients during the summer and wrote during the winter months. He edited such health magazines as *Der Naturarzt (The Nature Doctor)* and *Der Hausarzt (The House Doctor)*, and was editor of *The Vegetarian.* He wrote various vegetarian cookbooks and pamphlets in defense of vegetarianism. In his most important work on this subject, *The Paradise of Health—Lost and Regained,* Hahn attempted to prove that the meatless diet was the diet which Nature had provided for humans and which was most suitable for them. For support he cited many outstanding personalities from Pythagoras, Plutarch, Newton, John Milton, and Benjamin Franklin to Shelley, Byron, Sylvester Graham, and Russell T. Trall. He researched a vast amount of medical literature. He felt a pure vegetarian diet stimulated the activity of the colon and promoted detoxification. Meat on the other hand, overacidified the organism and left uric acid in the body, thus contributing to rheumatism, gout, and stones in the bladder. Based on the structure of their teeth and digestive tract, Hahn believed that humans were originally fruitarians and that they switched to meat only after the influence of environmental catastrophies. Hahn also objected to meat-eating on moral grounds. If everyone had to kill the animal which he eats, Hahn argued, many people would become vegetarians to avoid the horror of animal slaughter. Hahn also argued that the production of vegetarian food was much cheaper than that of flesh food and that a given amount of acreage could support many more vegetarians than meat eaters. In short, Hahn anticipated all the arguments of modern vegetarianism.

Hahn's *magnum opus* was his *Praktische Handbuch der Naturgemässen Heilweise* (*Practical Handbook of Natural Healing)* published in 1865. The first part is devoted to health and its preservation through natural living and the second part to diseases and their natural treatment with detailed prescriptions concerning diet and water applications. Hahn wrote somewhat immodestly if not correctly in the preface to the second edition, "With respect to dietetics as well as to the healing methods of the future, I am far, far in advance, not only for decades, perhaps even for centuries" (cited in Rothschuh 1983, 26).

In his treatment methods, Hahn preferred mild applications such as ablutions, sitz baths and half baths over the stronger full-body baths, affusions, douches, dry sweat packs and steam baths. He even rejected the sunbath which then became Rikli's important discovery. Like Kneipp later, he encouraged barefooted and bareheaded walking. He tried to avoid the healing crises Priessnitz and Schroth were famous for and complained that most nature cure establishments were too harsh in their treatment methods, not only ignoring the patient's inner healing instinct, but also each patient's different vitality and power of reaction. He placed little value in gymnastics, considering them unproductive compared to gardening. Exercises reminded the patient too much of his illness, while garden work distracted him and strengthened his body and mind at the same time.

Hahn was a serious, reserved, and scholarly person who liked to be alone in his study or to stroll through the beautiful park of his sanitarium where he with great love and care had himself planted the trees and shrubs. He died of colon cancer on March 3, 1883, at age 59, completely destitute, after sending a moving appeal to his followers not to abandon his family. A raw granite block at the park's entrance, engraved with his name, was the only memorial left to him. When Philo vom Walde sought out Hahn's widow, he found her and her family living in a squalid apartment under the roof in St. Gallen. She bitterly complained that nobody remembered her husband anymore and that the whole world only talked about Kneipp as if he had invented the water cure (1898, 91).

Hahn's contribution is "that he considered a vegetarian diet as equally important as water for the treatment of the sick" (Brauchle 1951, 173). Therefore he was more than a water doctor; he was a nature doctor and dietician. He felt that nature cure required principles and methods of the utmost clarity and simplicity and he rejected any complicated medicines, methods, or technical apparatus. He believed that the means of true nature cure could easily be obtained from Nature anywhere and at any time. Hahn held the very modern belief that the nature doctor should be an educator who brought the knowledge of healthful living and natural treatments to the people so that they would realize they were responsible for their own health. "Theodor Hahn became the leading propagandist of natural health and healing methods in the second half of the 19th century," wrote Rothschuh. "He started out exclusively with the water cure but with his addition of dietetics and vegetarianism to nature cure, he pushed its influence into the beginning of the health and life reform movement" (1983, 79). Unlike Priessnitz and Kneipp, Hahn never had enthusiastic followers from America who spread his fame there. He preserved and extended Rausse's work; he helped establish "Nature cure" as a term and concept; and he refined the philosophy of nature cure and expanded its practice to include dietetics. Though little known, Hahn deserves recognition for the important role he played in the development of naturopathic medicine.

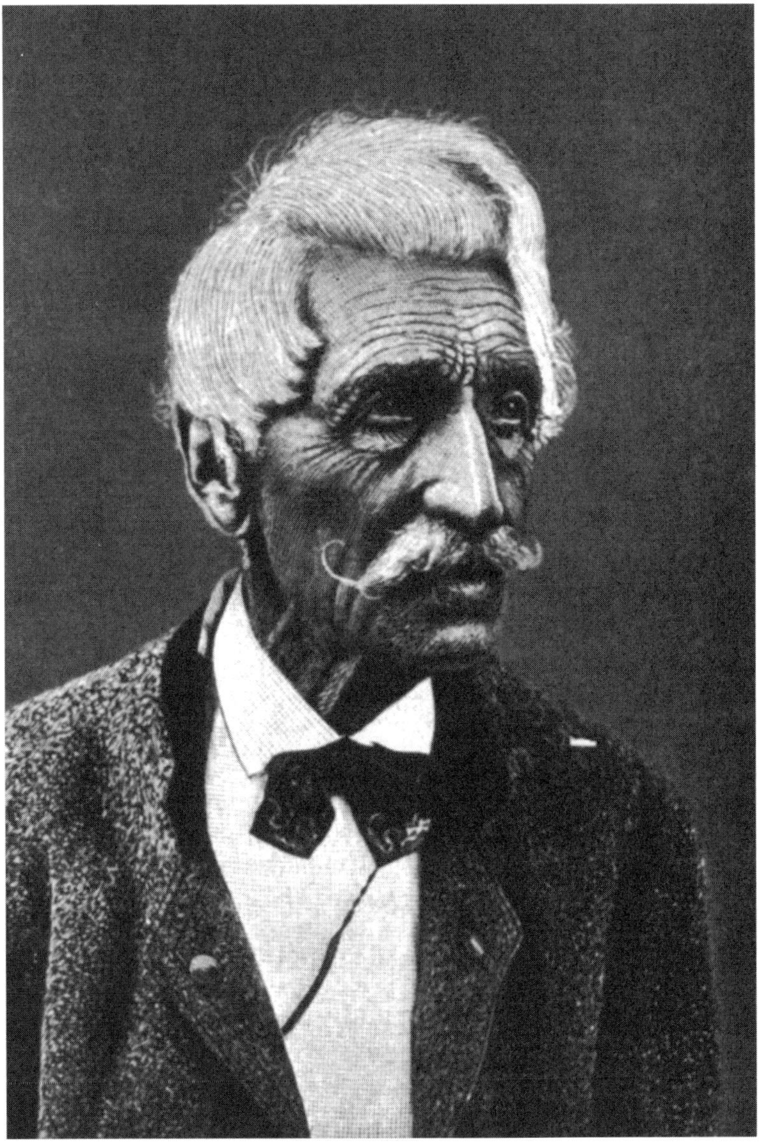

Arnold Rikli
(Brauchle 1933,37)

Discoverer of the Atmospheric Cure

Arnold Rikli

(1823-1906)

The great "sun doctor" and the father of the "atmospheric cure," Arnold Rikli, is little known in the U.S. None of his writings have been translated into English and hardly any literature exists about him in English. His famous saying, "Water is good; air is better, but light is best of all," was the motto of his nature cure establishment in Veldes. It's widely quoted here but few people know any more than that about him. Benedict Lust paid a brief tribute to Rikli as "the first to call the attention of the world to the value of the light, air and sunbath" (Lust 1900, 5). It is unfortunate that Lust didn't make it to Veldes when he toured the famous establishments of the great European nature cure pioneers in 1926.

> This is the only place I had to cut out of my program, but surely on my next trip to Europe I will also visit this way off place, because Arnold Rikli is also one of the great pioneers who gave the world the atmospheric-heliotherapeutic light, air and sun treatment (Lust, 1927, 272).

Rikli was a gifted and prolific author. He wrote a number of books, the best known being *The Basic Doctrines of Nature Cure including The Atmospheric Cure, Let There Be Light and Words of Farewell*; and numerous articles for *Der Naturarzt (The Nature Doctor)*, the most important German nature cure journal. Like Rausse, he minced no words with respect to the medical profession that dogged him constantly:

> A privileged caste always develops an egotistical interest in making the public depend on it. Therefore, the majority of the privileged priests in charge of the public health have become frauds instead of teachers. The proof is that health conditions are worst where many privileged physicians practice. Therefore, down with all privileges. They plunder the public welfare and are a curse for all of humankind (Rikli 1868, 26).

Rikli was a zealous explorer of health who constantly tried to perfect new methods, experimenting on himself before applying them to his patients. He must be regarded as a great nature cure pioneer of the same rank as Priessnitz and Kneipp.

Arnold Rikli was born February 13, 1823, at Wangen-on-the-Aare in the canton of Bern. He was the fourth of six sons of the owner of a dyeing factory. His birthplace, a stately mansion in the rustic Bern style, is still standing and bears a memorial plaque from the Swiss Association for Public Health. Until the age of seventeen, Rikli was educated in private institutions in Switzerland and Germany. Although talented and eager for knowledge, he revolted against the rigid educational system and his despotic teachers, seeking escape in the intensive exploration of nature. Even as a young child he was drawn to nature:

> When I was a boy, I took the highest pleasure and delight in bathing. My mother could not inflict a more severe punishment on me than to forbid me to bathe in the river. I also felt a strong urge to sunbathe, especially during springtime. Even then it was dawning on me that sunbaths must have an enlivening and strengthening effect. Therefore I wandered the southern slopes of the hills on beautiful March days and at the edge of a forest uncovered myself and lay down on my clothes in the sun (Brauchle 1951, 208).

Rikli was brought up to believe that exposing the body to the open air was dangerous, so even his first experiments with sun and air baths required a form of rebellion.

Rikli never studied physics and chemistry at a university. His parents wanted to employ him in their factory as soon as possible and so permitted him only technical training. At age twenty he became a foreman in his father's company. At the same time, on an educational trip, he discovered Carl Munde's *Memoirs of a Water Doctor* (1844) and Luigi Cornaros' famous Renaissance classic about longevity (1558), *Discorsi de la vita sobria (Discourses on a Sober and Temperate Life)*. From then on he obtained as many works as possible about water cure, especially those about Priessnitz and by Rausse. He read these books eagerly and tested the different applications they described on himself.

There is disagreement whether Rikli, like Priessnitz, Kneipp, Just and other nature doctors, converted to nature cure after it saved his life. Turner says, "Dying of dysentery, he saved his life with the aid of a hydropathic manual" (1967, 262). Gray says he was a notable exception to this tradition:

"It was not so with Rikli, for he possessed both health and strength from his boyhood up" (1904, 154).

He married at twenty-one to free himself from parental domination, a happy marriage which lasted for 58 years. He also took the risk at twenty-two of starting a business with his two brothers. In 1845 they founded a new dyeing factory in Seebach, Austria, that soon employed 300 people. But it cost the brothers a fortune, and since they had not chosen their father's career of their own free will, they didn't have the motivation required to deal effectively with the problems of a new business. Also, Arnold was seeking fulfillment in another area:

> My entire life became so embittered that I strove for another career to separate myself from this partnership. This new career could be nothing other than the one to which I felt an irresistible inner call—the water cure or, in a broader sense, the nature cure. I went on to explore everything about this new, young science . . . . Thus I started to treat our sick workers with hydriatic applications (Levental 1977, 395-396).

His early success soon made it evident that Rikli was a born healer. His reputation grew quickly and attracted other sick people to him who entrusted even the most serious illnesses to his care.

Rikli went bathing in the river year round and constantly tried new treatments on himself. His self-experimentation with frequent applications of icy mountain water may have gone too far because he developed a nervous insomnia which he was only able to cure with warm baths. This led to his realization of the importance of the principle of "contrast" which played a crucial role in his healing system. Rikli used the contrasting weather cycles to explain it saying, "Atmospheric variations are of profound significance for any understanding of natural law" (Detmar 1951, 31). He searched for a suitable way to use heat along with cold for the cure of the sick. He found steam to be the best method for treating colds and other diseases which ran their course without fever. After experiencing steam baths, he invented the bed steam-bath in 1847. He described its construction and use in a long article in *Der Wasserfreund (The Water Friend)*, and justified the introduction of external heat into the "cold water cure."

> We imitate the chilly stage of the acute healing process of nature by making the different cold water applications to produce varying degrees of reactionary warmth. It is rare, however, that we achieve increased fever temperature. We are therefore justified in imitating nature in its contrast stage by producing an acute artificial heat . . .

Beilage zu № 6 des „Wasserfreundes."

Rikli's *) Bett-Dampfbad.

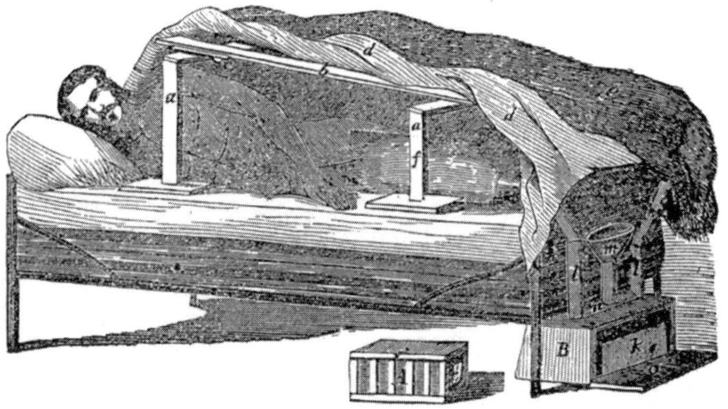

Rikli's bed steam bath
(Archive of the Eden Foundation, Bad Soden)

> The steam bath has proven a most suitable method, it results in a redness, swelling of the body, and increased pulse and breathing rate which is most appropriately defined as artificial fever . . . .
>
> We would not like to be a water doctor if we could not apply this versatile measure. Without it we would be completely helpless and have to give up in the face of many illnesses . . . . The cold procedures are more effective when employed with steam and sunbaths, because the contrasting applications lift each other up and achieve much faster results in most cases.
>
> So-called cold water establishments which only apply the principle of cold are irrational, because the true water cure encompasses all degrees of temperature which can be tolerated by the human organism. This includes the steam and sunbath. Therefore we call it simply the water cure (not the cold water cure) (Rikli 1861, 87-90).

At the same time Rikli experimented with steam, Johann Schroth in Lindewiese was enriching nature cure with warm baths and hot compresses.

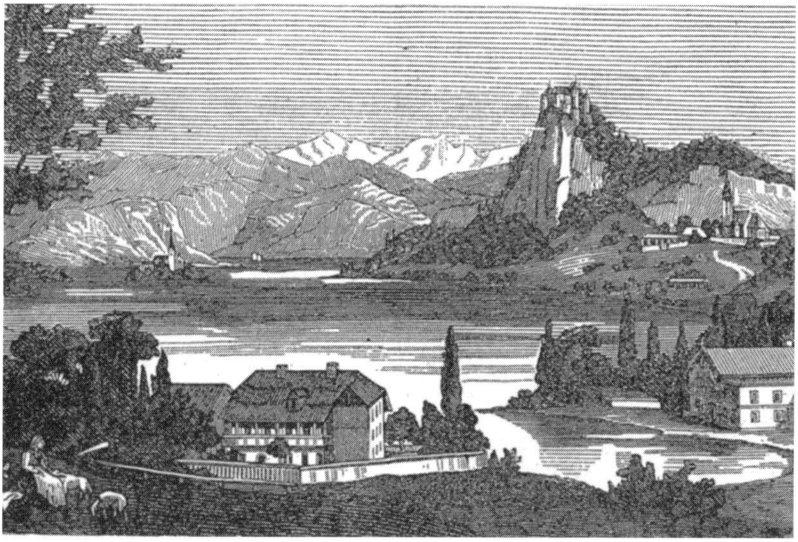

Rikli's nature cure establishment in Veldes, Slovenia
(Archive of the Eden Foundation, Bad Soden)

Kneipp made his first acquaintance with water treatment three years later. "Thus, it is Schroth's and Rikli's achievements to have introduced warm baths and the use of steam into nature cure" (Brauchle 1951, 209).

Rikli's spectacular success as a healer convinced him to abandon his original profession and devote himself to the treatment of the sick. He fell ill with pleurisy in 1852, but cured himself with natural treatments, and on the advice of friends, went to Veldes in Slovenia for his convalescence. Veldes' magnificent location on a beautiful lake, its mild climate and pure alpine air, inspired him to establish a nature cure sanitarium there. In 1854, he left Seebach forever and moved with his family to Veldes.

Rikli practiced in Veldes every summer for the next 50 years. He started modestly with a few patients who had not been helped by regular physicians and were so desperate that they didn't mind being considered "crazy" for turning themselves over to such a weird nature doctor as Rikli.

> Even in later years Rikli's patients were called "Rikli nuts" and Rikli himself the "king of fools." It took decades for his "cure" to receive any attention from the sophisticated public. Until then

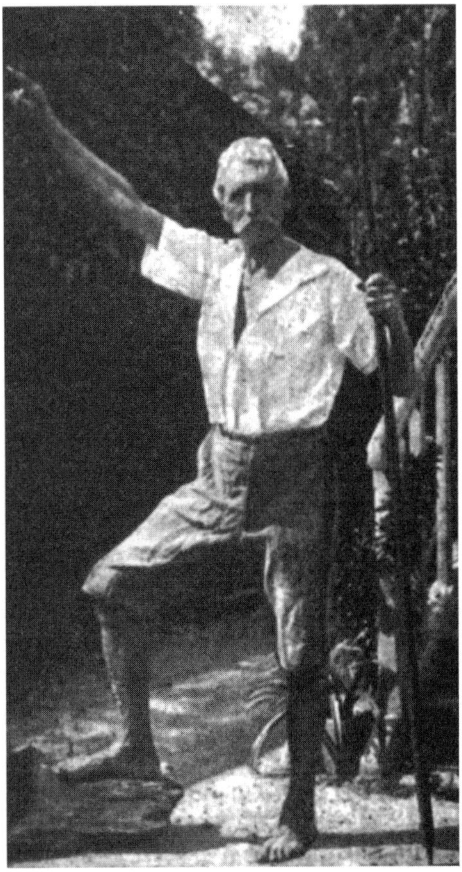

Rikli in his air bathing suit (Archive of the Eden Foundation, Bad Suden)

> Rikli was avoided as an odd fellow and looked down upon, even by other nature doctors. His struggle was difficult, not only because his methods were new, but also because the Slovenic population, which did not take much of a liking to this peculiar foreigner, caused him many difficulties (Anonymous 1906, 129).

During the winter months Rikli practiced in different towns, Ljubljana and Trieste, because he had to provide for his large family. While Veldes was frequented mainly by chronically ill patients, Rikli had the opportunity to treat acutely ill patients, suffering from smallpox, typhoid fever, etc., in Trieste. Zdenk Levental writes:

> There his infinite self-confidence tempted him to treat—not always successfully—the most serious acute cases, including smallpox. This cost him some of his own children whom he had cared for himself, blind to the tragic dangers of such an attitude,

as is evident from the notes in his diary (1856-1863) about the early deaths of these children (Levental 1977, 396).

Unfortunately, we have no access to this diary held by the Rikli family, and we are dependent solely on Levental's interpretation. We can't determine the fairness of his implication that Rikli's treatment methods caused the death of his children. Another viewpoint was offered by Matthäus Schmidtbauer, an ardent Rikli partisan. He emphasized the many skirmishes Rikli had with the medical establishment.

> Such quarrels embittered Rikli's life to the extreme, but this bitterness reached its culmination when his favorite son whom he had chosen as the successor of his establishment became martyr of the horrors of vaccination. Can it be a surprise that this irreplaceable loss broke Rikli's heart? Rikli hated the medics from the depths of his being—and we can completely understand why (Schmidtbauer 1892, 228).

Rikli endured considerable harassment and persecution from the medical profession. In thirty-five years he had to appear in court seven times to defend himself against charges of quackery.

> Each time he emerged as the victor against his jealous medical foes. When his patients testified that he had alleviated illnesses which could not be helped by the physicians, the judge remarked: "Then we must be glad to have such a man in the country!" Rikli ended this hate campaign by transferring the medical direction of his establishment to a licensed physician or "proxy." In this way the witch-hunt of the medics could no longer find a target (Schmidtbauer 1890, 72).

When he started in Veldes, the cold water cure, as practiced by Priessnitz and Rausse, was still an important part of the treatment program. By 1865, Rikli began looking for alternatives to the harsh cold water applications. He started experimenting on himself by exposing his body to the air, winds and storms in all possible temperatures and weather conditions. In his *Basic Doctrines of Nature Cure including The Atmospheric Cure* he gives a vivid description of his heroic feats:

> In the 42nd year of my life I began taking light-air baths for at least two hours every morning. No weather, as bad as it might be, could hold me back. During winters in Trieste, we undertook the air bath tour up the Karst mountain, 500 meters high. Only someone familiar with the awful winter storms of the Adriatic bay

> knows what it means to climb the Karst peak in light-airbath attire every day.
>
> It was not unusual for the trees to be covered with ice from top to bottom due to freezing rain. In eighteen years, I completed over 3000 atmospheric baths in every conceivable weather condition which resulted in unprecedented colds, compared to which the common colds of normal life are a joke. However, I did not suffer the slightest harm; in fact, I never felt healthier and more vigorous (cited in Schmidtbauer 1906, 126-127).

In an article describing the sun as the original source of all life, Rikli concluded that man was less a water creature than a light-air creature:

> Man is not born in clothes but is destined to live like a walking plant in light and air. Indeed, he is the noblest light-air-creature on earth . . . Light and air, the finer fluids of life, are completely adequate for our organism and can never do harm if the balance between cooling and warming is handled appropriately. On the contrary, light and air will tremendously enhance the development of body and mind (Rikli 1896, 177-178).

As early as 1869 he proposed his thesis of the superiority of air and light to water in *Thermodietetics:*

> The light and airbath cure leads to a faster more efficient restoration of a human being than any method of water cure no matter how refined it might be. A human being is not a fish. Water is not our highest element of life . . . Light and Air are our highest, most delicately organized life-vessels. All organic life would degrade and die in the shortest time without them (Rikli 1869, v).

Rikli introduced airbaths in 1865, after he had satisfied himself that they were beneficial. He prescribed them for his patients to take each morning in lieu of cold ablutions. In 1869, he began building a colony of air huts, which were "a blessing which only someone who spent a few nights in such an air hut can fully appreciate" (Schmidtbauer 1902, 66). In addition, he created large light-and-air parks. In 1895, a new "cure house" was built and in 1899, two new large bathing establishments began operation. Dr. A. Laab, the physician directing Rikli's establishment during this time, described it like this:

> Five cozy light-air bath parks, three on the mountains, two in the valley; two colonies of air totaling 44 in all; a spacious, modern, tasteful, and well equipped bathing establishment with three sunbathing galleries and installations for all possible appli-

> cations of steam and water; a bright and airy "cure salon" with a spacious kitchen and pantries; a dining hall for 120 persons, covered, but open on all sides; finally, a large number of health-seekers from all corners of the world, increasing yearly. Here they strengthen their exhausted nerves and harden their pale, flabby skin by taking daily light- and-air baths of one to five hours—not in Parisian but paradisiac fashion—in God's free, magnificent nature which stimulates the mind and heart; here they cleanse their sluggish blood through the incomparable sunbaths; here they refresh their weak, overworked bodies by walking barefoot, wearing garments as light and permeable as possible; by taking numerous water applications here they fall asleep deeply in air huts and strengthen their intestines by a natural, predominantly vegetarian diet; here they widen their narrow chests by rowing on the lake, stretch their limbs with gymnastics, take in the pure mountain air in deep breaths by climbing the many hills; here they confer happily with other patients, full of new hope for a recovery they have not found elsewhere; here one can closely observe the methods of cure and objectively evaluate the results; and without doubt one would have to concede that Veldes is a precious pearl (cited in Schmidtbauer 1903, 122-123).

Rikli emphasized the importance of walking barefoot long before Kneipp did. However, he advised against constantly walking barefoot in the dew. Only a portion of his parks was maintained as lawn, the rest being covered with dry sand. He considered it necessary in air bathing for the bare feet to touch the ground, to achieve a sufficient "drainage" effect.

> It is well known that some people catch cold when walking barefoot on cold wet ground and contract so-called disease-symptoms such as diarrhea, cough, stuffed nose, etc. which in reality have no other purpose than the expulsion of waste by the organs' healing power . . . therefore the cough is not the disease, but a curative reaction against the disease . . . .
>
> It is extremely injurious to harden the head by keeping it bare, and on the other hand to keep the feet covered all the time, as people suffering from headache are prone to do . . . .
>
> The balance of circulation between the head and the feet and between the intestines and the skin is the most important principle for the preservation and restoration of health (Rikli 1869, 12-14).

Rikli rarely advertised his establishment and in later years agreed only reluctantly to some publicity at the urging of his patients and medical staff. Nevertheless, the flow of patients increased tremendously over the years. They arrived from all the corners of the world, well-known personalities and physicians being among them.

> They placed the greatest trust in Rikli, the experienced nature doctor who was so conscientious and ready day and night to assist his patients by word and deed. Rikli was a passionate healer who lived only for his vocation. Nothing else gave him so much joy as his successful cures (Schmidtbauer 1906, 129-130).

Rikli took part in everything at Veldes, walking barefoot into the mountains with his patients as "virtue company," lightly dressed with a small triangular loin-cloth. He was a shining example who encouraged everyone with his enthusiasm. In this way he achieved a high "cure morale" in Veldes.

> I will lead you through the mountains of Upper Carniola with greater boldness than an imperial captain his troops. If you prefer to take the light bath while ploughing or swinging a hoe instead of climbing the mountains, I will give you that opportunity. All of you will be surprised how you will return home refreshed in body and spirit and filled with a new sense of life's worth and purpose (Rikli 1869, 120).

Although the cure cost 105 gulden, not a low price at that time, Rikli had many regular guests who returned every year attracted by the robust vitality Rikli enjoyed.

> Not only was the sun of Veldes shining but also our Arnold Rikli. It was his radiant health which made such a deep impression on his guests. He lived 83 active years, a sign that he was on the right path of health (Keller-Jakob 1950, 12).

Rikli's aversion to fanaticism, his flexibility and moderation were exemplified in his attitude toward vegetarianism. When he was 38 years old, he converted to a vegetarian diet under the influence of Theodor Hahn. He felt much healthier and lived happily on the regime for the next 12 years, often eloquently expressing his enthusiasm for the diet in his writings. However, after he had been a vegetarian for 15 years, his health deteriorated. He began to experience an almost uninterrupted rectal catarrh, an unnatural weakness, a deterioration of his mood, a miserable appearance, an abnormal loss of body heat, increased heart palpitations during mountain climbing and brittle fingernails. In addition, he developed an aversion to fruits and an irresistible craving for cheese, fat, sugar, meat and spicy food. At first he was at a loss to explain the decline of his health, adamantly resisting the idea that his vegetarian diet caused it. Having bragged so much about the benefits of the vegetarian lifestyle, change was painful. However, he was finally forced to give in to his cravings for meat and stimulants, and he returned to a mixed diet, eating a daily small portion of meat and partaking of wine, beer, coffee and tea again as well. After two years on this diet all his problems disappeared. He could come up with no other explanation but that vegetarian food was excellent as a temporary therapy but not suitable as a permanent diet for everyone:

> Despite my experiences I still recognize the principles of the vegetarian diet as useful and ennobling and continue to prescribe it for the majority of my patients; I only reject its abstract use without consideration of the patient's constitution, custom, occupation, etc . . . . There is no doubt that it can produce marvelous results in some cases; however, this does not prove that it is advisable in every situation. A diet which might be right for the blacksmith may not be appropriate for the tailor (Rikli 1879, 86).

In light of the benefits he enjoyed and observed in others from a mixed diet, Rikli asked:

> Why must the vegetarian be locked in the cool, sulky mood which a vegetarian diet eventually produces. Everything changes, everything rises and falls in this world; this is a natural law! Monotony is boring, even detrimental to human health . . . . Why should not the vegetarian be permitted to break out from his perpetual cool mood and warm and cheer himself up with a daily glass of wine.
>
> The super-vegetarians totally misunderstand human nature when they proclaim that man shall live by bread and fruits alone. Children who receive only Graham bread grasp greedily for excessive amounts of white bread at every opportunity. (Rikli 1879, 88).

Fearless of the consequences, Rikli left the Vegetarian Association in 1878, and explained his reasons in *Der Naturarzt.* "The Paulus of vegetarianism had become a Saulus" (Brauchle 1951, 217). Rikli's step caused an uproar in the vegetarian and nature cure press. He was called a traitor to the sacred cause, torn to shreds editorially and expelled from their ranks. Dismissing their attacks with gentle sarcasm Rikli wrote, "I still hope to make a tiny contribution to human society for a few years, despite my excommunication by the super-vegetarians and despite my small consumption of meat and wine" (Brauchle 1951, 217-218).

We cannot know whether Rikli's health problems were due to vegetarianism in general or only to the special version, but we can admire his readiness to change a long-held conviction in the face of new evidence, even at the cost of his reputation.

Rikli published numerous articles about his methods in the nature cure journals. The following account gives a good picture of his practice:

> J.P., a M.D. from H., started the atmospheric cure in Veldes during the middle of June and made the following confession: 'I am in the 67th year of my life. I have been suffering from a seriously ill stomach for the last 25 years . . . (with) pressure over the stomach and acidity after every meal. It totally embittered my life and gave me sleepless nights. From time to time I suffered from severe spells of dizziness and for over 50 years from otorrhea. In earlier times I used countless allopathic remedies against my afflictions . . . The homeopathic Nux brought only momentary relief . . . Several times I tried seaside resorts and repeated countless cold water cures . . . I also visited the nature cure establishments of Waldesheim near Düsseldorf and Chemnitz in Saxonia, all without any success . . . '
>
> The essence of my prescriptions for this patient consisted of a daily light-air bath at 5 o'clock in the morning, lasting from 15 minutes to 4 hours depending on the weather; the same in the afternoon from 2:30 to 5 o'clock if a sunbath was not scheduled for that time. Sunbaths as often as possible, in the morning over the whole body except for the head, in the afternoon merely the lower part of the body half an hour long. The first one was followed by a half-bath between 22 to 20 R [Reaumur = 26 to 24 C] for 4 minutes and then an ablution of the legs between 14 to 8 R [17 to 9.5 C] for 1 minute. In the afternoon three different alternating applications: first a warm sitz-bath from 31 to 29 R [37 to 35 C] duration of 40 minutes followed by cool ablution to the lower part of the body between 22 to 20 R [26.5 to 24 C] for 1 minute; second an ablution to the upper part of the body 22 R [26.5 C] for 1 minute followed by a cold gown friction to the lower part of the body between 14 to 10 R [17 to 12 C] for 3 minutes; third a cold leg bath between 18 to 16 R [21.5 to 19 C] — 14 to 12 minutes long. Every second night abdominal bandage of 18 R [21.5 C] or leg packs of 10 R [12 C]. The patient received a vegetarian diet during the first treatment period; however, since it did not suit him well, he was given a mixed diet with slightly fewer vegetables during the second period. He also had to observe two weekly

> thirst days to induce more warmth in the stomach through more intense contraction. Without doubt, the atmospheric baths (light-air and sunbaths) were the most important elements of the treatment, for they quickly gave this elderly gentleman a much better appearance and a more cheerful mood.
>
> The patient underwent the treatment for 50 days, the stomach pains stopping in the last three weeks. At the end of February 1891 I received the following news from him:
>
> 'In consideration of the fact that I am now 68 years old and that I tried all possible kinds of "cures" against my obstinate stomach ailment and my periodic severe spells of dizziness, I have to regard the effect of your prescriptions as half a miracle. Indeed, I have never felt so well and strong for many years as during this harsh winter. If I use the necessary caution and abstain from certain foods, such as whole wheat bread, milk and cabbage, I feel perfectly healthy and can sleep without difficulties in the night, while I felt miserable before my cure at Veldes, no matter how carefully I lived because I felt stomach pain without exception after each meal' (Rikli 1896, 174-175).

Rikli tried to influence other water doctors to follow his example:

> My esteemed colleagues hopefully won't consider it self-aggrandizing if I urge them to lobby for the establishment of public light-air parks with sunbathing galleries. It would enormously benefit our good cause if water doctors everywhere introduced light-air baths and sunbaths to counteract the fast-spreading misery of nervous afflictions. The water grind must be replaced with the light-air cult (Rikli 1896, 178).

Rikli exhorted his colleagues to include light, air and sunshine in their treatment programs and challenged the people in general to get rid of their prudish, suffocating clothing and open the windows of their musty rooms. In his brochure, "Let there be Light!," he offered the following health catechism for parents:

> Discard your out-dated concepts of "bad air" and the "dangerous heat of sun." On the contrary, introduce your children to these highest elements of life methodically. If you want to raise a stronger and more vigorous race than the present pitiable one, obey the following rules:
>
> 1. Every day an absolutely naked air bath of a half to two hours, in a warm room during winter, and during the warmer season, in a garden park or woods.

> 2. Light clothing in general, barefooted and bareheaded as much as possible.
>
> 3. Keep the youth outside as much as possible, even in harsh weather. If they happen to cool off too much, give them sweat baths.
>
> 4. Each month two to four cleansing baths, the best are bed-steam baths (if sun sweat baths are not possible).
>
> 5. Nourishing, simple, vegetarian diet consisting mainly of milk, flour and fruits (Rikli 1911, 37).

Some have suggested that Rikli's light-air-sun ideology may have been a precursor to the twentieth century leisure cult of nudism, but he used the light-air- and sunbath only for therapeutic purposes. He was not motivated by the later "body beautiful" considerations of physical culture, or the ideology of naturism that condemned modern civilization and advocated a radical return to nature. He also avoided the excesses of later-day sun-bathing fanatics, and the danger of skin cancer. He used the sunbath to complement the cooling light-air bath he considered too one-sided. His sunbathing started in the late morning and consisted of a "direct sunbath" of approximately forty minutes and an "indirect light-warmth-bath" of twenty minutes. The first was a direct exposure to the sun; during the second the patient reclined on a platform, protected from any draft by wooden walls, wrapped in a blanket in order to sweat. The time span of each application was extended or shortened according to the patient's constitution and the prevailing weather conditions. Each sunbath was concluded with a mildly cool half bath or an ablution of 22 to 27 Centigrade lasting five minutes.

Rikli, like Priessnitz and Rausse, believed that the treatment of a sick person had to be individualized and that a diseased organ could only be influenced by treating the entire organism:

> Since each individual forms a complete whole, and each disorder also affects the whole, the entire organism has to be taken into account to improve the problem. A merely local treatment proves the physician's shortsightedness and must be declared a bungling patchwork (Brauchle 1951, 212).

The principle of contrast was Rikli's most original contribution to nature cure philosophy. Monotony in treatment methods meant atony, stagnation and death. Priessnitz had best results when he used the contrast principle by having his patients sweat before receiving cold water applications. Without variety, Rikli believed, there could be no enlivening, strengthening or development. For him, polarity influenced all phenomena of life—the polarity of cold and warmth, night and day, rain and sunshine, summer and winter.

"These atmospheric changes reflect natural laws and are absolutely necessary as stimuli for the plants, animals and humans living on earth." Changes are necessary in the atmospheric realm and in everyday life. Rikli believed that every change in lifestyle provoked a "new movement" and therefore had curative effects. Thus, even changes on the emotional level in the form of entertainment, music, dance and enjoyment of beautiful natural sights were needed to balance the monotony of everyday life. "The truth," Rikli noted, "lies in the observance of these contrasts" (Brauchle,1951, 212).

Toward the end of his life, Rikli published his *Words of Farewell to My Esteemed Colleagues and Followers.* The following quotes from this document reflect the optimism, fighting spirit and enormous self-confidence which as an old man he still possessed:

> I have fought like a brave soldier for our noble cause and suffered many difficulties and injustices, especially as creator of the atmospheric cure; on the other hand, I have also been acknowledged with warm thanks and leave this world satisfied that my work was not in vain and convinced that nature cure will open the way for a grand reformation for all humankind . . . (Rikli 1903, 205).

> The fundamental antagonism of orthodox medicine against all the disease symptoms through which Nature attempts to rid our bodies of toxins has brought unspeakable suffering upon humankind, far more than all the horrible wars . . . The people would be healthier if we had no physicians . . . (207).

> Is it surprising when we nature doctors follow the great teachings of Nature and achieve much better results than our adversaries? (211)

Rikli died April 30, 1906, at age 84, from the infirmities of old age. A more detailed account of his death comes from his former secretary in a letter dated May 17, 1906.

> Mr. Rikli did not die from cancer as you assumed. Why should he perish from such a horrible illness when he lived so hygienically? As you know, Rikli suffered from chest pains from his youth on. They only vanished after hemorrhoids emerged. From then on his well-being depended on their regular bleeding. A year ago this bleeding took an unusual route, i.e. through the bladder; for 5-6 days dark blood was passed painlessly with the urine. This year (1906) the bleeding stopped entirely, the acid blood flowing into the muscle tissues and causing a rheumatism

> of the thigh and the back with such pain at times that he had to be lifted up and laid down. The sunbaths brought him relief, more so than the cold packs . . . . The disease matter then entered the lungs and heart . . . . The difficult breathing and cardiac weakness grew worse in the following days . . . . In the last week the bladder also failed and the urine had to be removed artificially. It must have passed into the blood, because the decline came so rapidly; until this point he was mentally alert, but from then on he had only a few clear moments. His last words were "cold friction" when he was already covered with the sweat of death. This was the end of the great man (Schmidtbauer 1906, 127-128).

His son, Oskar, managed Veldes until 1918, when the break-up of the Austrian empire occurred. One of Rikli's enthusiastic patients, the Swiss industrialist and senator, Isidor Grauer-Frey, founded the nature cure institution, Sennrüti, in his Swiss home town, Degersheim (St. Gallen), in 1904. It was closely patterned after Veldes and still exists today, although Rikli's "atmospheric cure" is no longer practiced there.

Even representatives of the medical profession grudgingly acknowledged the pioneering role of the "lay-healer" Rikli as a light and sun therapist. The Swiss surgeon, Oskar Bernhard (1861-1939), used the sunlight of the high mountains in his clinic at St. Moritz with success in the treatment of tubercular lesions and for the purulent non-healing wounds of many World War I soldiers. In an essay on the "History of the Sunlight-Treatment" (1919) he wrote:

> A Swiss so-called nature doctor, Arnold Rikli . . . intensively took up the sun-therapy . . . establishing a real institution for its application. It is to Rikli's credit that he advanced the sun treatment and awakened the interest of physicians in it. Unfortunately, there was no scientific basis for his endeavors (Levental 1977, 400).

Auguste Rollier (1874-1954), another Swiss physician, visited Bernhard and was astonished at how rapidly wounds healed in the high mountains. In 1904 he established a sanatorium in Leysin, which, like Veldes, was located at a very high, sunny, protected location on Lake Geneva. He used sun therapy with great success on thousands of patients with extrapulmonary tuberculosis. Unlike Bernhard, who used only local applications of sunlight, he was convinced that tuberculosis was a generalized condition which required generalized sun therapy like Rikli's. Rollier combined this treatment with breathing exercises and a vegetarian diet. He also established an "Ecole au Soleil" where children, predisposed to tuberculosis, could be educated in an ideal environment, and a "Colonie de Travail" which added occupational therapy to the convalescent regimen. By 1938, his sanatorium had 36 buildings. Rollier, in his classic work *Heliotherapy,* gave due credit to the "sun-doctor" Rikli.

> We must not forget Arnold Rikli, who, though he was not a medical man, understood the importance of the sunbath, and opened a clinic at Veldes for a "cure athmospherique," which included sunbaths (Rollier 1923, 2).

In his *History of Ultraviolet Therapy* Sidney Licht, editor of the renowned *Physical Medicine Library,* wrote that "although Rikli's sanatorium was popular and prosperous, the movement did not spread" (Licht 1967, 203). This might have been true in some areas but not in Germany and Switzerland where around the turn of the 20th century the different nature cure associations competed with each other in establishing light and airbaths in many large cities.

> The air and sunbath idea was propagated by the nature cure associations and eventually gained general recognition with the result that air-and sunbathing have become a common activity. We owe it all to Rikli (Keller-Jakob 1950, 10).

Physicians of today who are interested in the therapeutic use of light haven't completely forgotten Rikli. The following news item appeared in a recent issue of *Naturheilpraxis.*

> Prof. Hans Meffert and Dr. H. P. Scherf of the Charité, Humboldt University in Berlin, are the winners of the 1991 Arnold Rikli Award for their research on the biopositive systemic effects of optic rays on humans. This award will be presented by Prof. E. G. Jung, M.D. of Mannheim, to the prize-winners on the occasion of the 2nd International Arnold Rikli Symposium, October 13-15, 1991, in Atlanta, USA . . . (Naturheilpraxis 44 (1991):884).

In 1886, the nature cure physician Heinrich Lahmann went on a tour of the most important nature cure establishments of his time, and Veldes received his strongest praise:

> I consider the effect of light on the skin extremely beneficial, and I give first prize to the sun as the best source of warmth. Therefore I regard Rikli's sun, light and air-cult as an excellent addition to the nature cure method (Lahmann 1886, 150-151).

Lahmann went on to follow Rikli's example at his sanitarium, Weisser Hirsch, near Dresden, where he regularly prescribed sun and airbaths for his patients. The same was true of the various "Jungborns," established by Adolf

Just, Emanuel Felke and Benedict Lust, with their air huts and light and airparks.

When the *New York American* of 23rd October 1922, hailed the physicians of Beth Israel Hospital for their great discovery that the sun's rays can cure tuberculosis of the glands, bone and skin diseases and speed up the healing of surgical wounds, Lust commented:

> The physicians of the Beth-Israel Hospital ought to punch themselves and find out whether they are awake or not. Heliotherapy was discovered by Arnold Rikli, N.D., who established the first institution for heliotherapy at Veldes, Krain, Austria, in 1848. The sun treatment has been used in Europe in all drugless institutions ever since for the cure of tuberculosis and many other diseases .... It has been taught in the American School of Naturopathy, 7 West 76th Street, New York City, ever since its establishment in 1896. Today there are hundreds of drugless institutions in the United States where this treatment is used successfully. Dr. Lust's health institutions, Yungborn, in Butler, N.J., and Tangerine, Florida; Dr. Lindlahr, Elmhurst, Ill.; Dr. Strueh, McHenry, Ill., and Dr. Schultz, Los Angeles, Calif., own probably the largest and most important institutions of this kind in the United States.
>
> It is indeed gratifying that the Rip Van Winkles of the Beth-Israel Hospital are awakening (1920, 558)

None of the later great nature cure institutions would have been possible without Rikli's model in Veldes and without his dictum: "Water is good, air is better, but light is the best of all!"

The World's Most Famous Nature Doctor

Sebastian Kneipp

(1824 - 1897)

One hundred years ago a large American newspaper surveyed its two million readers to determine the best-known people of the time. Most famous was the president of the United States. Second most famous was the Chancellor of Germany, Bismarck. Third was one of the founders of naturopathy, Sebastian Kneipp, a priest at Wörishofen, Bavaria (Burghardt 1988, 4).

How could a humble priest in an obscure mountain village become one of the most famous people in the world: by treating thousands of sick people with natural remedies such as pure water, fresh air, exercise and herbs and by teaching millions of others about these remedies through his popular health writings. His method was originally known as Nature Cure. Transplanted to the United States almost a century ago by his disciple Benedict Lust, who added homeopathy and manipulative therapy, it soon became "naturopathy" and evolved to the naturopathic medicine we know today.

Sebastian Kneipp was born May 17, 1824 at Stefansried, a tiny Bavarian hamlet. He was the son of a weaver and grew up in such poverty that his mother had to cut up her black wedding dress to make a suit for his confirmation in the church. Although ridiculed by his richer peers when he wore it, he recalled, "This suit delighted me more than anything else would have, for young as I was, I fully understood the sacrifice on the part of my mother" (Lust 1900, 34).

From the earliest age he desired to become a priest, but his family could not afford to give him the necessary education. If God had wanted him to become a priest, they told him, he would have provided money for his training. Kneipp took up weaving at the age of eleven; by age twelve he could make five yards of linen daily. He continued to seek every opportunity to gain the priesthood but was repeatedly rebuffed. The passport he obtained as a teenager said "weaver apprentice," but, as he wrote, "something very different had been inscribed on the leaves of my heart.. With unspeakable pain and longing I wished to become a priest" (Kneipp 1893, 2).

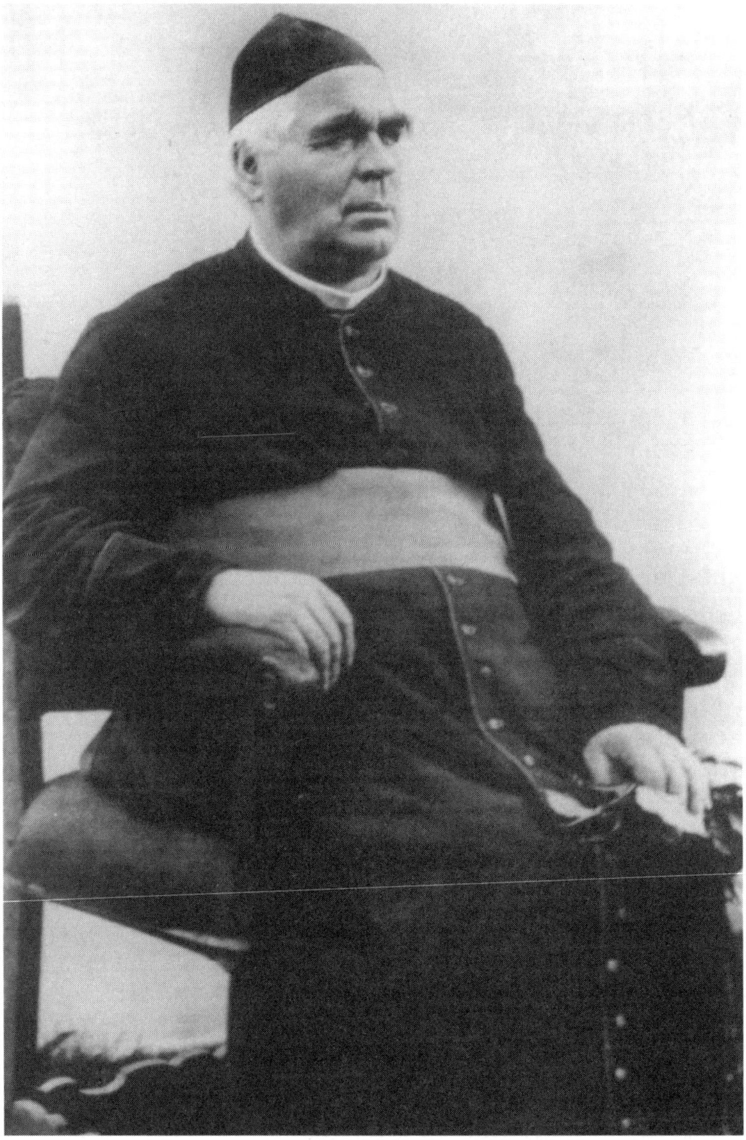

Sebastian Kneipp
(Mariafai 1987, 87)

A sympathetic chaplain, Dr. Matthias Merkle, finally agreed to prepare him for his entrance exams. Due to lack of funds his diet during his student days was poor. A typical menu was "three kreuzer's worth of lung and one kreuzer's worth of bread for dinner" (Lust 1900, 36).

His body had already been weakened by tuberculosis of the lungs contracted from working long hours in his father's damp weaving room. So desirous was he of religious orders that he further ruined his health in rigorous study to pass his exams. At one point, when he was going home for a vacation, his landlord told his father, "Weaver, you are fetching the student for the last time" (Kneipp 1893, 4). The doctors concurred. "In the opinion of two distinguished physicians," Kneipp wrote, "I was in 1847 on the brink of the grave; they had indeed given me up" (Kneipp 1889, ix).

His desire for knowledge made the young Kneipp a voracious reader. Even in illness he was "fond of dipping into books to amuse and distract my thoughts." "Chance threw an insignificant little volume in my way," he wrote, "a treatise on cold water cure." This book, which he found in the Court Library at Munich, was Johann Sigmund Hahn's *Lectures on the Wonderful Healing Power of Fresh Water* in Oertel's new edition (1833). He went on:

> This little book was the first straw at which I grasped; soon it became the staff on which the patient could lean; today I regard it as the lifeboat sent by a merciful Providence in the hour of my greatest need (Kneipp 1893, 3-4).

Too poor to afford further professional medical help, Kneipp treated himself with cold water according to this book. Although the prescriptions were most exceedingly violent and severe, he endured six months of self-treatment. He noticed no dramatic change for the better but was encouraged that his disease had not gotten worse.

In the winter of 1849, two or three times a week he sought out a lonely spot at the Danube and bathed in the icy water for a few minutes. Again he found no harm in this water treatment; in fact, he noted a small benefit. The following year he helped cure a fellow student who was being refused holy orders for health reasons. Taking the cold water treatments together, they both improved significantly. Of course, their nude nocturnal river bathing in the dead of winter was open to misinterpretation by the townspeople, and when his superiors found out about these water treatment activities, Kneipp was ordered to stop. He still stole out nightly through a basement window to spray himself with a watering can, and eventually his recovery was complete.

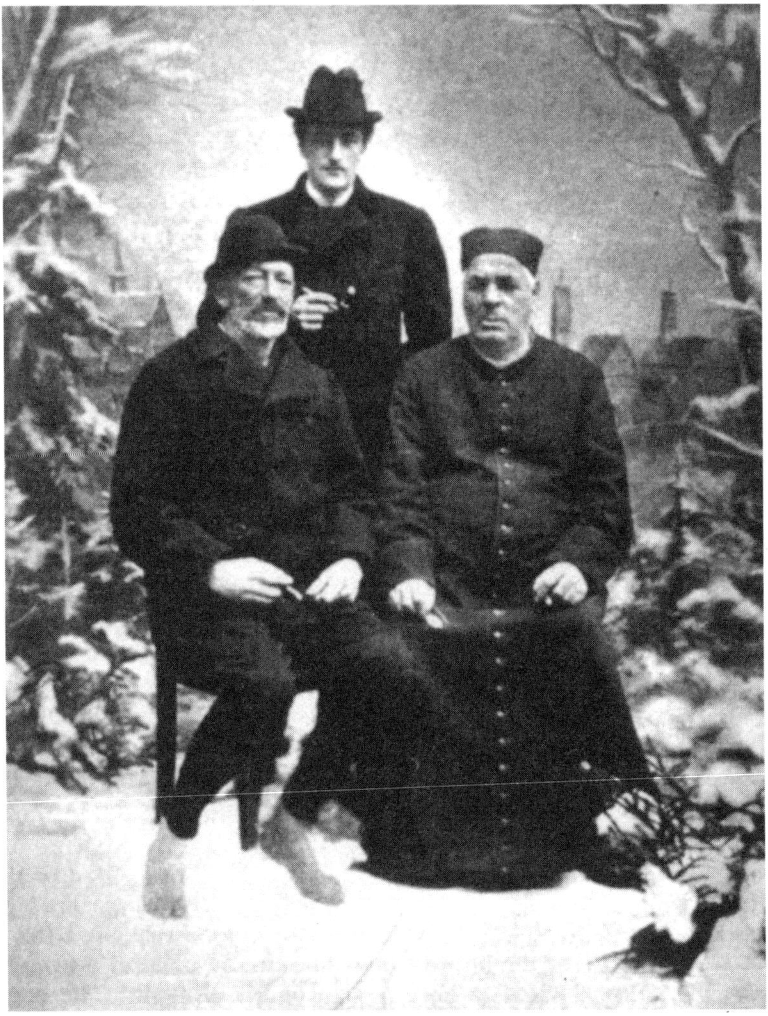

Father Kneipp with Emperor Franz Joseph and Archduke Ferdinand of Austria.

Finally on August 6, 1852, Sebastian Kneipp was ordained a priest and was assigned as chaplain to various parishes. Moved by the misery of his ill parishioners, he treated them with a modified cold water system—not so harsh as he had endured. As early as 1854, he became known as the "cholera vicar" because of the many lives saved by his treatments in the village during an epidemic. The growing fame embarrassed his Dominican masters and neighboring farmers complained because their crops were often spoiled by hosts of barefoot morning walkers. Finally his bishop forbade any more healing. Kneipp did his best to obey, but one night, after repeatedly refusing the requests of a dying woman for treatment, he could not sleep. Finally he got up, saying, "I'm going to see the woman, and stick to the work of curing the sick from this time on" (Lust 1904, 146).

One source suggested that Kneipp was ultimately sent to Wörishofen in 1855 to be spiritual father of the convent there as punishment for his healing activities. Wörishofen was such a tiny, remote and poverty-stricken village it was felt the water priest could get into little trouble there. Moved by the great need of the area, Father Kneipp immediately founded a school and orphanage for the poor children. He headed the renovation of the village church and showed the local farmers new, more productive agricultural methods. Although he became famous years later for his water cure writings, his first publications were practical, straightforward instructions in crop management, animal husbandry and beekeeping. Early in his career, Kneipp took a sick heifer on the verge of death from a nearby farm "to experiment a little." To everyone's astonishment the heifer not only recovered, but also won first prize at the next agricultural fair in Munich. When asked what "prime elixir" he had given the animal, Kneipp replied, "I fed him a decoction of hayseeds and that cured him" (Muller 1917, 142).

In time the parish flourished, and as the fame of Father Kneipp's healing methods spread, he began to attract patients from all over the world. The original villagers of Wörishofen, which was on its way to swelling to a population of 24,000, were not overly enthusiastic about these developments, but went along with them out of respect and affection for Father Kneipp. By 1880, there was little the church hierarchy could do but to accept Father Kneipp's healing ministry and make him priest of the village.

Father Kneipp was confident he could help his sick parishioners back to health because he firmly believed that God, in nature, had provided remedies for nearly every human ailment. He believed that disease originated in deranged blood—either that which circulated imperfectly or that which contained poisonous elements. Water healed by dissolving and removing toxins from the blood, restoring normal circulation and strengthening the entire system. It acted "like oil on the wheel of a rusty machine" and

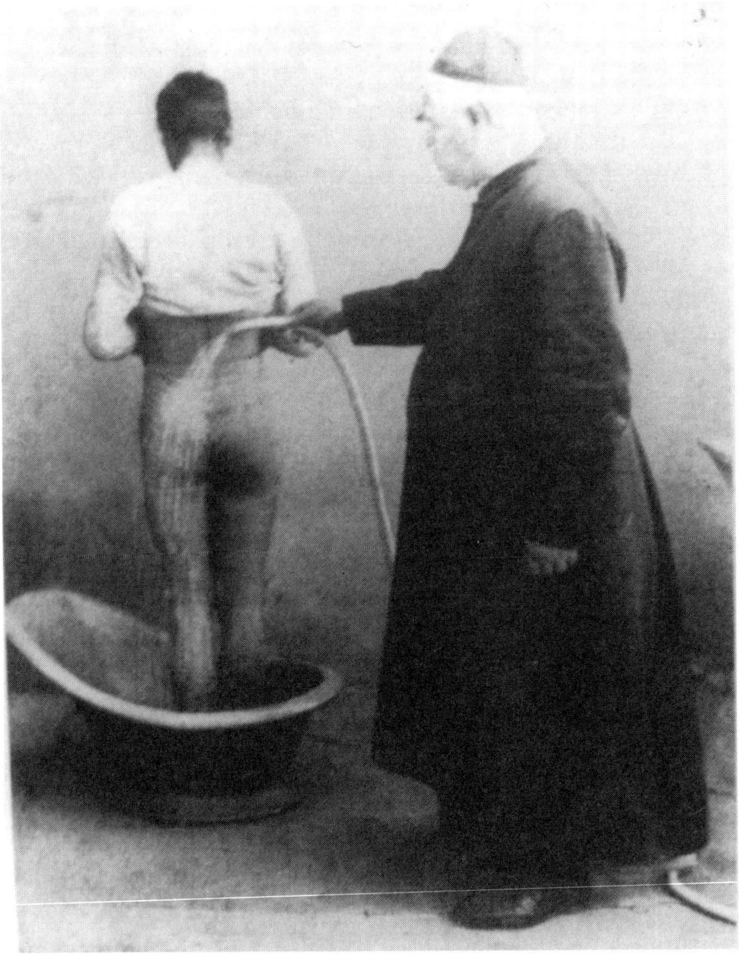

Thigh spray with hose applied by Kneipp
(Mariafai 1987, 39)

removed "unhealthy secretions, as a winnowing machine removes the chaff" (Kneipp 1893, 153). This seemingly outdated humoral concept of disease is not so far off from the view of a modern holistic physician who wrote, "Blood is the principal carrier of healing energy" (Weil 1988, 61).

The healing effect of water in conjunction with herbs reflected the universal harmony Kneipp saw in the purpose of God's creation. As he wrote, "My whole effort has been to point out and explain what the Creator offers us in Water and in Herbs" (Kneipp 1894, v).

Father Kneipp's treatment methods were distinguished by two things: individualization and gentleness. Although he never examined a patient by auscultation or percussion, he achieved remarkable clinical success. He would keenly observe the patient's complexion, weight, posture and demeanor, and assess for toxicity, anemia, nervousness, etc., and adjust the treatments accordingly. If the patient was weak, anemic, or nervous, only one part of the body was treated with water at a time. "Patients are too often treated in a stereotyped general fashion, " he wrote, "and far too little stress is laid on the peculiarities of each separate case" (1893, 5). Or in the words of one of his admirers, "No one knew better than he how to individualize and to adapt the temperature of his procedures to the individual, i.e., to the status of vitality of his patient" (Winternitz 1909, 221).

The following delightful case history from *My Water Cure* illustrates how Kneipp treated even a local affliction by strengthening the patient's entire organism:

> William, a boy of 9 years of age, had diseased eyes. He could no longer read and scarcely distinguish persons, the poor little one was more than half blind. His parents had spent a fortune for the cure of these eyes but without result. The whole body of the child was just as impaired as the eyes. His hands and feet were always cold, his stomach without appetite, his body emaciated, his stature drooping and depressed. Wretched are not only the eyes, wretched is the whole little man.
>
> In 4 months William was restored to perfect health of body and eyes. The little one had to take 2 warm baths weekly. 4 times weekly I had a shirt dipped in cold salt water and put on him. He remained in it for 1 to 1 1/2 hours. Moreover I let the boy walk barefoot in wet grass or when it was raining. After the first 4 weeks William took 3 to 4 baths of 15 R [18 C] every week; the baths were of only 1 minute's duration and always followed by exercise. They were continued for several weeks. The boy also washed his eyes twice daily with alum-water (a saltspoonful of alum in 1/4 pint of water). As the body revived and recovered his health, the eyes, too, became better. At last they shone in the blooming face of the boy as if they had never suffered from the least disease (1896, 277).

Kneipp utilized wraps, compresses, packs, baths and steamings, but his major contribution to hydrotherapy was his discovery of the healing power of the cold gush or pour. This was an affusion to a specific part of the anatomy, e.g. the knee, often administered from a watering can or unnozzled hose. He made these applications gentle by keeping them very short. Many lasted for only a minute which could be timed by his watchless peasant patients by "reciting two Paternosters" (1893, 17). He experienced the harsh cold water applications during his earlier self-experimentations and felt that such a "horse cure" would only bring the cold water cure into discredit. It attests to his greatness as a healer that he was not rigid but always willing to learn from his experiences and refine his methods.

> For 30 years, I have tried every single application upon myself. Three times — this I acknowledge openly — I found myself induced to change my system, to loosen the strings, to descend from strictness to softness, from great to still greater softness. According to my present conviction, now fixed for 17 years and tested by innumerable cures, he who knows how to apply the water in the plainest, easiest, and most simple way, will produce the most profitable results (1896, 6).

It should be pointed out that to Kneipp "gentler" meant shorter and over a smaller area but not warmer. "The colder the water the better," he maintained even to the end of his career, often mixing it with snow when possible.

Lust wrote about Kneipp's system that "it is as simple as his success is great" (1900, 4). That certainly applied to the diet he gave his patients. He advocated "a dry, simple nourishing diet, free from all spices and condiments; and as a beverage, the pure crystal element which the Creator has so lavishly provided" (1893, 10). However, he was no Puritan and did not object to an occasional taste of wine or beer.

As regarded dress, Kneipp said, "I cling to the old adage—the best for everyone is homemade and homespun" (ibid., 11). Like Priessnitz before him, he eschewed wool in all forms in favor of linen. Kneipp recommended the wearing of mesh garments made of porous linen or vegetable fiber next to the skin, as it caused a gentle friction (which stimulated circulation) and held sufficient air in the meshes to protect the body against excessive heat or cold. He was against heavy clothing, even in winter, for he felt it weakened the body's own heat-generating capacity. He campaigned strongly against the evils of the corset. As Lust pointed out, Kneipp established "a world industry for health underwear, porous clothing and footwear "(1927, 11).

Kneipp's mother was an experienced herbalist, and when he was a child, she took him with her to the meadows and taught him the herbs for various conditions. Under this influence Father Kneipp became the first to introduce herbalism into nature cure. This is one of his greatest contributions to naturopathic medicine. However, this innovation was not universally acclaimed at the time. "Even the best representatives of the nature cure movement did not understand Kneipp," wrote one historian. "His originality was doubted and his introduction of herbs condemned" (Bohn 1922, 217).

Philo vom Walde, a great champion of Priessnitz, typified the criticism aimed at Kneipp for mixing water and herbs. "Kneipp's herbalism," he wrote, "is a great set-back in the development of the natural healing system; if this part of his system becomes dominant, then the water itself will soon be of secondary importance again" (1899, 138). Lust always staunchly defended Kneipp against such charges and found them "unduly severe."

> It is true that humble water is always in danger of being obscured by glamorous herbs and other more attractive treatments, but it would be fairer to praise Kneipp for directing attention anew to water therapy which was on the verge of slipping into oblivion than to criticize him for linking it to other therapies which enhance its utility (1918, 211).

Kneipp himself seemed to have anticipated these objections against his "herb cure" when he wrote:

> I have long deliberated before I resolved to add this apotheca to the applications of water, which in themselves are sufficient, lest these remedies which assist the water by operating inwardly, could be looked upon as a vote of mistrust in the water (1896, 122).

Kneipp used herbs like the water with the same aim "to dissolve morbid matters in the interior, to evacuate them, and then to strengthen the organism." He believed "that both cures, the interior and the exterior, harmonize and work together with perfect unity." Again, he cautioned against their overuse confirming his great wisdom as a healer: "Whoever is of the opinion that he ought to use interior remedies often and in great quantities, is likewise mistaken. Always and in all cases keep to the golden principle: the gentlest application, be it exterior or interior is the best" (ibid., 122-123).

Kneipp used herbs externally in the baths he administered, oat straw being a favorite, and internally as teas and tinctures, chamomile and rush being frequently used. He introduced the internal use of herbs for those patients who didn't like or couldn't tolerate the water treatments. He often recommended nettles (Urtica sp.) in his health lectures, which he gave 365 days per year to his eager patients who numbered as many as 1,500-1,800 per session. After his death, Kneipp's herbs became proprietary formulas, and dozens of genuine "Kneipp Remedies" ranging from "Kneipp's Ear Oil" to "Diabetic Tea" became available from an exclusive pharmacy.

Kneipp's knowledge of herbs was empirical but sound:

> For long years, I have examined and experimented, dried and cut up, boiled and tasted. There is not one little herb, or powder, which I have not myself tried and found good. My only wish is that my old acquaintances may be respected again (Kneipp 1896, 122).

Many of his herbal therapies have since been validated by modern researchers. Of bilberries Kneipp writes:

> Obstinate diarrhoea may be relieved by a spoonful of bilberry extract, taken in a gill of warm water, and repeated after 8 to 10 hours. It will hardly be necessary to repeat the dose a third time (Kneipp 1893, 82).

This is uncannily echoed by Rudolf Fritz Weiss, one of the world's most respected medical authorities in botanical medicines:

> Dried bilberries are quite effective against diarrhoea. A fairly concentrated decoction is made from them, and patients are given this by the tablespoon or in a wine glass (Weiss 1988, 191).

Kneipp had an almost brotherly love for "his little acquaintances." His jubilant praise for their virtues reminds us of St. Francis, who had similarly praised God's creation:

> How good is God! Oh that we could recognize it! Let us search for the little herbs which announce themselves by the smelling bottles attached to them by the Creator, the aromatic wholesome scent; and let us, when gathering them, glorify with filial gratitude our infinite Father, who is in Heaven! (Kneipp 1896, 123).

Another testimony of Kneipp's love for herbs was his *Plant-Atlas* with its true-to-life illustrations of medicinal plants. He issued it at the request of his publisher, Josef Kösel, who had it translated into several languages.

In 1927 Benedict Lust made a pilgrimage to Wörishofen and received treatments similar to those given during Father Kneipp's heyday. He was wakened early in the morning for a cold, full-body ablution, then allowed to return to bed for 10 minutes to warm up. After warming up he was dressed in sandals and clothes of porous linen and sent outside to walk for 20-50 minutes in the dewy grass (nasses Graslaufen). This was topped off by soaking the feet in a lively brook and then walking briskly to the dining hall for a simple breakfast of whole wheat toast (with no butter) and malt coffee. After the meal, walking was resumed followed by various douches, gushes, sitz baths and vapor baths, depending on the condition of the patient. Sun and air baths were taken in the late morning. Lunch, consisting of a hearty vegetable soup, a meat substitute and baked potato, was followed by a rest in individual quarters. In the early afternoon sun and air baths were renewed, followed by appropriate douches and baths. A mid-afternoon social hour was observed with a coffee substitute, zwieback and sour milk as a refreshment. Nature walks followed, then a simple supper. After an evening concert everyone retired. If bad weather prevented outdoor activities, health education lectures took their place (Lust 1927, 59-66).

Father Kneipp's friends and supporters begged him to write down his experiences using the healing power of water and herbs. In 1882, he published *My Water Cure*, which he dictated to a secretary provided by an abbot who was impressed with his work. Kneipp turned out to be an effective, even elegant writer. His book took Germany by storm and was an instant international best-seller. It was translated almost immediately into fourteen languages and went through 100 printings, 18 in a single year. One reason for Kneipp's success as a writer was that he wrote in a down-to-earth style which spoke directly to the hearts and minds of common people:

> I have had a peculiar affection and care for the poorer classes, the sick country-people who are so often neglected and forsaken, and to them especially I dedicate my little book; therefore the language is plain and clear. I have purposely tried to use familiar language instead of giving a dry, inefficacious skeleton (Kneipp 1896, vi).

Kneipp's next book was *Thus Shalt Thou Live!* (1889) which was translated into nine languages. This work offered his teachings about how to lead a healthy life with special consideration of diet, dwellings, sleep, clothing, exercise and care of the body and soul. Then followed *Baby Kneipp Cure* (1891), *My Will* (1894) in collaboration with Dr. Alfred Baumgarten and *Codicil to My Will* (1896) with assistance of Bonifaz Reile.

Kneipp believed that bracing and strengthening our power of resistance was the best way to prevent disease. "Going barefoot" was among his favorite means to achieve this, especially going barefoot in dewy grass, on wet stones and even in fresh fallen snow or wading in cold water. In *My Will*, he praised the benefits of going barefoot:

> Those who go bare-foot never suffer from cold feet which is the result of poorness of blood and too little of it . . . . I recommend going bare-foot not only as a relief, but as protection against many

> diseases peculiar to those who lead a sedentary life, in which the brain has too much to do and the body little (1897, 26-28).

Kneipp originally published these books hoping that by explaining his methods in detail the people would stay at home and treat themselves and not come to him. Ironically the effect was exactly the opposite. The popularity of his books swelled the ranks of his patients by thousands more. Forced to see as many as 200 patients per day, Father Kneipp became one of the busiest doctors of all time. In his own words, "The sick came in such numbers that we knew not what to do with them" (Kneipp 1894, viii). One of his medical critics described Kneipp's "mass processing" of patients as follows:

> The most varied and complicated diseases, forming a clinical material that would be the envy of a professor, are subjected after two or three questions to a treatment differing only in the smallest details. A diagnosis is neither made nor attempted. "What do you complain of," is the parson's question. "I have headaches;" "I suffer from spasms;" "I have an eruption;" "I suffer from bad digestion;" "I cannot sleep;" etc. These replies are followed rapidly as thunder follows lightning by the prescriptions, "*Rückenguss*, two seconds, *Schenkelguss*, three or four; *über nasse Steine laufen*" (translated, cold stream upon the back; upon the thighs, three or four seconds, walk upon wet stones). The prescription is written in a little book which is given to the patient. No precious time is wasted on notes, records of results, effects of the douches, and "wet" meanderings.Thirty or forty patients are thus dispatched in an hour (Baruch 1895, 522).

Kneipp was besieged by so many patients from all over the world that he had no other choice than to limit each patient contact to a minimum. Soon after 7 a.m. the regular stream of patients arrived and until night, as a rule, there was not one moment's pause in the succession of people. One can only admire the stamina of a man who was quite advanced in age.

All who came in contact with Father Kneipp were impressed by the strength of his presence and bearing. According to Lust, Kneipp was a "very simple man," with great "personal magnetism that created confidence and love and made people willing to obey him promptly and unquestioningly" (Lust 1904, 145). Even one of his critics, a physician who after a visit in Wörishofen concluded that "the great majority of really sick people find neither improvement nor restoration here," couldn't avoid being impressed by Kneipp's majestic appearance:

> A splendid and expressive peasant head, with shrewd eyes brightly shining beneath white, bushy eyebrows; a pleasing attractive face, uniting goodness, shrewdness, dignity, and inspiration in beautiful harmony. The head, which is covered by heavy silver-gray hair and surmounted by a small cap, rests upon a strong, broad shouldered body of handsome proportions.... Such a man must awaken confidence, which is heightened by the mild voice and Bavarian dialect with which the prescriptions are dictated to the two priestly secretaries. If one may deduce the presence of talent from a man's exterior, it must be confessed that rarely has Nature endowed a man with so many points indicating the true physician as this remarkable priest possesses (Baruch 1895, 522).

Kneipp was not only a gifted writer but also a born orator. His immensely popular daily Public Lectures, held before large crowds of "cure guests" in the wooden "promenade hall" of Wörishofen, were transcribed and edited by his secretary Prior Bonifaz Reile and published in four volumes (1896-98). After patients had founded Kneipp Associations in many towns, his friends urged Kneipp to go on lecture tours to spread his teachings. The visits of the seventy-year old Kneipp to many European cities turned into triumphal processions. As many as 4,000 jammed the lecture halls on his speaking tours, captivated by "the perfect and fearless confidence which inspired every word" (Lust 1904, 148).

Kneipp was well-known for his impartiality. The richest Croesus and the poorest beggar were treated alike. A European princess who registered at a fine hotel in the region of Wörishofen and sent a special messenger to Father Kneipp offered him a huge sum if he would come to the hotel and treat her. The priest sent back word that if the princess would come to his home in the mountains and stand in line with the waiting peasants, she would be treated free. Kneipp had little patience for those who were lazy or thought they were better than others. The piercing gaze of his eyes often gave discomfort to those who had not followed his instructions or who had something to hide. If necessary, he did not mince words, although his sense of humor always shone through. A typical example is his reply to a wealthy and overweight man who was describing his daily opulent eating, "I tell you what's wrong with you, you need a second stomach!" (Schomburg, 1981, 91). His prescription for a lady who could not be stopped in her long litany of complaints was: "Three douches on her mouth!" (Riedel 1985, 53).

Despite sternness, Father Kneipp was famous for his charity. Although Kneipp could have gotten millions, he treated all his patients for free. In addition he established three charitable institutions: the Sebastianeum, a sanatorium for sick priests, the Kneippianum for poor patients, and an asylum for sick children and orphans, now called Kneipp Children's Sanatorium. Kneipp was able to do this with the support from his congregation, gifts from rich patients, and royalties from his books. However, he was not above a little benevolent extortion. When a prosperous restauranteur, cured by Kneipp, asked what he owed, the priest inquired how business was. When the man replied, "Oh, the restaurant is doing fairly well," Kneipp said, "Well, then you have to give two marks for my poor children in the asylum" (Muller 1917, 141). But Kneipp was indifferent to material wealth. When one of the Rothschilds offered him 50,000 florins if he would go to Vienna to treat him, he didn't even answer the letter. When an Austrian prince gave him a purse of gold in appreciation for a successful treatment, Father Kneipp put it in his deep pocket. Later, when a Romanian woman asked him for fare back to Bucharest, he "dived into his pocket and handed her the purse he had just received from the Archduke, which contained 800 marks" (Lust 1904, 149).

One of Kneipp's most loyal supporters was the Archduke Joseph of Austria-Hungary who came to Wörishofen in 1893 when 70 years old suffering from severe sciatica. After Kneipp brought him relief, he returned many times for the cure, even after Kneipp's death. The Archduke was a great propagandist for Kneipp and also did much for Wörishofen. He donated thousands of trees and shrubs for the new "cure park" and helped finance the construction of a railroad. Due to the Archduke's influence, the Pope awarded Kneipp with the honorary title of "Papal Secret Chamberlain."

Despite Kneipp's successful career as a healer he was first and foremost a priest and wanted to devote his life to the salvation of immortal souls. He was forced to spend much of his time in "the care for mortal bodies," but he never neglected his priestly duties. He rose at 5 a.m. and worked until 10 p.m. every day to make room for all his activities. As a priest he was quite liberal, frequently inviting protestants, Jews, and Armenians to his services. He was accompanied in most of his duties by a small white Pomeranian dog named Spitz, who could be kept out of church only with great difficulty.

Kneipp did not want to be a physician. To him it was an annoying inconvenience. He earnestly wished a medical doctor would relieve him of the burden. After a rocky start, his career as a priest was a success. Not only did his parish become a model of a prosperous, efficient charity, but on October 17, 1893, Kneipp received the Papal Secret Chamberlain nomination with the title Monsignore by Pope Leo XIII, whom he met and eventually treated with cold water. The Pope was the only person Father Kneipp left his parish to treat. Although he was frequently called upon to treat royalty and high dignitaries, Kneipp made them all come to him except the Pope. Kneipp was very shy in first meeting the Pope, but he soon warmed up to the occasion. As Kneipp later confided to Lust, "You see, first he was the Pope, and afterwards I was the Pope" (Anonymous 1931, 109).

Kneipp died June 17, 1897, at the age of 76, as penniless as when he entered the world. "A malignant malady, an insidious formation on the bladder, carried off the hale and vigorous old man in the course of six months" (Lust 1918, 212). Dr. Alfred Baumgarten, his close associate, detected the large tumor in the lower abdomen, but Kneipp rejected his recommendation to call a surgeon. He tried to cure himself with wraps and cold sitz baths. Even when Dr. Fritz Bernhuber, a surgeon and his first medical assistant, confronted him with the full truth of his condition, Kneipp clung to his self-treatment. Joseph H. Kaiser, a prominent modern Kneipp physician, commented, "The tragedy was that he did not see or did not want to see the limits of nature cure" (1975, 26). Still, who can definitely say whether he was wrong in adhering to his principles and whether the crude surgery of his time would have extended his life or only prolonged his suffering.

The news of Father Kneipp's death spread quickly around the world. Newspapers were printed with a black edge. Telegrams of tribute and condolence came from all over the world and flags flew at half-mast. In spite of heavy rain storms 6,000 people followed his funeral procession, among them over 100 priests. He was "deeply mourned by the many thousands whom he had succored, as well as by all the friends and followers of the natural healing art" (Lust 1918, 212). In *My Water Cure* he had written: "And when one day my friends of the water cure are told that I have departed this life, I beg of them to send me a refreshing 'Our Father' in the place where the physician of physicians heals and purifies the souls in the fire cure for eternal life" (1896, vii-viii). His wish is being fulfilled even today by the grateful patients who still visit the mausoleum erected by the town of Bad Wörishofen for its most famous citizen.

Many predicted a quick end of Kneipp's healing methods after his death, but able successors carried on his work. One was Prior Bonifaz Reile, a male nurse from the Hospitaler's order, who had been a devoted and energetic secretary since 1892. Reile became head of the Sebastianeum and one of the leading forces behind the Kneipp Association, which was founded in December 1890 by former patients to promote Kneipp's work. Reile was also authorized by him to compile and edit *The Great Kneippbook* (1903), which became the nature cure bible in many German homes. It still exists today, completely rewritten by a team of Kneipp physicians (Kaiser 1975).

Kneipp had sought the assistance of physicians from early on and was able to establish excellent relationships with medical doctors who studied and verified his system. In fact, no other lay healer attracted as many followers from the ranks of the medical profession than Kneipp. In the preface to *My Water Cure* he wrote:

> My earnest wish has been that a professional man, a physician, would release me of this heavy burden and oppressive work, and I should feel so happy if at last these professional men would begin to study the system of hydropathy thoroughly and put it in practice under their inspection (Kneipp 1896, vi-vii).

He sent a petition to the Bavarian king in 1892 requesting the establishment of hydrotherapy departments at the state's universities.

Unfortunately, his last years of life were overshadowed by a bitter rivalry between Prior Reile, his lay successor, and his medical successor, Dr. Baumgarten, chief physician of the Kneippianum, both men having strong personalities. Reile stayed demonstratively away when 24 physicians founded the International Society of Kneipp Physicians on February 2, 1894 under Kneipp's chairmanship. This rift between the lay and medical organizations prompted Kneipp to appeal for unity in his last book, *Codicil to My Will:* "If the Doctors and Association find themselves in accord and mutually support each other then both sides will experience the greatest success from my method. This is my heartfelt wish" (1896, vi).

Kneipp's first medical assistant had been Dr. Fritz Bernhuber, a surgeon from the nearby town Türkheim, who joined him in 1887. When he set up his own Kneipp cure establishment in the nearby Rosenheim, he was followed by Dr. Franz Kleinschrod (1860-1934) in 1890 and Dr. Alfred Baumgarten (1862-1924) in 1892. These two physicians tirelessly promoted the Kneipp cure in innumerable books and articles.

Dr. Kleinschrod's conversion to nature cure shows how Kneipp could turn a disbeliever into a believer. The young doctor had treated a peasant woman with a serious long-standing foot ulcer "scientifically with phenol and iodoform" without result. When she returned after six weeks, he found her foot completely healed. She told him that she had gone to Father Kneipp. Puzzled and humiliated, he went to Kneipp to find out how the charlatan had done it. After a kind welcome Kneipp told him:

> You see, Doctor, you have treated only a single part and almost nothing done for the healing. The woman suffered badly from varicose veins which impaired the blood circulation and were an impediment to the healing process. I treated the foot with steeped hayflowers which promote healing. I tried to stimulate

> the blood circulation with gushes and to produce an elimination with wraps and teas (Wolf 1965, 88-89).

This experience opened the young doctor's eyes to a completely new principle of healing which did not suppress symptoms. Kleinschrod contributed the practice of the "hay sack" to Kneipp therapy, hayflowers filled in a porous sack being steamed and applied as a pack on the affected part. This proved especially effective for painful spasms of inner organs and for chronic rheumatic diseases. The Kneipp-haypack or Herbatherm is still available as a ready-made health product from the Kneipp Works in Würzburg.

Dr. Alfred Baumgarten became Kneipp's intimate friend and scientific adviser during the last five years of his life. Baumgarten deserves much of the credit for the continuation of Kneipp's work and the development of Wörishofen into a world spa. Only two days after Kneipp's death he continued Kneipp's public lectures, appealing to his listeners to unite so that Kneipp's legacy would succeed. Dr. Baumgarten was one of Kneipp's first biographers (1898) and wrote the first scientific treatise on Kneipp's hydrotherapy (1909). In size and depth it compared to John Harvey Kellogg's *Rational Hydrotherapy* (1903). In the preface he strongly defended Kneipp against the acrimonious attacks of Professor Wilhelm Winternitz, Dean of Scientific Hydrotherapy at the University of Vienna, who hated the "miracle man of Wörishofen" and accused him of pure plagiarism.

Dr. Baumgarten's prophecy that Kneipp's work was the beginning and not the end of a development became true. During his lifetime Kneipp hydropathic institutions were springing up like mushrooms out of the earth, and Wörishofen eventually grew to become the most fashionable and frequented spa in Europe. When Lust visited Wörishofen in 1927, he was "happy to find the Kneipp cure just as enthusiastically and honestly carried out as in the days of Kneipp himself" (Lust 1927, 111).

In fact, Father Kneipp's work has come through two world wars intact, and his "influence survives into this age of antibiotics" (Turner 1967, 264), largely due to the activities of the Kneipp Association, which has been coordinating and promoting Kneipp therapies since 1890. The International Society of Kneipp Physicians, founded in 1894, guaranteed professional training in Kneipp's methods. Its scientific journal, *Zentralblatt für das Kneipp'sche Heilverfahren (Central Organ for the Kneippian Healing Methods),* was published from 1894-1911. After World War II, Dr. Christian Fey (1901-1961) and Dr. Josef H. Kaiser (1906-1992) were the two physicians most instrumental for the development of modern Kneipp physiotherapy and the renewal of the Kneipp movement. Both were awarded the Sebastian Kneipp Medal in 1976; Dr. Fey posthumously. Today, Kneipp doctors are organized in the Kneipp Physicians Union which consists of over 1,000 doctors who have received post-graduate training in Kneipp's methods. Many of them teach at the Sebastian Kneipp School, where Kneipp bath masters and massage therapists are trained, and at the Sebastian Kneipp Academy. Both are located in Bad Wörishofen. The Academy offers continuing education for Kneipp physicians and health courses for members of the Kneipp Association and its affiliate, the International Kneipp Confederation, with more than a quarter million members, the largest health promotion organization in the world. In 1980, W. Brüggemann edited a modern scientific textbook on Kneipp therapy which was published by Springer Verlag; in 1981 the scientific journal *Kneipp Physiotherapie* was founded; and in 1990 the annual Sebastian Kneipp Prize in the amount of 20,000 German Mark was awarded to a physician who "investigated the effect of symptomatic treatment with herbal steam inhalants on patients with common colds" (*Erfahrungsheilkunde* 39:544). The popular *Kneipp-Blätter,* founded in 1891, continues to have a large readership.

No other nature doctor has inspired so many biographical writings. The "Bibliography of Kneippliterature" (1974) by Judith M. Mariafai, late librarian of the Kneipp Archive, lists 30 biographies, novels, collections of anecdotes and poems and even a comedy about Kneipp. The popular priest became a folk hero. Yet Kneipp, who had a great influence on the health consciousness of millions, far more than many prominent physicians in standard histories of medicine, completely escaped the attention of most medical historians.

There are dozens of Kneipp health resorts and spas in Germany today. Bad Wörishofen accommodates about 70,000 guests, representing over one million nights lodging per year. It is a virtual hydrotherapy town. It has over fifty Kneipp doctors, eighty masseurs, and 120 trained bath attendants. A Kneipp museum is one of its tourist attractions. And in the U.S., *The New Yorker* magazine regularly runs advertisements for Kneipp Herbal Baths featuring a comely woman luxuriating in a tub under the heading "I bring nature into my bath."

While he was alive, Kneipp suffered the ruthless exploitation of his name for commercial purposes. He also lamented about real estate speculation in Wörishofen and tried to intervene against unscrupulous businesses which usurped his name for dubious health products. He authorized only a few companies after establishing quality standards with their owners to use his name as a trademark for such products as Kneipp bread, Kneipp cereals, Kneipp sandals, Kneipp malt coffee and Kneipp herbal extracts. The "Kneipp craze" gave rise to an entire souvenir industry.

> Kneipp's person and name had an especially beneficial effect on the business of photographers. Kneipp was sent in thousands upon thousands of pictures all over the world and there is no doubt that this helped fill their purses . . . In Wörishofen his portrait can be found on wallets, visiting cards, notebooks, paperweights, brief cases, vases, baskets, etc . . . . There is no item or knick-knack imaginable which was not imprinted with his effigy or his water applications . . . This unique man provided thousands of people with work and a livelihood. Here we have the reason for his tremendous significance for our national economy (Verus 1897, 116-117).

A modern Kneipp physician, Dr. Joseph H. Kaiser, warned against several dangers to Kneipp physiotherapy, including an inflation of Kneipp institutions, production of Kneipp objects and Kneipp merchandise which have nothing to do with the Kneipp therapy, inclusion of methods which are completely incompatible with it and which can often be found in the advertisements of sanatoriums where the name "Kneipp" is only used as marketing gimmick, and the renunciation of a holistic approach (16).

Kneipp's influence in the U. S. has not been so deep or long-lived as in Europe. The first American institution to use Kneipp's system was established in 1892 by Father Rauber in Dansville, Wisconsin. Two years later Dr. Joseph Joch, a theologian-physician trained by Kneipp, established the St. Francis Sanatorium in the same town. In 1893, Mother Alexia established an "American Wörishofen" in Milwaukee which grew into a Kneipp clinic, treating 80 patients at a time. In the same year Reverend Father Rougé of the Mount Carmel Orphan Asylum founded the New Orleans Kneipp Water Cure where he influenced Otis G. Carroll to enter the natural healing profession. Other Kneipp sanatoriums were founded in Cleveland and Peoria in 1894 and in Newark and Poughkeepsie in 1898. Most of these early Kneipp establishments were staffed by members of religious orders whose fundamental purpose was Christian missionary service to the sick and suffering. The best and most long lived example of this was the Kneipp Springs Sanatorium in Rome City, Indiana. Founded in 1894 by Dr. William Giermann in a 180-acre site, it was taken over in 1901 by the Sisters of the Precious Blood under the direction of Mother Mary Emma Nunkist. For 50 years it treated an average of 2000 patients each year, going out of existence in 1977. Except for Kneipp Springs and the New Orleans Water Cure, the impact of these sanatoriums was strictly local. Individuals who read Kneipp's works were often inspired to try out his water treatments at home, as when Mark Twain's mother practiced the Kneipp water cure on him, but the more general influence of Kneippism has been in health and diet consciousness. Others must be credited as well, but what Lust wrote in 1927 could be repeated today:

> We Americans are drinking Postum and eat Grape Nuts; we are ordering bran and fruit muffins and bran for breakfast food; we eat whole wheat bread, whole wheat crackers, fruit and nuts and honey cakes—how few people think that it was due to the genial originator, Monsignor Sebastian Kneipp, the father of the Water and Nature Cure (Lust 1927, 11).

Kneipp's most specific influence in the U.S. has been on naturopathic medicine. Not only did he inspire Benedict Lust and Henry Lindlahr to become naturopaths and establish his healing principles in this country, but he saved them from life-threatening illnesses so they could accomplish this task. The hydropathic movement in the U.S., inspired by Priessnitz a generation earlier, had prepared the ground, and Kneipp's Nature Cure, transplanted and augmented with other natural therapies by Lust, and established on a scientific basis by Lindlahr, blossomed into naturopathy, which over the course of the twentieth century evolved into naturopathic medicine. It is ironic that naturopathy has eclipsed Kneippism in this country. As one critic suggested:

> The success Lust achieved in America, coupled with his confrontial style, antagonized traditional allopathic American medicine. Because of Lust's earlier association with Kneipp, most of Kneipp's American critics directly associated Kneipp with Lust's Naturopathic cause. This was unfortunate since Kneipp's basic and complementary principles contain many practical methods worthy on their own merits (De Vierville 1991, 76).

The Kneipp system was not widely accepted here because America never developed a spa culture like the one in Europe which provided the environment most suitable for Kneipp's water applications.

Although Kneipp never claimed to be the originator of a special method of cure, he raised hydrotherapy to a new level by introducing new treatments, most notably the "Kneipp douches" or gushes which allowed individual variations to suit the unique aspects of each case. He also moderated the intensity of the more heroic water applications. Before Kneipp, compresses and packs were applied daily for three to six hours. Kneipp's packs only lasted one hour and were given only two or three times per week. Before

Kneipp, cold baths were sometimes given for fifteen to forty-five minutes, or even hours. He reduced them to three minutes, then to one minute and finally to ten seconds.

Hydrotherapy was central to Kneipp's healing system but he augmented it with four other categories of therapies which may be described as holistic. These were exercise therapy in the form of walking, running, gymnastics and light sport supplemented by various forms of massage; diet therapy in the form of a wide variety of wholesome natural foods without one-sidedness or fanaticism; herb therapy in the form of tinctures, teas and bathing lotions; and "order" or regulative therapy in the form of proper organization of daily life with due regard to the biological rhythms, the balance between work and leisure, stress and relaxation and the harmony between the mental, emotional, physical, social, and ecological planes. In short, "he asked for a different life, not for better pills; he asked for the active patient and rejected the passive one" (Schaefer 1982, 680).

He was widely loved and respected, but not without his detractors. In spite of his famous patients like Emperor Francis Joseph, the Pope, and the Archduke of Austria, Kneipp was looked upon with suspicion by physicians. Legal action was taken against him a number of times, but he was never punished because he used only simple home remedies of harmless herbs and water. As one historian noted, "Doctors and apothecaries tried their utmost to discredit Kneipp as a humbug, but his cures were a sufficient answer" (Turner 1967, 266).

Kneipp was once summoned to the district office and confronted with evidence of quackery. When he said, "I am not a quack," the official was quite surprised. "You are well-known as a quack," the official said, and cited three cases Kneipp had cured. Kneipp answered, "If it is your intention to sue me because I cure people, then I proudly admit that I cured many who could not find help elsewhere or who had no money." Kneipp defined a quack as someone who pretended to heal but could not. When he was dismissed, a few curious people were waiting outside to ask him how things went. "Pretty well," he answered, but he was still indignant at being called a quack. "It is just this official who could use such a quack as me," he said, "because his looks tell me his condition is very critical." Indeed, in a month the official suffered a stroke and died, and Kneipp was convinced he could have prevented this misfortune if he had been given the opportunity.

Kneipp was understandably suspicious when another official from the same district office brought his sick wife to him. "One official condemns me for practicing quackery," he said, unable to restrain himself; "the other official brings his wife for treatment." He took pity on the woman who was so weak she could hardly stand and so depressed it was impossible to get a word out of her. Kneipp prescribed water treatments and a simple diet for her, and she returned in two weeks joyful and well. She told Kneipp how her doctors, who had pronounced here incurable, had wanted to give her drugs when they saw her improving to speed her recovery. She refused. She had also been told that she could no longer have children, yet after a year of following Kneipp's method, she gave birth to a healthy boy. Her husband warned her to keep silent about her wonderful cure because he was afraid it would get Kneipp in trouble again, but the woman refused. "If a complaint is made against this gentleman," she replied, "then his first penalty amounts to seven gulden. I have them already put aside. Don't even bother to summon him. All you want is the money anyway. I want to tell the entire world that it was the water which made me healthy" (Kneipp 1979, 27-29).

Kneipp fared well in his conflicts with authorities but also faced strong criticism from other quarters. Devotees and relatives of Priessnitz took Kneipp to task for not crediting Priessnitz as the originator of his system. Philo vom Walde acknowledged that "Kneipp's merits as a health educator are infinite," and admitted that he was a "genuine good Samaritan, a strong personality, the representative of a great cause," but he concluded that he was "no great man," because he was too timid to acknowledge his great predecessor and "life savior." He boldly contended that "we have nevertheless to trace back the entire Kneipp movement to Gräfenberg. Both systems resemble each other exactly, only the names have been changed" (Vom Walde 1899, 112-113).

For these critics, the identity of the "insignificant little volume" from which Kneipp gleaned the knowledge to cure himself of his tuberculosis was crucial. Kneipp never mentioned the title of the book and only once mentioned the author's last name, Hahn, in a discussion with a Dr. Bilfinger. Bilfinger assumed he meant *Lectures on the Wonderful Healing Power of Fresh Water* by Dr. Johann Sigmund Hahn, which Kneipp had in his library. Vom Walde contended that this book was so rudimentary that it would have been useless to Kneipp. If Kneipp could cure himself through Johann Sigmund Hahn's book and founded his system on it, he would "indeed have been a great man," Vom Walde admitted. "Only a genius could form a statue from this raw boulder" (ibid., 117).

Vom Walde believed the little book was actually *Instructions for the Use of Water Cure*, begun by J. H. Rausse, Priessnitz' former patient and student, and completed by Theodor Hahn. Vom Walde's argument is apparently supported by Prior Reilly, Kneipp's successor, who identified the book as Theodor Hahn's. Lust also declared the book as Theodor Hahn's (Lust 1900, 36). Vom Walde concluded:

> Without Priessnitz no Rausse and Hahn; without both of them no Kneipp and without Kneipp not the thousandfold blessing which he brought to mankind! He should have laid down a small branch from his crown of laurels at Priessnitz' monument (Vom Walde 1899, 122).

In this controversy, Dr. Richard Kapferer of Wörishofen gained the upper hand and even convinced the Priessnitz partisan, Dr. Franz Schönenberger, that the book which Kneipp had discovered in the Munich library in 1849 was indeed Johann Sigmund Hahn's. It could not have been the Rausse/Hahn book because their work was published a year later in 1850. However, it was not the original 1738 edition but the "completely revised and modernized" 1833 edition, made "more practically useful" by Eucharius Ferdinand Christian Oertel (1765-1850), Priessnitz' admirer and the first great propagandist of water cure. By recognizing that the go-between was not Theodor Hahn but Professor Oertel, Schönenberger modified Vom Walde's statement above.

> After all, Kneipp is at least partially dependent on Priessnitz .... Therefore we can say: Without Priessnitz and Dr. Johann Sigmund Hahn's book no Prof. Oertel and without Prof Oertel no Kneipp (1931, 261).

Colonel Hans Ripper, Priessnitz' son-in-law, wrote an "Open Missive Letter to Father Kneipp" in 1893 bemoaning Kneipp's failure "to mention, even by a word, in any of the twenty-two editions of your work, *My Water Cure,* the founder and inventor of the water cure, Vincent Priessnitz." Although respectful in tone, Ripper's letter pulls no punches in its attempt to redress the wrongs against Priessnitz' honored memory. "You tell the world nothing new in your book," he asserted. "By ignoring your great and far-famed predecessor, you do not, believe me, reverend sir, add to your own greatness" (Metcalfe 1898, 119-129).

It is easy to understand the indignation of Ripper and others for Kneipp's apparent slight of their hero, Priessnitz. But, their focus on the egotistical aspects of competition for fame misses the point. Kneipp was an honest, humble and very practical man. It is unlikely that Kneipp would have been unfamiliar with Priessnitz' work and it is curious that he mentioned him only a single time to say that a Priessnitz bandage applied all night increases inflammation rather than diminishes it. The criticism implicit in this statement may suggest the answer. Father Kneipp's treatments were characterized by increasingly gentle applications. His system was a refinement and expansion of Priessnitz'. He might have found the harsh treatments described in the Hahn book and the heroic therapies associated with Priessnitz offensive and possibly harmful, and might not have wanted his work associated with Priessnitz in any form which may have invited prejudice against his system. He had enough problems as it was. The final word on this issue should be given to Dr. Bernhard Detmar:

> Priessnitz practiced for about thirty years, Kneipp for about forty. Priessnitz treated altogether 40,000 patients, Kneipp many times that figure. Both men had great successes, and both were world-famous. Both were men of intuition and genius, gifted with an outstanding capacity for sharing the thoughts and feelings of others, as if they were their own. Both made fresh, cold water the basis of their treatment. Both were philanthropists, and were inspired by love of their fellow-men and sympathy with those who suffered. Both were strong-minded personalities who rejected compromise. They are together the most outstanding representatives of natural healing methods so far (1951, 100).

The two great American authorities on hydrotherapy, John Harvey Kellogg, M.D. and Simon Baruch, M. D., were highly critical of Kneippism. Kellogg regarded it as a revival of the "rude practices of ignorant English peasants a century and a half ago" (Kellogg 1903, 28-29). It is likely that he was influenced in his negative view by his teacher and friend, Professor Winternitz, who felt antipathy toward Kneipp. Kellogg offered a negative version of Kneipp's sojourn to the Vatican.

> Pastor Kneipp, the Bavarian water cure empiric, a few years ago being called upon to visit the Pope, who was suffering from chronic rheumatism, was received with great honors, but the first cold bath given the aged prelate, entirely unaccustomed to such heroic treatment, occasioned such an exacerbation of his suffering that the poor priest was peremptorily dismissed in disgrace. Had the patient been a sturdy young German peasant instead of a feeble Italian gentleman, the prescription might have succeeded better. A similar lack of discrimination, whether by a charlatan or a legally qualified practitioner, is always attended by disastrous results. The untoward effects thus produced should not, however, be attributed to scientific hydrotherapy but must be charged to the stupid audacity of quackery (ibid.,23).

Kellogg does not identify the source for his story, but in light of the detailed account offered by Baumgarten, it is not highly credible. Nonetheless it does reflect his concern that water treatments should be gentle and adapted to individual cases, which would agree with Kneipp.

America's foremost representative of scientific hydrotherapy, Dr. Simon Baruch (1840-1921), was also critical of the Kneipp Cure. In a 1895 article, he tried to counteract Kneipp's success for the sake of his own "scientific hydrotherapy."

> We already have in this city and elsewhere blatant imitators who vaunt the miraculous effects of the Kneipp "system" as panacea. These pages would not be occupied by a reference to this subject at all had it not come to my positive knowledge that intelligent physicians in this city have permitted themselves to be gulled by these quacks, and have actually prescribed the "Kneipp cure" to be administered by these uneducated men. One prominent physician has even sent a patient to an institution for scientific water treatment in this city, with a prescription for the Kneipp treatment (525).

Baruch considered Priessnitz and Kneipp to be impediments to progress in hydrotherapy and accused them of discrediting it with their heroic methods and their attacks on the medical profession. In his view, the history of hydrotherapy proved "that although water is an orthodox remedy, advocated and lauded by coryphei of medicine like Hippocrates, Galen, Celsus, and Asclepiades, whenever the empirics have trumpeted its virtues to the world, physicians have abandoned its use" (524). This sounds like a reversal of cause and effect. As we have seen, it was Priessnitz and Kneipp who elevated hydrotherapy to a new level of sophistication and effectiveness and it was thanks to them that some of the best physicians rediscovered its usefulness.

Despite these negative voices, Kneipp remains an influential figure in the development of rational health care. As an author who sold millions of books, a doctor who treated hundreds of thousands of patients, and as an innovator who defined natural health practices from herb baths to underwear, his importance to the history of naturopathic medicine is unsurpassed. Even today his dictums carry great authority. His medical philosophy is summed up by his motto: "Individualize in practice. Save the little energy there is and add to it little by little, because vitality cures" (Lust 1926, 9). His attitude toward service is summarized in his farewell admonition to Benedict

Lust in 1896 when charging him with the mission of bringing his treatments to the United States:

> Never forget the poor. They also have a right to the benefits of my method, and, if you always take care of them, you, and all your practitioners in the U.S.A., will always be prosperous and have God's blessing (ibid., 8).

The First Big City Nature Doctor

Louis Kuhne

(1835-1901)

Besides Kneipp, the German nature doctor who had the greatest influence on Benedict Lust and Henry Lindlahr was Louis Kuhne. Kuhne's writings helped Lindlahr to turn his failing health around. Lust was so impressed with Kuhne's two books that he reprinted them, promoted them, and used them as textbooks in his American School of Naturopathy.

Kuhne was the first big city nature doctor. While Priessnitz, Schroth, Hahn, Kneipp and Rikli founded their health resorts in the country with beautiful surroundings, Kuhne operated his establishment in the city of Leipzig. "Thus he became a model for all those natural healers whose field of action was the large city where the demand for a more natural life and treatment was greatest" (Brauchle 1951, 293). Henry Lindlahr followed Kuhne's example when he established his sanitarium in Chicago.

Louis Kuhne was born March 14, 1835 in Lössen near Delitzsch in Saxony where he grew up and attended the village school. When 14 years old, he was sent to Leipzig to apprentice in carpentry, after which he wandered through Germany and Austria working as an itinerant carpenter. At the age of 27, he set up his own business as a tool-maker. Before Kuhne, woodworkers purchased the necessary steel and produced their own tools. Realizing that homemade tools often turned out less than perfect, Kuhne was inspired to found a new trade, manufacturing quality carpentry tools. Soon his simple tool-shop became a factory, and Kuhne became well-known and quite wealthy as a tool-manufacturer.

> His enemies liked to call him "the former carpenter," but they usually concealed the fact that he had worked his way up to being a factory owner. By the same rationale a physician could be called "the former medical student" (Hering 1901, 177).

Kuhne explained how he made the transition from tool manufacturing to natural living in his work, *The New Science of Healing*. Like other nature doctors before him, Kuhne felt a special love for nature early in life:

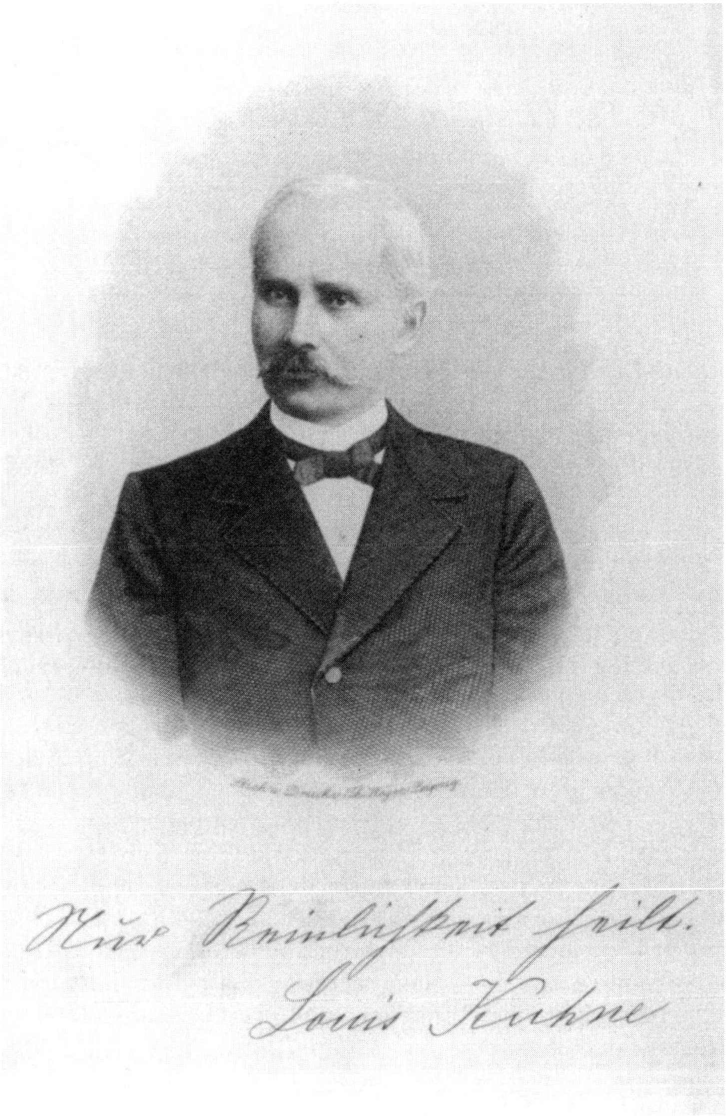

Louis Kuhne
(*Kuhne n.d.*, frontispiece)

> There was no greater delight for me than to observe the life of the field and forest and the conditions under which plants and animals live and thrive; to trace the workings of our great mother, Nature, on the earth and in the sky, and to apprehend and establish her immutable laws (Kuhne n.d., 2).

It was also the inability to find medical help for his own poor health that led him to nature cure. His father had died of stomach cancer and his mother, ailing for many years, had repeatedly warned him against "the doctors," whom she blamed for her own misery. When twenty, he began experiencing pains in his lungs and head. He read about the local nature cure society and began attending meetings, especially after a compress, which one member recommended, had an immediate beneficial result.

In 1868, Kuhne's brother became so ill that the simple prescriptions of the Nature Cure Society could not help him, so the brother consulted Theodor Hahn, and returned in a few weeks much improved. This convinced Kuhne even more firmly about the superiority of nature cure methods.

In the meantime Kuhne's own condition had grown much worse:

> Hereditary cancer had appeared in the stomach; the lungs were partially destroyed, the nerves of the head were so irritable that I found relief only out of doors in the fresh air (Kuhne n.d.,3).

When all the baths, packs, enemas, douches and other natural methods he had learned only gave him temporary relief of the pain, he resorted to the method which had worked so well earlier, when faced with an inadequate method of tool production. He invented a whole new system.

> At this period, through observations made in free nature, I discovered the laws upon which the method of cure now practiced and taught by me is based. I commenced, as a trial, with a course of cure for myself, and constructed the most practical appliances I could for the purpose. The experiment succeeded. My condition improved from day to day. Others who followed my advice and observed the same course were also satisfied (Kuhne n.d., 4).

Kuhne was not a modest man, and his claim to have discovered the true origin and cure of disease was met with skepticism, by both established medicine and by representatives of the nature cure method. Only "by effecting a large number of striking cures," could he "prove the superiority of my system over allopathy, homeopathy and the earlier hygienic method" (Kuhne n.d., 5). After much soul-searching, he gave up the factory which he had successfully operated for 24 years and devoted his managerial skills to

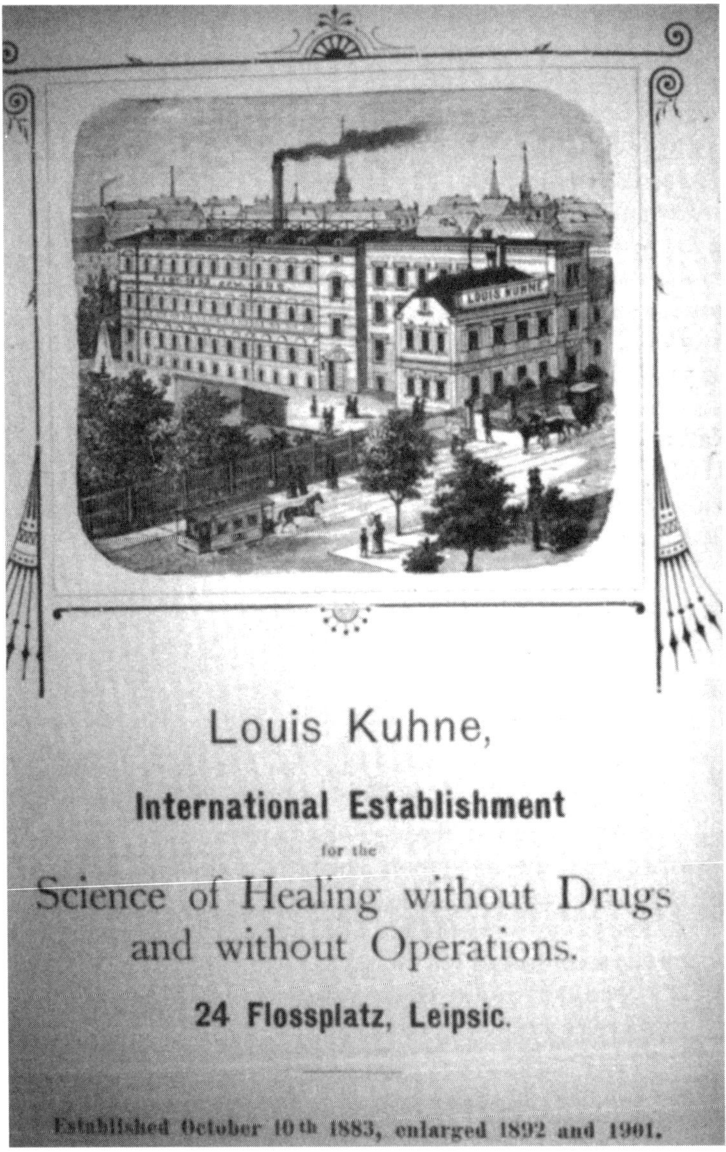
Louis Kuhne,

International Establishment

for the

Science of Healing without Drugs and without Operations.

24 Flossplatz, Leipsic.

Established October 10th 1883, enlarged 1892 and 1901.

(*Kuhne n.d.,* back of title page)

the new healing methods he had discovered. On October 10th, 1883, he opened the "Louis Kuhne International Establishment for the Science of Healing without Medicine and without Operations" in Leipzig. Although patient flow was sparse at first, it increased to the point where additions to the sanitarium were necessary in 1892, 1901 and 1904. In his own words:

> My method of curing and new system of diagnosis, the Science of Facial Expression, proved successful in thousands of cases, and I was able to save many from serious danger by foretelling future illnesses (Kuhne n.d., 5).

In 1894, he published *The New Science of Healing* which was almost as popular as Kneipp's *My Water Cure* of a few years earlier. Patients from all over the world were attracted to Kuhne's establishment, even more than had visited Priessnitz' Gräfenberg at its busiest time.

This book was translated into many languages, twenty-four according to Brauchle and over fifty according to Lust. Lust reprinted the work in 1917 under the title *Neo-Naturopathy: The New Science of Healing,* writing a new preface:

> It was in 1888 that I first heard of this work by Louis Kuhne, and it became the inspiration of my life work. I feel today that it is the very cornerstone of Naturopathy, and that every honest investigator will approve its teachings. In publishing this treatise, my aim is to prove Naturopathy a logical and exact science . . . and to make the drugless doctor a bigger and a better doctor, and the patient more appreciative of the merits of natural healing (Kuhne 1917, 4-5).

Perhaps even more important was the reaction of Lust's great contemporary, Henry Lindlahr, to Kuhne's book.

> At the age of thirty-five I was a physical and mental wreck. One day I confided my deplorable condition to a visiting friend. He brought me a book, saying that its perusal might do me some good . . . . When I read the book, it seemed to me as though a great light was rising before me and illuminating my darkened consciousness . . . and the next morning in the bathroom and at the breakfast table I began the practice of the natural regime, and carried it out from that time on to the best of my ability. The results were most gratifying (Lindlahr 1918, 34-35).

Kuhne's book even influenced Mahatma Gandhi (1869-1948), an ardent advocate of nature cure methods, which he used on himself and recommended to his countrymen. Gandhi founded the Nature Cure Centre at

Uruli-Kanchan, Poona District, in 1946. "The writings of Kuhne, Just and Father Kneipp are simple, popular and useful for all," he wrote. "It is our duty to read them" (Gandhi 1954, 10). He spoke specifically about Kuhne and hydrotherapy:

> Hydrotherapy is a well-known and ancient form of therapy. Many books have been written on the subject but in my opinion the form of hydrotherapy suggested by Kuhne is simple and effective. Kuhne's book on nature cure is very popular in India. It has been translated in several languages of India (Gandhi 1954, 10-11).

Kuhne believed his system was so unique that he called it the "New Science of Healing without Drugs and without Operations" to distinguish it from allopathy, homeopathy and the earlier nature cure methods. He was ever critical of allopathy.

> In fact, I consider the whole scheme of poisoning patients by medicine, lately so decidedly on the increase, as one, if not the chief cause that thoroughly healthy persons are now hardly to be found, and that chronic diseases are multiplying with fearful rapidity. The proper and timely intervention of the new art of healing will render surgery almost wholly superfluous (Kuhne, n.d., 7).

His judgment about homeopathy was milder but not completely positive.

> Homeopathy I welcome as a brave ally in the crusade against the fatal faith in medicines. With its minute doses wherein the chemist is unable to discover a trace of the drug; and the stress which it lays on the choice of a proper diet, it forms a transition, a stepping-stone, to the new art of healing. With reference to diet, however, it formulates no fixed, clear principles, and my experience proves even its minute doses of medicine to be not altogether harmless (Kuhne n.d., p.7).

Kuhne reserved the greatest praise for "the natural method as hitherto applied, which far excels the other systems," but with reservation:

> I have found it necessary, however, to follow more the great discoverers and founders of the system - Priessnitz, Schroth, Rausse and Theodor Hahn - rather than its later representatives. The latter, in their excessive zeal for individualization, run the risk

> of degenerating into artificiality and deviating from the clear and simple paths of nature (Kuhne n.d., 7-8).

Still, he criticized the founders for their lack of insight into the true nature of disease and their bewildering array of superfluous water applications: "The New Science of Healing simplifies the application of water as much as possible" (Kuhne n.d., 8). He also criticized their diet which seemed to him to be unregulated and without any guiding concept. He favored a low sodium vegetarian diet: "Food precisely in the form nature gives it to us," he wrote, "is always the best for the digestion" (Kuhne n.d., 125). Therefore, he reasoned, "all foods, the fermentability of which we alter by artificial preparation, or suppress by means of salt, sugar or cooking, are difficult to digest" (Kuhne n.d., 126). He considered raw food to be the most digestible and nutritious. He also preferred unripe fruits to ripe ones because of their cleansing effect. Since even a healthy stomach could digest only a certain quantity of food, he believed excess intake created toxins which, if not excreted, would be subject to fermentation. This fermentation raised the temperature of the blood and resulted in fever. Fever could therefore only occur when foreign matter was present and the natural exits for such waste as the bowels, urinary tract, skin and lungs were deficient. According to Kuhne, bacilli were the product of fermentation and therefore disappeared of themselves when fermentation ceased and the system was restored to health. "The question is not how to kill the bacilli, but rather how to remove the cause of fermentation, the foreign matter" (Kuhne n.d., 29).

Kuhne defined disease as "the presence of foreign matter in the system" (Kuhne n.d., 18). His gift for simplification, his striking illustrations taken from the animal and vegetable kingdoms and his logical thinking captivated the minds of many people who were disillusioned with orthodox medicine. A prime example was his doctrine of the "Unity of Disease" which stated:

> There is only one cause of disease, and there is also only one disease, which shows itself under different forms. We therefore ought not, strictly speaking, to distinguish between different diseases but only between different forms of disease (Kuhne n.d., 32-33).

Henry Lindlahr later expanded and refined this concept in his book *Nature Cure: Philosophy & Practice Based on the Unity of Disease & Cure* (1913).

Kuhne's next book was *The Science of Facial Expression* (1902), reprinted by Lust in 1917. E. Hering considered it Kuhne's most important work. According to Kuhne it was "the result of thirty years of observation and the conclusions drawn have been proved correct in thousands of cases" (Kuhne 1917, 88). He based his new system of diagnosis on the premise that diseases revealed themselves by changes in the body, most easily discernible in the face and neck where the morbid encumbrances were most evident. Kuhne claimed his system made other methods of diagnosis superfluous and allowed him to foretell future illnesses. His method of diagnosis and its value was not verified by others, though we know that Felke used it. Brauchle believed the expert could gain some valuable clues from Kuhne's facial diagnosis, but that it could never replace a careful physical examination (Brauchle 1951, 295). Like iris diagnosis, or iridology, discovered by the Hungarian Ignatz von Peczely (1826-1911), Kuhne's facial diagnosis was an attempt to diagnose health problems by a simple, non-invasive method and to detect predispositions to diseases before they manifested pathologically. Unlike von Peczely, whose work was taken up and refined by Lindlahr, Felke and modern naturopathic practitioners, Kuhne never found many followers.

Kuhne's therapeutic measures were of striking simplicity. They consisted of steam baths, sun baths, friction hip baths and friction sitz baths designed to enhance elimination of poisonous substances from the body. *The New Science of Healing* contained 133 testimonials of grateful patients who were supposedly cured from such afflictions as breast cancer, impotence, migraine, rheumatism, syphilis, epilepsy, asthma and general debility. The following is illustrative of his approach:

> In the middle of July 1889, the four-year old son in a Leipsic family got the whooping-cough. At the beginning of August the sickness had reached its height. Then the baby daughter, aged two, also took ill. For ten days the illness became worse and worse, and during this time the child could take no nourishment. At last, the parents, who till then had been using the natural method of cure to the best of their knowledge, applied to me. I took over the case. The little girl had lost so much strength that she could no longer stand. I ordered four friction sitz baths daily, the children then to be put to bed, or given a sunbath to bring out the perspiration . . . After only a few weeks of energetic treatment, both children were out of danger, and in two months they had fully recovered (Kuhne n.d., 54).

Kuhne is less well remembered for his doctrine of the Unity of Disease or *The Science of Facial Expression* than for his invention of the friction hip bath and the friction sitz bath. These measures might not be the cure-alls which he claimed them to be, but they have powerful, stimulating effects, and are still used by nature cure practitioners worldwide. Gandhi considered them "the most important of Kuhne's contributions to hydrotherapy" (Gandhi 1954,11). Then he described the friction hip-bath as follows:

> The tub should be filled with fresh cold water . . . After the patient is comfortably seated in the tub, gentle friction should be applied to his abdomen with a soft towel. This bath can be taken for five to thirty minutes. When it is over, the body should be rubbed dry and the patient put to bed.
>
> Hip bath brings down the temperature in high fever . . . It relieves constipation and improves digestion. The patient feels fresh and active after it . . .
>
> I have tried hip baths on a fairly large scale. They have proved efficacious in more than 75 cases out of 100 (Gandhi 1954, 11-12).

The friction sitz bath, which consists of the application of gentle friction to the external genitalia by means of a soft, wet linen cloth dipped into cold water, produces even stronger effects than the friction hip bath. According to Kuhne:

> It is only at the genitals that the entire nervous system can be influenced. Here is, in a sense, the root of the whole tree of life. By washing in cold water, not only is the morbid internal heat diminished, but there is also a marked invigoration of the nerves; that is, the vitality of the whole body, down to the minutest part, is stimulated (Kuhne n.d., 113).

In an obituary, E. Hering praised Kuhne as a person of great benevolence, honesty, tireless energy and perseverance:

> He knew no obstacles when acting according to his convictions; he feared no one. His energy was combined with a simplicity and unpretentiousness which he preserved until the end of his life (Hering 1901, 177).

Kuhne needed a strong character to survive the attacks from the medical profession. One enemy circulated a letter to physicians throughout Germany soliciting reports about negative experiences with the Kuhne Cure. Several physicians who received these requests found them in bad taste and forwarded them to Kuhne. The persecution of Kuhne culminated in a lawsuit brought against him by the medical profession. In 1901. *Der Naturarzt (The Nature Doctor)*, the chief organ of the nature cure movement in Germany, carried the following notice:

> Louis Kuhne of Leipzig . . . was charged with fraud in several hundred cases. The prosecution contended that he inflicted great harm with his "friction sitz baths" and strict diet regimes, a charge which was not based on the denunciations of patients but

> rather on those of medical doctors. The trial lasted 4 days. Prof. Dr. Trendelenburg, Dr. Lahmann, Prof. Flechsig, Dr. Katz, Dr. Winsch and others were called as expert witnesses . . . Not one single punishable injury of his patients could be proven against Kuhne. All witnesses testified in his favor. Of course, he was acquitted and the public treasury had to bear the costs (*Der Naturarzt* 1901, no.3, 70).

The Dr. Lahmann mentioned was Heinrich Lahmann, M.D., the first great scientific nature physician, who founded the large nature cure sanitarium Weisser Hirsch near Dresden. Dr. Katz, who also testified, was the surgeon-in-chief of the Prussian army, who, during the Franco-Prussian war, became convinced that antiseptics were causing more harm than good and abandoned them for natural methods. Despite professional and social ostracism, he became a staunch advocate of natural healing and founded a nature cure sanitarium near Stuttgart which he directed until his death (Lust 1918, 446). Wilhelm Winsch, M.D. (1863-1946) was cured as a student by Kuhne of a serious stomach ailment after all allopathic treatment had failed him. Winsch later wrote *About Heat Culture,* advocating warm water treatments and fever therapy as an alternative to the cold water cure, especially for many asthenic and neurasthenic patients who shied away from nature cure because cold water was too harsh for them (Brauchle/Groh 1971, 108-110).

These three physicians were ideal witnesses on Kuhne's behalf, because they used methods similar to his in their own practice. Kuhne himself used the trial as an opportunity to defend his theories in public. The lawsuit increased his fame and made him a martyr for the cause of nature cure. But the stress from this legal battle may have ruined his health and ultimately caused his death. Kuhne turned over his health establishment to his son in 1899, but continued to advise patients while writing a new work. The news of his sudden death on April 3, 1901 shocked everyone as he had been in perfect health in spite of his 66 years. According to Hering:

> Kuhne had just come through a period of great excitement. It was not the six days of the trial itself so much as the preceding weeks which had drained him. He had to make several long trips during the coldest part of winter, because his presence during the interrogation of prosecution witnesses was absolutely necessary. On one of these trips he caught a bad cold . . . . Several days before his death he fell sick with influenza. As soon as he recovered he succumbed to a cerebral stroke. No doubt, the strain of these last weeks was responsible for this devastating outcome (Hering 1901, 177-178).

Hering ends his tribute to Kuhne with the words:

> We can only hope that Kuhne will be judged in a more objective way after his death and that he will receive the appreciation which he deserves—as a man of noble character and rare gifts who made sensational discoveries without any scientific training (Hering 1901, 179).

During his lifetime it was impossible to judge Kuhne objectively since the medical profession rallied against him and he generated controversy within the nature cure movement. In-fighting between different nature cure groups was not unusual with so many strong personalities and their enthusiastic followers. The lengthy feud between the Priessnitz and the Schroth camps is only one example. However, no other nature doctor received more criticism from his nature cure colleagues than Kuhne. They accused him of being a charlatan, a swindler and a boaster. A more negative report on the Kuhne hearings, emphasizing the testimony offered against him, was given by *Der Natur und Volksarzt (The Nature and People's Doctor)*, a publication of medical doctors who practiced natural therapeutics:

> Kuhne prescribed out-door movement and friction sitz baths for the appendicitis of the 11 year old sister of the cartographer Michael of Trier. The result was that the patient died after five days. Prof. Trendelenburg called the treatment by letter of such a serious condition to be down-right unscrupulous. Dr. Lahmann agreed that this patient was harmed by the Kuhne Cure.
>
> According to Prof. Trendelenburg Kuhne did not practice what he preached in his works . . . . Kuhne could not have employed his science of facial expression as a diagnosis for most of his patients, because he had not seen them, treating most of them by letter, as he had testified himself. How mechanical must Kuhne's treatment by letter have been . . . . His secretary Hoppe wrote 6-8 recommendations per day on preprinted forms which were almost the same for each inquirer . . . .
>
> Nevertheless, Kuhne was acquitted because it could not be proven that he disbelieved in his own doctrines, although there was a justifiable suspicion of fraud, and his prescriptions were clearly irresponsible . . . . This deplorable acquittal turned into a wonderful propaganda opportunity for Kuhne, as Dr. Lahmann pointed out with regret, because the cases presented were so badly chosen (Boden 1901, 51-52).

Even more disturbing, if true, are the "Disclosures about the Kuhne Cure" by J. G. Brockmann who claimed to have been the first deputy of

Kuhne's establishment. He asserted that Kuhne could not have written *The New Science of Healing*, because Kuhne only attended a small Prussian village school and received no formal education:

> Page 1-110 (IV.-VII. edition of his textbook) are the results of different educated friends of Kuhne, among them the eloquent lawyer Lothar Volkmar (editor of Kuhne's magazine *The New Science of Healing*). The main part of Kuhne's textbook, pp. 111-520, flowed exclusively from my pen . . . .
>
> Since there was too little time, many inconclusive case histories had to be used so that the most important evidence for the correctness of the theories left nothing to be desired in terms of superficiality . . . . I treated approx. 25,000 patients according to Kuhne's methods. We were successful with approx 8,000 of these, while 17,000, i.e., more than two thirds, not only were not helped, but even got worse . . . . I realized that the successes were more the result of diet than the baths and that they were similar to those achieved by the famous Professor Sylvester Graham many years ago in America. The whole diet of the Kuhne Cure was nothing more than an imitation of the regime of this American professor.
>
> The friction sitz bath has a harmful effect on most men because it increases the sex drive in a most unprecedented way. The result is not only destruction of the nervous system but also quite often a lung disease . . . .

Brockmann concluded his article with a description of the harm he had inflicted on himself using the friction sitz baths:

> At the end of the fifth year I had to give up my large practice in Kuhne's establishment due to enervation. I was incapable of speaking to anybody, so irritating was my cough. Further, I had not enough strength to climb the staircase to my apartment . . . If I had only continued the Kuhne Cure for a few weeks more, I would no longer be among the living (Brockmann 1895, 81-86).

Matthäus Schmidtbauer, a staunch advocate of Rikli's sun and air bath, cut Kuhne to pieces with unrelenting sarcasm. Kuhne was a plagiarist of the first rank who appropriated the achievements of the great pioneers as his own inventions. Schmidtbauer pointed out that the doctrine of the Unity of Disease was first proposed by Rausse long before Kuhne "simplified it ad absurdum." Like other Kuhne critics, Schmidtbauer was most irked by Kuhne's indiscriminate recommendation of the friction sitz bath as a cure-all. "But we must warn all humankind against this hydropathic homeopath . . . Kuhne should have called his friction sitz bath "homeopathic sitz bath" since only the smallest part of the body can be moistened during this bath" (Schmidtbauer, 1897, 49). Possibly the friction sitz bath was rejected by some nature cure apostles, not so much because it was harmful, but because it offended their Victorian sexual mores.

Some of these polemics were justified while others stemmed from envy of Kuhne's success. Kuhne's books reveal his propensity for exaggeration and oversimplification. As one of his detractors pointed out, the hereditary stomach cancer which he cured in himself may have been a stomach ulcer. Maybe Kuhne was a mixture of genius and charlatan, but his simple, convincing methods converted many people to nature cure and inspired future nature doctors for generations, while most of his critics have been forgotten.

The greatest praise Kuhne ever received was from Alexander Rosendorff, M.D. (1871-1963), who ran a successful practice based on Kuhne's principles for 50 years. "It is astonishing with what intelligence and strict logic he established a healing system a hundred years ago which still has its value today and which will probably have it for all future time" (Rosendorff 1964, 49).

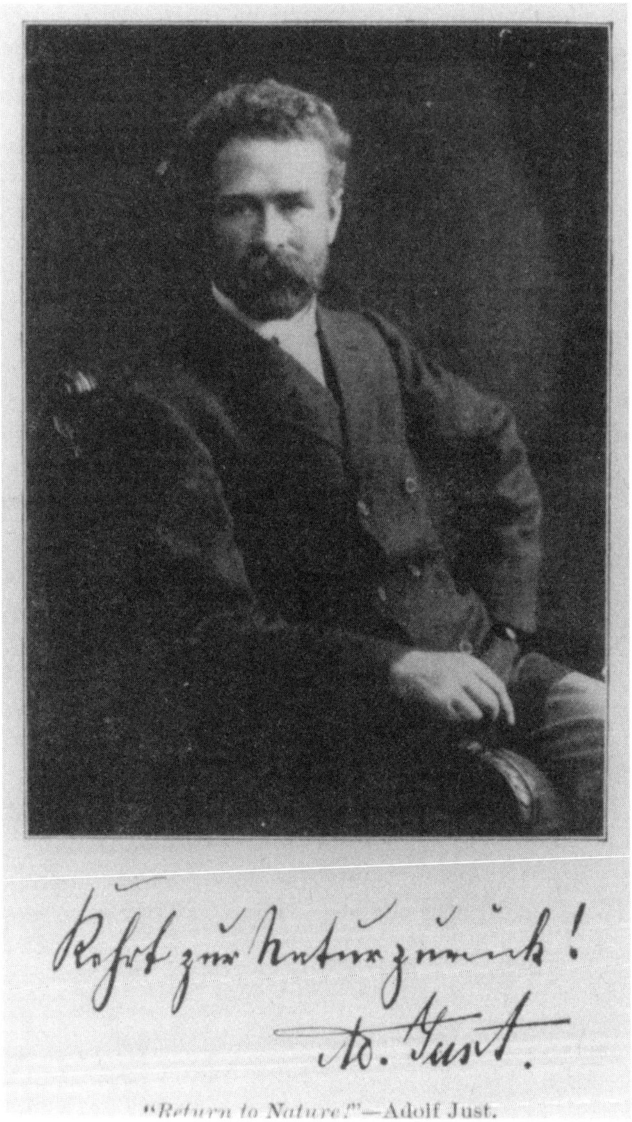

Adolf Just
(Just 1903, frontispiece)

Return to Nature!

Adolf Just

(1859-1936)

Adolf Just was an enthusiastic follower of Jean-Jacques Rousseau (1712-1778) and his philosophy of Naturism. He adopted Rousseau's battle cry "Return to Nature!" as the title of his main work and filled the book with statements reminiscent of Rousseau.

> Man originally came from the hand of the Creator absolutely healthy and good, without any blemish in body and soul (Just 1903, 1).

This corresponds to Rousseau's famous words at the beginning of *Emile* (1762): *"Tout est bien sortant des mains de l'auteur des choses, tout degenere entre les mains de l'homme"* (Everything is good as it leaves the hands of the Author of things; everything degenerates in the hands of man) (Rousseau 1979, 37). Just shared Rousseau's contempt for civilization and science and indulged in the same romantic idealization of nature.

> The voices of nature have always been true to man, but science is the cunning serpent in paradise which deceived man from the start, led him astray, and gave him false instruction.
>
> Men who no longer listen to the voice of nature become the victims of a thousand different diseases and miseries. But the creatures of pure nature on the other hand, the animals of our forests, are free from sickness and from everything else as well that corresponds to the sins and vices of mankind.
>
> In all cases, and in all diseases, man can recover and again become happy only by a true return to nature; man must today strenuously endeavor, in his mode of living, to heed again the voice of nature, and thus choose the food that nature has laid before him from the beginning, and to bring himself again into the relation with water, light and air, earth, etc., that nature originally designed for him (Just ibid., 4-6).

Just strongly influenced Benedict Lust, who translated and published an early edition of *Return to Nature!* and modeled his naturopathic sanitarium in the scenic Ramapo Mountains of New Jersey after Just's Jungborn in the Hartz mountains of Germany. Lust added a chapter about his "Yungborn" to *Return to Nature!*.

> In its course of development, slowly casting off all its former defects, the Nature Cure Method has attained the stage of the uttermost simplicity and perfection in the Jungborn. I founded and established the Jungborn according to views that are fully and particularly described in the book "Return to Nature," and indeed from the first day of its appearance it met with a most enthusiastic reception (ibid., 297).

The American Yungborn ("Jungborn" means "Fountain of Youth") offered the same facilities and therapy program as its German counterpart; parks with light-air cottages for sun, air and rain baths, earth baths, earth compresses and the Just fruit diet. On the last pages of *Return to Nature!*, Lust advertised his naturopathic health store as the American depot of Jungborn articles, porous reform clothing, air shoes, clay packs and Jungborn Bread. He visited Just and his Jungborn in 1906 and 1926, and "each time it was an inspiration to us" (Lust 1936, 69). On his last visit, he presented a lifetime membership in the American Naturopathic Association to Just, and conferred on him the honorary degree of Doctor of Naturopathy.

Adolf Just was born in Lüthorst, near Hannover in North Germany, August 8, 1859; the oldest of twelve brothers and sisters, five of whom died in childhood. His father was an innkeeper and small farmer and had great difficulty supporting his large family. Young Adolf grew up in the isolation of a simple country setting attending the village school. Prepared by the village pastor, a great nature enthusiast and follower of Rousseau, he later attended secondary school in Goslar.

Adolf was a lively, imaginative child, full of love for nature, but also beset by inner struggles. When older, his oversensitive nature led to attacks of neurasthenia and possible episodes of psychosis with religious hallucinations. "If the career of most nature cure practitioners is determined by the experience of physical illness," wrote Brauchle, "then the driving force behind Just's return to nature was psychic distress. The predominance of his own psychic difficulties gives his nature cure system quite a special flavor" (Brauchle 1951, 297).

In 1882, Just passed his high school examination in Goslar, but was unable to study of mathematics as he had hoped to, due to his poor health. Seeking a practical career, he became an apprentice in a bookstore in Leipzig, the German publishing center. However, a nervous breakdown forced him to return home and he sought recovery by doing simple farm tasks.This strengthened him enough so he could start his own book business in Brunswick, maintaining it successfully for twelve years.

However, he suffered from repeated bouts of neurasthenia. Medicine proved useless, and a fattening diet combined with daily warm baths made his condition worse.

> In my sufferings I naturally consulted, first, the old-school physicians. I called on celebrated doctors and university professors, but they could not help me. In the direst distress and despair I finally lost my high opinion of science. What did I care for science; in my despair I wanted help and nothing but help (Just 1903, 2).

Only the Priessnitz wet sheet packs, recommended by a psychiatrist, gave him relief. At the same time he heard about Kneipp and started to walk barefoot. While this had a relaxing effect on his brain, the Kneipp cold gushes were too strong for his nerves. He used the Kuhne friction sitz bath with soothing effect, but found Kuhne's fat-free vegetarian diet to have a deleterious effect. Then he discovered Rikli's light and air cures which later played an important role in his own system. But, since none of these methods produced a lasting cure, Just was compelled, like Kuhne, to create his own system.

> I placed my greatest hope in the nature cure method . . . . But finally my confidence was undermined and shaken. The realization of my hopes for a complete recovery was still delayed. Besides, I saw so much quarreling and controversy among the individual champions of the nature cure method (ibid., 3).

Finally Just concluded that he could only recover through a direct and intimate contact with nature. With a few like-minded people he attempted to live a truly natural life in the von Pawel Woods near Brunswick, trying out on himself all the future Jungborn cure methods. Here he built his first light-and-air hut where he spent many nights. He also went on long barefoot hikes into the Hartz mountains, taking his special bath in a babbling creek. One of his early patients who accompanied him remembered:

> He was a keen observer of people, animals and plants. He loved the silence and the solitude of the forest; he took lonely hikes for days observing fruit trees, shrubs, the wallowing of wild boars in the mud and other such events as nature had to offer. He drew quite a few conclusions from animal behavior for the treatment of

> illness and later announced them to the world with great courage. His fellow-citizens jeered at Just as "the crazy bookseller " (R. Just 1934, 86).

The wonderful results of his return to nature elated him.

> I soon recognized how wisely and easily Nature communicates her rules and prescriptions to him who harkens at her voice. When I arranged my mode of life according to her after such a long time of sickness and anguish, I perceived a real feeling of health, strength and freshness of youth, happiness and joy of life, repose and peace of the soul; a beatitude as never divined before. I had found the fountain of health (Just 1910, 643).

His recovery inspired him to write *Return to Nature!* and to establish a sanitarium in the Hartz mountains, in the beautiful valley of the Ecker, between Harzburg and Ilsenburg.

> Here was the opportunity given to exhausted and suffering humanity to use the remedies of Nature exactly according to her prescriptions for a real, thorough strengthening of its health and the curing of its maladies. An entire return to nature was made possible here . . . . I called this institute "Jungborn," after the legendary fountain of youth (Just 1910, 643).

Just encountered many difficulties before he was able to open the Jungborn as a "Health Resort and School for Natural Healing and Living" on June 21, 1896.

> From the first day on he had to fight against many strong opposing forces . . . . Moreover, banks did not give any credit for this "dubious matter." However, in an almost superhuman effort he prevailed against a world of enemies and overcame all obstacles which were put in his path. (Rudolf Just 1934, 70-71).

He published the first edition of *Return to Nature!* in celebration of this event. The book was a guide to the nature cure methods practiced by Just, and at the same time an indictment of modern science and its alienation from nature and a manifesto for the return to nature as the only salvation from the ills of modern civilization. Following Kneipp's *My Water Cure* in 1886 and Kuhne's *The New Science of Healing* in 1893, it was the last nature cure best-seller with worldwide success. It went through many editions and, according to Lust, was translated into English, French, Spanish, Italian, Hungarian and Polish. "It has brought to millions of people throughout the world a message of health and happiness, and has prolonged the life of thousands" (Lust 1936, 69).

Lust's translation of the fourth German edition in 1903 was followed by H. A. Nesbitt's translation of the seventh German edition, published in England in 1912 and double in size. The earlier edition was less burdened with philosophical reflections, polemics, and quotes from the Bible and Goethe. The later edition suggests Just was trying to find support for his nature religion in the teachings of Christianity, where his tormented soul sought peace:

> My great longing drove me towards real healing and redemption. I therefore plunged deeper and deeper into the secrets of nature and of God . . . . I earnestly turned against the original evil, the just cause of all sickness and trouble: sin. I clung with my whole heart and will to Jesus the Saviour, and thus came for the first time into true communion with God (Just 1912, 433).

Unlike nature doctors before him, Just was not only concerned with health reform but also with the reform of other aspects of human life which he wanted to bring into harmony with nature. In a special issue of the "Jungborn-Blätter" honoring Just's 75th birthday, his brother Rudolf wrote:

> How greatly this man toiled! Night after night he wrote on the new editions of his books. Whatever the issues of importance to the public welfare were, he confronted them all: disease, immunization, vivisection, agriculture, alcohol, nutrition, clothing, housing and education (R. Just 1934, 73).

Just condemned everything that was not in accordance with a natural life: polluting automobiles, closed-in modern housing, deforming styles of dress and modern chemical agriculture. For every problem of life, he tried to find a natural and simple solution, including funeral procedures.

> In nature, animals who die are devoured by beast of prey. Their bodies thus serve as food for other creatures . . . . I believe that the best and most natural way of proceeding is to give back the corpses of our dead to the earth without any coffin. The body would then dissolve into earth in the simplest and quickest way, without the evil arising from the process of decay, such as injurious gases (Just 1912, 200).

His comments about education speak to the heart of any restless student.

> Much of our completely useless talking, disputing, writing, studying, meditating, investigating, etc., ought to be discontinued. Instead, we ought to approach Nature, devote ourselves to the pleasures she offers, practice brotherly love, and in this way gain joys and rich blessedness which will always promote health and elevate mind and soul (Just 1903, 260).

His greatest contempt was directed against medical science, especially vivisection and vaccination:

> It seems to me that vivisection more than anything else tramples under foot all the nobler impulses of man . . . .
>
> I have frequently shown how all vaccine poisons . . . destroy more and more all health among men, and are largely the cause of the misery that is abroad in the world (Just 1903, 256-257).

He also rejected any form of examination and diagnosis, because they might instill a state of unrest and excitement in the patient:

> My observations of so many invalids have forced upon me the conviction of the injury and danger caused by diagnosis . . . . The patient can never become really healthy till he has entirely forgotten every diagnosis of his illness (Just 1903, 28).

Nor did he have high regard for homeopathy.

> The homeopathic drops are quite innocuous, but they leave no room for nature and God, and in this lies the danger of homeopathy (Just 1912, 298).

Even the old nature cure methods did not escape his criticism if they used the forces of nature only as drugs.

> I do not wish to consider water, light, air, earth and diet as a kind of medicine. My task is principally to point out how men may break with so many absurdities and unnatural proceedings . . . . Men will be astonished how even severe maladies pass away and . . . how the whole of existence may be made easier and more beautiful by a simple natural mode of life (Just 1912, 13-14).

He also rejected warm baths, vapor baths, electric light baths, and massage.

> It is especially dangerous when these entirely artificial means are regarded as natural remedies . . . . Men are thus finally deceived and led astray (Just 1912, 59).

Even gymnastics did not meet his approval.

> I for my part cannot see anything natural in all this artificial bending, winding, straining, stretching; in these gymnastic feats indoors . . . . To the physical culturists, therefore, I would say: "Return to Nature!" Come forth from your musty, dusty rooms and halls, out into free nature! (Just 1903, 261).

Despite his criticism of the nature cure methods which preceded him, Just's philosophy of health was almost identical to Kuhne's doctrine of the unity of disease and cure. Disease was caused by the introduction of unnatural food into the body. Insufficiently digested, it became "foreign matter" which "enters into fermentation, and becomes the cause of all disease, all pain and suffering of man" (Just 1903, 24). Negative emotional influences could also cause disease by disturbing the nervous and digestive functions and thus contributing to the formation of foreign matter.

The aim of the cure was to lower the internal heat caused by fermentation of foreign matter. This was achieved by the application of cold to the abdomen, and to the sexual organs, the center of the nervous system, and by stimulation of the patient's vitality through water, earth, light, air and correct diet, so it could throw off the foreign matter through the skin, urine and stool. So firm was Just's confidence in the benevolence of nature that he believed acute diseases were favorable healing events which became dangerous only when the patient was shut off from fresh air and treated with suppressive medicines.

> Yes, the acute diseases, typhoid fever, cholera, and what not, which are mainly brought on by taking cold, and which are still today terribly dreaded by mankind, are wholly without danger. They prove to be of the greatest benefit when correctly treated (Just 1903, 109).

Just, however, contended that patients could avoid such unpleasant healing crises altogether if they carefully followed his prescriptions.

> Among the many young and old people who . . . started going barefooted, taking the new bath in the open, sleeping in an open light-and-air hut or entirely in the open air and on the bare ground, and walking about naked, not one such crisis appeared (Just 1903, 111).

This quote names the important treatment methods used by Just. The "natural bath" or "new bath" strongly resembled Kuhne's friction hip-bath, except that the bather used his bare hands instead of a cloth to rub the body. Just claimed he got the clue for this bath from watching wild animals cool their sexual organs in the mud or water. He boldly stated that the natural bath united most of the nature cure methods of his day such as barefoot walking, light-and-air baths, abdominal compresses, Kneipp douches and massage.

Just followed Rikli's emphasis of the light-and-air bath over the water bath. Since man was born without clothes, Just argued, going naked was fully in accordance with nature:

> Going naked temporarily, even in the room with as many open windows as possible, but better still in the open, in the woods, proves of wonderful benefit and efficacy, and is more strengthening than any other means (Just 1903, 55).

Just believed that the first concern of a nature doctor called to a sick room should be to free the patient from bed clothes and take him into the open air. If this was not possible, to let him lie naked in the room with the windows open, from one to three hours in summer and from fifteen to twenty minutes in the winter, even on the coldest days.

The main attraction at the Jungborn was the large, magnificent light-and-air parks with their light-and-air huts and cottages where the patients lived. Built according to Just's design without walls or with only lattice walls, they offered free access to light and air, yet protection against the rain. They were supplied with curtains for stormy weather, and by means of straw and special partitions, could be made habitable even in snowy winter weather. The separate parks for ladies and gentlemen were enclosed by fences and thick bushes where the patients could take their light-and-air baths naked and undisturbed. An early Jungborn patient who later became head of the ladies' park, wrote:

> When I arrived, I was completely surprised by a sight which was beyond my imagination. I saw a group of female figures, picturesquely grouped on the meadow, in all shades from the usual light color to pink, Indian bronze and mulatto brown. I hesitated to accept their friendly invitation and to join them but after only an hour, having lost all self-consciousness, I was lying among them with indescribable pleasure. ..
>
> Now and then a rain bath offered a pleasant change. Forgetting all our worries, we lived like children in a paradise, enjoying games, singing and exercises. There were no rules, no system; everyone sought out for himself what would be most beneficial and wholesome, completely giving himself over to Mother Nature (R. Just 1934, 89).

Just always emphasized the patient's freedom to choose what suited him or her best. The nature doctor's highest mission was to teach people to be responsible for their own health.

> It is of course always easier and pleasanter to let others think for us . . . . But if people wish to pursue a course that will certainly lead them to true health, to the springs of life, each must be his own doctor (Just 1903, 37).

Just's most original contribution to nature cure was the discovery of the healing power of the earth or geotherapy.

> Water applications have been long in vogue since Priessnitz, Kneipp, Kuhne, and others. To combine rubbing with the bath has also already been taught . . . . Going naked was preached long ago by Rikli . . . . But the earth power and its application has been overlooked entirely (Just 1903, 101).

Again, Just got his inspiration from the animal kingdom, observing that when hares and deer lay down to rest, they carefully cleared away all the wood, leaves and even snow to be in touch with the earth. He believed that "animals and men are but moving plants." Since man dwelled on dry land, Just credited earth with a greater healing power than water. "I believe that the roebuck observed by Priessnitz would have done much better if he had laid his wounded leg in mud instead of water" (Just 1912, 84). He also referred to the Greek myth of Antaeus, son of the earth goddess. In combat with Hercules Antaeus weakened when he was lifted from the earth, but regained his strength as soon as he was allowed to touch earth again. Finally, Just cited Jesus, who supposedly walked barefooted and commanded his disciples, "Carry neither shoes!" (Luke 10:4). Just wrote: "Going barefooted, without sandals, if possible, ought to be the foundation of every nature cure" (1903, 93). As one patient noted: "When Mr. Just referred to the special healing power of the earth, all the patients would enthusiastically walk around barefooted the next morning" [R. Just 1934, 91]. Just also convinced his patients to sleep naked on the bare ground.

> All diseases, especially the nervous troubles of our age, would entirely loose their power if patients slept on the earth at night . . . . Whoever has not tried it, can have no conception of how refreshing, vitalizing, and strengthening it can be (R. Just 1934, 87-88).

He constructed special sandbeds covered by porous burlap or linen to make sleeping on the ground more comfortable. He preferred that these beds be placed in the open, "for man is also influenced by a wonderful, mysterious curative power from above that seems to be especially active at night, invigorating and strengthening his entire organism while he is resting under the starry sky, under the great dome of heaven" (Just 1903, 103).

Just not only used the healing power of the earth in these general ways but also as earth bandages for specific conditions in lieu of water applications. After the successful self-treatment of a serious dog bite with the application of moist earth, he began to employ this remedy for all kinds of afflictions.

> For every injury of the skin, wounds of cutting, stabbing, burning, shooting, etc., for every boil or ulcer, every inflammation, stings and bites of animals, blood-poisoning, for all skin diseases, cancer, lupus, tetter, dandruff, eruptions, leprosy, for broken bones, etc., the affected locality ought to be bandaged with moist earth or moist clay (Just 1903, 120).

In 1918, the German High Command seized all the copies of his book *Return to Nature!* and prohibited its further distribution because of Just's recommendation to use earth treatments for war injuries in World War I. This was a blow to Just, but did not deter the physician Friedrich Wolf from using purified clay internally against dysentery and externally as an absorbent for purulent wounds on hundreds of war casualties (Wolf 1929, 333).

Earth bandages were made in the same way as the Priessnitz compresses, but Just claimed that they were "much more in accordance with nature and much more effective, since the earth will hold more water and retain it longer, and possesses a dissolving and absorbing power of its own" (Just 1903, 124). Brauchle pointed out that the once widespread knowledge of the healing power of the earth was lost with the emergence of scientific medicine (Brauchle 1951, 301). The Sicilian physician Dioscorides (circa 40-80 A.D.) recommended the healing earths from the Greek islands Lemnos and Armenia (Luvos) as remedies against deadly animal bites and dysentery. Galen (circa 130-200 A.D.), the most influential Roman physician, travelled to Lemnos to study its famous healing earth. Jesus' cure of the blind man in John 9:1 was a favorite of Just.

> And as Jesus passed by He saw a man which was blind from his birth . . . . When he had thus spoken He spat on the ground and made clay of the spittle, and He anointed the eyes of the blind man with the clay (Just 1903, 123).

Inspired by Professor Stumpf, who successfully used white clay (Bolus alba) in an East Prussian cholera epidemic, Just concentrated on the development of a more purified and effective healing clay for internal use. Just believed he found it in the diluvian sediment of the Hartz mountains. He used this "Luvos healing clay" with good results on his wife who suffered from chronic constipation. Neither the fruit diet nor earth compresses had brought her any relief, but the internal use of the Luvos clay immediately eliminated the problem. Just's pioneering role in the therapeutic use of earth is acknowledged by the French nature doctor Raymond Dextreit in his classic book on clay therapy *Our Earth, Our Cure* (1974).

Just was one of the first nature doctors to propose a pure raw food diet. He declared fruits and nuts as the most natural foods for man.

> In our part of the globe the berries of the forest were the original food of man; later he added the fruit of trees, and chief of all the nut; everything that tastes good in the raw, pure, unchanged state of nature (Just 1903, 135).

Since the discovery of fire enabled man to create civilization, Just viewed fire as the great arch-enemy of humanity which made man stray from nature. He pointed to the myth of Prometheus, which "tells us most impressively and beautifully how terribly the gods resented the discovery of fire by men, how severely man is punished for it, and how every evil has come into the world through fire" (Just 1903, 175). He painted a vivid picture of the advantages women would gain if they renounced the pernicious custom of cooking.

> Women need no longer ruin their health before the cooking stove, the source of poisonous vapors, where they acquire their many troubles and diseases; they will gain time for nobler occupations, can devote themselves more to their children and spend more time in God's beautiful, free nature; they need no longer prepare those viands, which for themselves as for their families are the cause of all diseases, and indeed of all unhappiness in the world. All members of the family will soon have a finer taste, be able to enjoy their food better, and will gain rare vigor and joy of life (Just 1903, 177).

Just's role as a pioneer of the raw food diet was recognized by Max Bircher-Benner, M.D. (1867-1939), the great Swiss food doctor, who gave the diet a scientific basis and proved its benefits on thousands of patients in his famous sanitarium in Zurich. Bircher-Benner wrote in the preface to the 12th German edition of *Return to Nature!*:

> We wish especially that medical students and young physicians take its content to heart. A fresh wind of renewal in health care is blowing from it. The man who wrote it did not learn this therapy but experienced it himself (Rudolf Just 1934, 104).

Mikkel Hindhede, M.D. (1862-1945), the great Danish nutrition reformer, commented along similar lines. "I am not completely in agreement with his theories," he wrote, "but I cannot refrain from admiring a man who found the truth about nutrition half a century earlier than the physicians" (Rudolf Just 1934, 99).

Just also believed strongly in the benefits of fasting, especially the morning fast. His patients "never experienced such unmistakable good results from the treatment as when they fasted until noon" (Just 1903, 181). But he advised against "any harshness or asceticism . . . . Everyone should try fasting and practice it according to his own knowledge and with entire free will." He also stressed fasting's ability to "awaken the full spiritual power of the man" (Just 1912, 112-113).

Just himself was deeply religious. One Jungborn building was a chapel. Its bell called the patients daily to morning prayers. He also gave two lectures each week and was a persuasive, charismatic speaker who made a lasting impression on his patients. One recorded some of his more memorable maxims.

> "Only God can cure."
>
> "First a person has to become healthy inside, then outside."
>
> "Everyone who wants health must turn to Nature. God is so close and so is a handful of earth, the water, the air and the sun."
>
> "Why are you so ill? Because you are too smart!"
>
> "Don't look at your bodily sores, at the ailments of your old age; look at God! Does not the old eagle fly through the air like the young one? Because he did not fall from Nature, but stayed with God's laws!" (R. Just 1934, 78-79).

Just's strongest criticism of the old nature cure method was its neglect of the spiritual dimension.

> It knows nothing of the wonderful curative effects achieved through soul influences, especially by fellow-feeling and love, that is cherished in the heart, and by true trust in God . . . . For this reason it is entirely powerless in many diseases (Just 1903, 234).

His favorite maxim was: "Every physician must also be a priest and every priest must also be a physician" (Just, R. 1934, 94). Just was the first nature doctor who considered the patient's spiritual care equally as important as physical care. Some of the astonishing cures reported in his book probably resulted both from the complete change of lifestyle at the Jungborn and the new outlook on life Just gave his patients.

Adolf Just managed the Jungborn for 12 years. In 1903, he married one of his patients, the daughter of an old farming family. She was devout, kindhearted and intelligent, and a great support. They had five children.

In 1906 the success of the Jungborn was at its height. There was not enough room to accommodate the influx of patients from Germany and other countries. His success caused an envious local physician to initiate a lawsuit against Just for using earth as a remedy. In defense Just declared:

> In this case I feel completely acquitted before God and repeat that I take full responsibility for my ideas. Twenty years from now, others might be condemned because they treated wounds without using clay (R. Just 1934, 72).

This lawsuit resulted in punishment for negligent bodily injury, and depressed Just so much he gave back the government concession granted for his establishment. He gave up the management of the Jungborn in 1908 and transferred it to his younger, more robust brother Rudolf, who ran it until he died in May, 1948.

Since Jungborn operated without a physician, the government urged Just to employ a physician as the number of patients increased. However, the Brunswick medical board passed a special resolution in 1904 prohibiting doctors from working with the "charlatan Just" (R. Just 1934, 71). After Rudolf took over, he assigned the medical direction to a certified doctor cured of a serious ailment while a Jungborn patient, who became the protector of the institution.

The Rudolf Just Jungborn Export House, started nearby in Stapelburg/Hartz in 1903 at Adolf's suggestion, was one of the first "reform houses," the German equivalent of a health food stores. It supplied everything necessary for the Jungborn natural life style, such "Adolf Just nutbutter," tropical fruits, vegetable coffee, porous bedding, linen underwear, air shoes and tubs for the natural bath. A small publishing house produced Adolf and Rudolf Just's publications as part of the thriving enterprise.

Adolf Just retired to the little town of Blankenburg/Hartz for reasons which reaffirmed his life-long concerns for natural health. He described it as a "lovely idyll" and "an El Dorado for the cultivation of fruit," and noted that it was "almost alone among the towns of Germany in having not a single factory" (Just 1912, 451-452). He purchased a piece of land to accommodate his new passion, experimenting with a natural fruit-culture method developed by the American Henry Martyn Stringfellow and perfected by the German Rudolf Richter.

Ten years later, after meeting the challenge of confiscation of his book in 1918, he devoted his full energy to the development of the healing agent he considered superior to all others, the earth. He established a successful family company for the preparation and distribution of the Hartz mountain Luvos healing clay which is still available from the "Healing Earth Company Luvos Just Ltd." in Friedrichsdorf today.

When his wife died in 1925, Adolf Just withdrew to a secluded private life in the beautiful tranquillity of Lake Starnberg, near Munich. He was cared for by his two daughters. He died January 20, 1936, "delivered from the plights of his earthly existence and the struggles of his tormented soul at the age of 77 years" (Brauchle 1951, 299).

Rudolf Just's description of his brother as a grateful, kindhearted man with a good sense of humor and cheerful outlook contradicts Brauchle's gloomy image of the "tormented soul:"

> He especially loved to tell funny stories from his life, and he had an enviable memory. I was the eleventh child of the family. He was 19 years older and my godfather. Since my father did not have the means to send me to high school, Adolf did it and became my mentor. He liked to give, and he helped his brothers and sisters by taking some of them in and employing them for his cause. After our father's death, he renounced his share of the inheritance.
>
> Every year during Christmas he asked for the names of the poorest people of Stapelburg and Ilsenburg and invited 60 to 80 poor mothers and their children to the Jungborn. Christmas carols were sung and they were treated with Jungborn-coffee and cake and presented with toys and useful gifts under the Christmas tree (Rudolf Just 1934, 73).

Brauchle's conclusion that Just suffered from episodes of psychosis with religious hallucinations might be exaggerated. Rudolf Just makes no mention of this. However, elements of fanaticism and obsessiveness can be detected in his writings. G. Hildebrand cites one example, Just's strange elevation of the Luvos healing clay into an almost divine substance. At first, the earth was nature's true remedy. Then Luvos became "the fulfillment of all his dreams and wishes," and the Luvos Healing Earth Company took on a "holy task and stood under the protection of God." Later he announced that the discovery of Luvos was divinely inspired. "I believe a soul called from the depth and was heard and answered by God." At the same time he indignantly condemned the "normal clay" and "all those who try to make money with it" (Hildebrand 1936, 75).

Adolf Just was the most radical and uncompromising naturist among the nature doctors. He deduced his system as much from philosophical speculations about nature as from practical experience. Brauchle forgave Just's rejection of all other healing systems "since his experiences were not extensive enough that he could judge everything in the right light."

> Just's success proves how intense the yearning of the people was to be saved from their physical and spiritual ills by a return to nature. In his Jungborn, Just created the outline of a paradisiac life which became a model for other nature cure establishments and which promised the poor exhausted big city dweller a true renewal of his energies (Brauchle 1951, 302).

Just himself considered the Jungborn "a model institution for the true natural life, where those who wish to make arrangement for such a life at home in their own gardens can find the pattern" (Just 1903, 9). Indeed, the Jungborn had many imitators all over the world, even in Australia, as this letter shows.

> Dear Mr. Just, Your book *Return to Nature !* was brought to my notice by some of my friends, and I am obliged to admit that at first I laughed at it. But I tried to test your ideas on patients in my institution, and I was astonished at their success. In my wooded park, thirty acres in extent, I have set up nature-beds, suitable to our warm climate. These are boxes a foot high, filled with earth and strewn with a soft kind of grass. These beds are made every day by watering the grass, and the patients assure me that they sleep as if they were in Paradise . . . . H. Letlang, M.D. (Just 1912, 77-78).

Just also warned against "the many disastrous and, I regret to say, dishonest imitations of Jungborn . . . . Our object is not to keep on founding institutions, but to make institutions superfluous" (Just 1912, 455). Many new establishments concealed their debt to Just's ideas. Honorable exceptions were Benedict Lust's and Emanuel Felke's Jungborns. A sign at the entrance of Felke's Jungborn read "System Adolf Just." In 1908, Felke wrote to Just, "I recommend your institution as *mater* and also as *optima omnium,* i. e. as the mother and also the best of all" (R. Just 1934, 96).

The physician Friedrich Wolf (1888-1953), a socialistic playwright, wrote a book, *Nature as Physician and Helper,* a nature cure compendium for the common man. He called for the establishments of nature cure parks for the lower classes patterned exactly after Just's Jungborn. In his manifesto "Create Nature Cure Parks!" he wrote:

> Mere prescriptions during out-patient care are not enough . . . . The body as a whole must be retuned during a nature

> cure. . . .It is something different to swallow a pill than to spend a night in an air hut and then to take a cool friction sitz bath in the early morning. The Jungborn physician himself must participate here! His example makes it easier! Such a Jungborn is not a cure-all automat, but a school for health training! (Wolf 1929, 589).

In an obituary of Just, Benedict Lust paid tribute to the man who inspired him to found the American Yungborn:

> Adolf Just really leaves us as a great teacher, a great humanitarian and a great example to follow. Whoever reads his book is carried away by its simplicity, sincerity as well as his love for his work. His soul speaks through every line. He was the first man to institute the sun and air cure on a big scale, advocating nude living while taking the Nature Cure with a natural diet (raw food diet); the use of sun, clay, water, human magnetism and true spirituality (Lust 1936, 69)

Just's most important contributions to naturopathy were his insistence on a raw foods diet, the development of earth therapy, the emphasis on spirituality and individual responsibility, the establishment of a model natural health retreat and the radical purity of his naturist philosophy. Modern naturopathic medicine might not agree with Just's wholesale condemnation of Science, Medicine, and Civilization, but it must acknowledge the prophetic truth of the following statement written by Just almost 90 years ago:

> Man has attacked nature the most by destroying and cutting down the woods; he has caused conditions, and especially dangerous climatic and aerial changes, which are today very detrimental to man and to beast. Many a country has by it become entirely inhospitable for man.
>
> The sick who has arrived at the end of all human perversities and errors must go again back to the woods. For in the woods alone he can regain his health, in the magic enchantment of the woods, in the rustling music of the forest, under the green shady canopy of the trees, through which the sun is lurking, to the frolicsome chirping of the birds his feeble pulses beat with greater vigor and the grave fetters of his sickness are more easily dissolved (Just 1910, 716).

The Clay (or Loam) Pastor and His "Jungborn"

Emanuel Felke

(1856-1926)

The spirit of the Jungborn as a natural health retreat is still alive, thanks to Pastor Erdmann Leopold Emanuel Felke. Thousands of patients visit Sobernheim/Nahe and Diez/Lahn in Germany each year, regaining health through the use of Felke's light-and-air parks, air huts, loam baths, friction sitz bath and special diets, offered in modern sanitarium facilities.

Felke became famous as the "Kneipp of Repelen," the little town where he established his first Jungborn. Like Kneipp, he was a clergyman who reluctantly became a nature doctor after his special gifts as a healer attracted many desperate patients. He was a good-hearted, folksy character, with kind, confidence-inspiring eyes. Also like Kneipp, he had a good sense of humor but did not mince words. Unlike Kneipp and other nature doctors, Felke was converted to nature cure through his success in treating members of his congregation during epidemics rather than through the experience of his own illness. His fame never reached the worldwide proportions of Kneipp's as he never wrote anything about his work. Like Priessnitz and Schroth, Felke was a practitioner but not a writer or teacher. We know about his methods only through his students and followers.

Felke was born in Kläden near Stendal/Altmark, February 7, 1856. His father was the rector of a training college for teachers. Magdalena Madaus (1857-1925), who had an honorary doctorate from Lust's American School of Naturopathy of New York, was also from Kläden. Her husband, a Lutheran pastor, was a colleague of Felke's, and their families maintained friendly relations. Udo Madaus, one of her grand-children, (and current vice-chairman of Madaus Ltd., a leading German producer of herbal drugs), tells the story about how this woman, after raising seven children, became a naturopathic practitioner:

> Her son Hans contracted polio when he was three or four years old. The physicians wanted to amputate a leg which was completely paralyzed. Since his mother Magdalena was a very resolute woman, she took the matter in her own hands and went

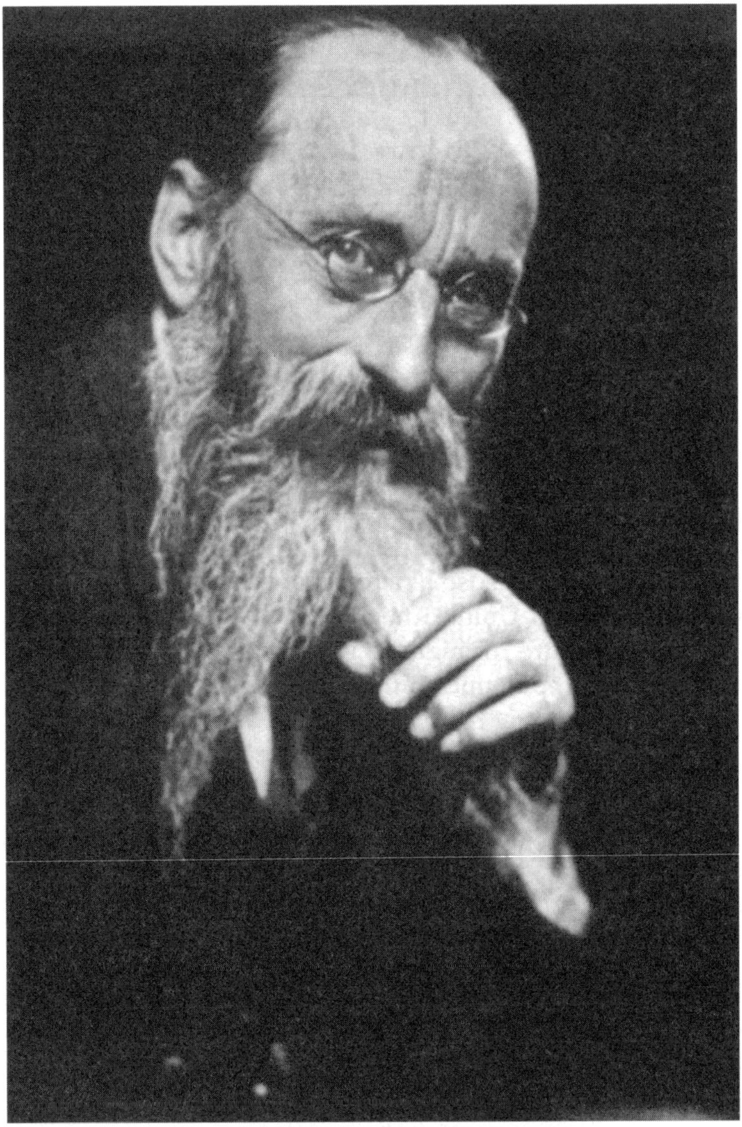

Emanuel Felke
(Schlau 1963, Frontispiece)

> to Pastor Felke. He treated Hans so well with massage, loam packs and gymnastics that the boy could walk again, which he was not able to do before as his brothers always had to pull him in a little wagon. Hans even did military service in World War I.
>
> After this success of Pastor Felke, Magdalena Madaus decided to become a naturopathic practitioner herself. She was Pastor Felke's apprentice for some time and later opened up her own practice—with great success. A large number of the so-called combination remedies date from the time before World War I when she had them compounded by a pharmacist in Barmen-Rittershausen. After the war her sons decided to take over the production of these remedies themselves. In 1919 the firm Dr. Madaus & Co. was founded in Bonn. It still produces the homeopathic combination remedies, now called oligoplexes. Magdalena Madaus also had a deep interest in iris diagnosis [which she had learned from Felke] and wrote a book about it (Madaus 1991).

Felke's father treated the illnesses in his family of nine children with simple homeopathic remedies and herbal teas, which made a strong impression on young Felke. Early in life he showed an intense interest in plants, especially in those used for healing. He also watched farmers treat injured domestic animals with loam poultices.

After attending gymnasium (high school) in Stendal, he complied with the fervent wish of his mother, daughter of a pastor, to study theology at the University of Berlin. However, he was more enthusiastic about lectures on medicine and science than theology. This conflict between theology and medicine would be characteristic of his life. "He wanted to assist the parishioners not only in their spiritual plight, but also in their physical distress" (Schicke 1985, 5). After passing the theological examination at the University of Münster, he became vicar in several parishes and gained a reputation as a captivating preacher and a caring pastor.

Felke gained a reputation as a healer for the first time in Cronenberg near Wuppertal. During a severe diphtheria epidemic in 1894, his congregation came to him for help, and he gave the sick children of the parish the homeopathic remedy, *Mercurius cyanatus*, with the result that none of the children died. In the neighboring villages, many succumbed to the disease. Others in his congregation who were sick, followed by people from villages near and far, sought his medical advice. Soon, he was unable to devote himself to his favorite endeavor, the scientific theological exegesis of the Bible. The only work he ever published was not about his healing methods but on the Song of Solomon and the Twenty-Seventh Psalm. As it was in his nature to help others, he could not refuse any who sought his healing skills though the church authorities took offence at the pastor's "quackery" and urged him to stop treating the sick.

At this point Felke decided to make a new start. In 1894, he accepted the position of pastor in Repelen near Krefeld (Lower Rhine Valley). He wanted to be nothing but a priest, but his reputation as a diagnostician and therapist followed him, and soon the sick besieged the parsonage. Felke never charged anything for his treatments, but it was the prospect of health, not the lack of a fee, which attracted so many patients. Success increased his interest in nature cure, and he began to study the treatment methods of Priessnitz, Kneipp, Rikli, Kuhne and Just. He was also influenced by the great nature curists and nutritionists Ragnar Berg, Max Bircher-Benner and Heinrich Lahmann. He sought to detect diseases and their causes in the earliest stages and became a master of facial and iris diagnosis. The originator of iridology, the Hungarian physician and homeopath, Ignatz von Peczely (1826-1911), published his only book, *Discoveries in the Realms of Nature and Art of Healing,* in 1873. The German translation of this book appeared in 1880 and reached Felke through a friend. The only written document left by Felke is the topographical drawing of an iris. Benedict Lust credited Felke with developing iris diagnosis "to the point of almost mathematical exactness" (Lust 1928, 44).

Felke realized that prescribing herbal teas, homeopathic remedies, diet and water applications was not sufficient. Inspired by the examples of Rikli and Just, he envisioned a therapeutic setting close to nature where patients could escape their accustomed environments and enjoy the benefits of light, air, sun and healthful food. Surprisingly, the residents of the small rural town of Repelen immediately warmed to their new pastor's idea. A delegation undertook the arduous and costly journey to the Hartz mountains to inspect Just's Jungborn. This visit resulted in the formation of the Repelen Jungborn Society, Ltd., with eighty-one associates, mostly members of a local homeopathic lay society. With a capital of 50,000 goldmark, quite a high sum, the group purchased sixty acres of land, which included a forested area and a dead channel of the Rhine abounding in fish. Two large light and air parks, one for women and the other for men, were created and surrounded with high wooden fences. Naked patients took light, air, water and loam baths and engaged in gymnastics twice a day. Felke himself often directed the male patients. Inside the two parks approximately 50 air huts with two or four rooms each were erected. To guarantee maximum access to fresh air they had no doors or windows, only curtains for privacy. An open wooden hall in the center of the park was used for walking during the day, for gymnastics during bad weather and for sleeping on straw mats at night. In the beginning the spa offered friction sitz baths in flat zinc tubs as the only cold water application. Felke also took up Just's earth-and-sand bath, but it was not until he introduced the loam bath in 1912 that he gained fame as the "loam pastor."

Even before the Repelen Jungborn was established, the number of patients seeing Felke had continually increased. He was visited by forty or fifty patients every day. When his Jungborn was completed, as many as 400 patients stayed in the park at peak times, though it also went through some difficult times. The police closed it numerous times at the request of the government in Düsseldorf on grounds of "endangering the morals."

The medical profession caused Felke even more problems, bringing sixteen lawsuits alleging quackery against him. In the most publicized case, the Great Felke-Process in Krefeld at the end of October,1909, twenty-four physicians appeared as expert witnesses for and against iris diagnosis:

> Twenty patients, unknown to Felke and completely wrapped up so that one could not tell whether they were male or female, were presented to Felke with the requirement that no questions were permitted.
>
> Among them was a patient with completely healthy feet who was seated in a wheel-chair to puzzle Felke! From the protocol:
>
> **Felke:** "Catarrh of the bronchi, lung problem. *Clinical diagnosis*: Pleurisy.
>
> **Felke:** " Tuberculosis of the left lung. *Clinical diagnosis*: Pulmonary tuberculosis.
>
> **Felke:** "Both kidneys are sick." *Clinical diagnosis:* Pyelitis.
>
> **Felke:** "Abdominal pain." *Clinical diagnosis:* Cancer of the uterus.
>
> **Felke:** "Leg area strongly marked." *Clinical diagnosis:* Complicated fracture of the lower leg.
>
> Of course, the press commented at length about the result of this process. They talked about the four wrong diagnoses, but they forgot to report that a multiple rib fracture diagnosed by Felke in one patient was only detected four weeks later! It should be remembered that Felke did not lose a single one of these processes nor was he ever condemned (Theegarten 1986, 15).

Instead of harming him, these legal proceedings enhanced Felke's reputation, as many of his patients testified in court on his behalf. News of his successes reached an even larger portion of the population. Despite its simple and improvised set-up, Repelen's Jungborn rapidly grew into a famous health center with a large influx of patients, many from abroad. In 1912, Felke felt compelled to give up his honorable office and pension as a pastor for the less respected job of a nature cure practitioner. He wearied of the unceasing attacks from church authorities against his work as a healer. In 1913, he built a larger and more attractive "cure house" with dining hall, kitchen and treatment rooms. Another impressive building housed the administration and the office of a physician who became medical director, as was decreed by the government. From then on, each patient had to be examined by the physician before beginning his "cure."

The outbreak of World War I in August, 1914, put a sudden end to the activities in Repelen. All patients left immediately, and the Jungborn turned into a military hospital, no longer accessible to civilian patients. Felke reestablished himself in Sobernheim/Nahe, where he moved in 1915 at the invitation of Andres Dhonau, a former patient. Dhonau, an enterprising butcher, cured of gout at Repelen in 1902, built a Felke-Jungborn in 1907 which rapidly grew into a successful establishment. With its marvelous Victorian "Kurhaus," it is today the oldest and most beautiful of the three large Felke sanitariums in Sobernheim, a small idyllic town in a wine-growing area of the Rhine. Felke found not only better climatic conditions than in Repelen, but also good soil for loam. It was an ideal place for the light-air and loam baths of the Jungborn cure.

Felke brought this previously unknown treatment into the limelight. The patients who arrived to undergo the Felke-Jungborn cure could hardly be accommodated in the hotels, private guest homes and cure-establishments. They slept on straw mattresses in wooden air-huts and enthusiastically followed the instructions of Pastor Felke who supervised the treatments with strict authority, tempered by benevolence and humor. One of Felke's patients described her first impression of him as follows:

> A clear blue September sky arched over the small house where Pastor Felke leaned out the window to greet me and press my hand. The impression which this powerful broad-shouldered figure made on me was so striking that I will never forget it. The broad forehead with its wonderful curvature over the temples was covered by a velvet cap which together with a long pipe gave his entire figure a cozy intimacy. And those lively eyes, which could look so deeply serious, yet so cheerful and mischievous, taught us that the heart beating in this unique man was feeling everything with us. The long, well-kept beard and the soft but firm hand resulted in an impression of paternal strength and maternal kindness . . . . Everyone who came to him left consoled; the vexed, careworn faces of workers brightened after his first kind words; the tense expression of suffering in the faces of the physically or psychically ill women disappeared after they sat in the room for a while. Even before he spoke, his magnetic radiation

> had such a soothing effect that it alone was sufficient to calm the overexcited nerves (Finger 1927, 18).

A good-humored, informal style pervaded the first floor of the "Hotel Schuler" (now Saarhotel) where Felke did consultations. Patients waited in the large dining-room. Felke could only handle the enormous crowd by calling in four patients at a time. He was in such demand that patients had to make appointments months in advance. Differences of rank were irrelevant to him.

> One day a lady of the imperial court came to him; as to everyone, he said to her: "Sit down on this chair!" The lady remarked with great indignation that she was a countess and a lady of the imperial court. "Well, then sit down on two chairs!" was Felke's answer which brought a smile to the face of everyone present (Brauchle 1951, 303-304).

Thanks to his skill in facial analysis and iris diagnosis Felke was able to assess the condition of a patient in a few minutes. He believed the findings in the iris revealed to him the condition of the patient's blood, and that he could identify the presence of mercury, quinine, iodine, opium, morphine and other drugs from the discolorations in the lacunae of the iris.

Felke's view of disease was similar to that of other nature doctors of his time, that blockages in the eliminative organs—skin, lungs, kidneys and intestines caused an accumulation of harmful substances. These blockages developed due to faulty nutrition, poisonous drugs, unhygienic living conditions, bad habits and hereditary taints. Andres Müller, Felke's assistant in Repelen, formulated his master's views.

> Since blood nourishes our body and permeates it to its most distant parts, it deposits either healthy or diseased substances according to its composition. Every chronic ailment is a disease of the total person, never only of a single organ. Thus the total illness must be approached with a total treatment, especially with respect to such natural factors as light, air, earth, water, diet and gymnastics (Müller 1904, 123-124).

According to Müller, Felke like other nature doctors aimed his therapies at producing a healing crisis, especially in chronic diseases.

> This may take place in such a stormy way that the healing power attacks the disease like a wild beast. When the healing crisis strikes, the cure should not be interrupted but rather vigorously pursued. During the healing crisis the entire body is affected, which proves that the entire body was diseased. However, the

> healing crisis does not have to tell us this first: Iris and facial diagnosis reveal it to us much earlier (Müller 1904, 124-125).

Without these diagnostic skills Felke could have never seen such massive numbers of patients. Only after analyzing the iris did he ask questions about the patient's complaints. Then he dictated to an assistant his prescriptions for various homeopathic remedies, herbal teas, loam and water applications and dietary changes.

His contemporaries described Felke as a modest man, and this is supported by one of the few quotations that we have from him: "If someone claims to know and to be able to do everything, then he is a conceited boaster. This is especially true in the field of diagnostics and therapy" (cited in Schicke 1985, 5). He treated all clergymen, all teachers, all independent artists, all the people of Sobernheim and all those who looked like they were poor for free. In some cases he even paid for their prescriptions and travel fare. His kindness, genuine joy of life, deep trust in God and intuitive link with nature played a considerable role in his success as a healer.

Felke is one of the few European nature cure doctors who visited America. A rich American named Henry Clay sent for Felke, having heard many good things about him and hoping for a cure. Felke undertook the journey and restored Clay's health. Deeply thankful, Clay asked Felke to stay, promising to build a hospital and church for him and to see that Felke's methods were taught at the university. Felke, however, was attached to his native country and declined the offer, returning home where "he was attacked as a quack, humiliated and dragged through the courts" (Brauchle 1951, 303).

The number of patients who consulted Felke has been estimated at nearly half a million. Despite his enormous popularity and the entire industry of reform articles that grew up around him—Felke underwear, Felke tooth paste, Felke mouthwash, Felke bathtubs, Felke loam, Felke coffee and Felke's homeopathic remedy kit, he never became rich. In fact, an irreparable breech between Felke and his former protégé, Andres Dhonau, occurred because of a new "cure house" which Dhonau completed in 1922. With its luxurious dining hall, reception rooms, kitchen and offices, it was too sumptuous and removed from nature for Felke. Ever modest, idealistic and perhaps without business acumen, Felke regarded the new building as an affront to his principles of "return to a simple and natural life." He practiced at other Jungborns, founded by former patients in Sobernheim and Diez/Lahn. He also visited his first Jungborn, in Repelen, every two weeks, after it was resurrected in 1924.

When Felke died on August 16, 1926 from a stomach ailment, he was as poor as a church-mouse:

> The life thread of the man who mastered every disease was cut off by an accidental blow to his stomach which caused such internal injuries that the seed of death was planted. Ignoring all his own pain and discomforts, his only thought was to use what was left of his life to help others (Finger 1927, 19).

His death was a hard blow for all Felke-Jungborns, because he had not arranged for a successor. The spa physicians in Sobernheim, familiar with the Felke Cure, continued his work there. In Repelen, his work was carried on by his son, a professor of medicine at the University of Rostock, with less success. The number of patients steadily declined. The mining industry drove the last patients away with its air pollution and its destruction of the idyllic landscape. The area where the former Jungborn once flourished was turned into a town park and named "Felke-Park."

Felke received numerous honorary tributes. Pope Pius X sent the Lutheran pastor his picture and gave a blessing as a sign of his gratitude for Felke's successful treatment of so many Catholics from all over the world. The town of Sobernheim, which Felke put on the map, organized a "royal" funeral for its honorary citizen. It placed a huge boulder from the nearby Soonwoods over his grave and decorated it with a plaque inscribed with his motto: "Despite of everything I will prevail!" (Menschel 1975, 9-10)

A facsimile of the old *House Rules,* in the prospectus of the Felke Curehouse Menschel, gives a good indication of what a health-seeker could expect while undergoing a Felke Cure.

6:30	Awakening at the sound of the gong
6:40	Felke sitz bath and early morning exercises in the air parks
7:00	Group gymnastics in the gymnasium
7:30	Herbal tea drinking together
8:00-9:00	Breakfast
9:00-12:30	Cure applications: Herbal baths, massages, packs, etc.
10:00-12:30	Loam and air baths in the air parks
12:30	Lunch—On Sundays and holidays at 12:00
13:30-15:00	After-dinner rest. During this time it is neither permitted to speak in the houses nor in the parks
15:00-18:00	Loam and air baths, cure applications
18:00	Dinner
22:00	Night's rest

Today the Felke cure program at the same establishment is less strict and more individualized. Felke sanitariums also offer month-long Felke Fasting Cures with herbal teas, freshly pressed juices and vegetable broth for cleansing, regeneration and weight loss. The therapeutic effects of the fasts are enhanced by the air-sun, water and loam baths, gymnastics, massages, manual lymph drainage, colonic irrigations, saunas, biological cosmetics, etc. Felke advocated a diet rich in raw fruits and vegetables. Patients suffering from cancer, intestinal problems, eczema and venereal diseases were fed only fruits, berries and nuts. Gravy was completely prohibited because of its uric acid content, which Felke considered a main cause for nervous irritation. For the healthy, he recommended a mixed lactovegetarian diet with occasional meat. He preferred raw milk and regarded cooked milk as "dead." When a woman asked him why he used this term, he replied, "Would you still be alive if you were cooked?" (Finger 1927, 17). Even for the healthy he recommended a fruit-only diet for fourteen days every three months, and fasting one day a month. He forbade salt, sugar, luxury food and condiments, but allowed the moderate drinking of beer and wine, which he considered beneficial. This enhanced his success in the joyous wine region of Sobernheim.

Felke gained fame for his loam bath and loam compresses which were a considerable improvement on Just's rather crude earth bath and earth compresses. They earned him the nickname "loam-pastor" (*Lehmpastor*) and "earth man" (*Erdmann*), "at first in derision by his traducers, but as the truly humanitarian character of the man and the greatness of his work became recognized more and more, the nickname became a badge of honor" (Lust 1928, 44). Felke was drawn to the loam bath, because it was so compatible with his theological thinking.

> We cannot proceed radically enough with the use of earth magnetism. The earth is the element closest to man, indeed, man consists of earth! The Lord says . . . "in the sweat of your face you shall toil until you return to earth, for out of it were you taken; you are earth and to earth shall you return." (Genesis 3:19).
>
> The more a person comes into intimate contact with the earth, the more he will have a share of that power which we call earth magnetism. This is the sum of the earth forces which influence the organic products of nature. When a person comes into contact with the earth, interchanges take place between the body and the earth. The latter draws diseased matter from the body and gives healthy matter back in return (cited in Schicke 1985, 6).

For the loam bath, low trenches, 120 cm long, 60 cm wide and 40-50 cm deep, were filled with loam, freshly dug and stirred into a mash with water. At Felke's time, the patients had to dig their own baths. Today, every patient is assigned his own bath for the duration of his stay and takes the bath for 30-45 minutes once or twice a day. The loam bath is a half bath. The patient spreads the loam mash upwards to the lower ribs. After the bath the patient roughly wipes the loam off and the remaining mud dries on the skin. During the ensuing gymnastics it generates a strong absorptive pressure. After the exercises the patient rubs off the remaining powder-like loam with self-massage, achieving an additional increase of blood supply to the skin, tissues and organs. Such a procedure could be quite a cheerful event when fifteen or twenty patients were sitting together taking morning loam baths. Originally the loam bath was taken in the open air. The bath's duration was adapted to the temperature and the patient's constitution. In modern Felke sanitariums the loam baths can also be carried out in floor-heated halls, independent of the weather.

It was not just the perfection of the earth cure that distinguished Felke from the other great European nature doctors, but also that he didn't limit himself to the classic nature cure of water, light, air, and diet. Like Lust and Lindlahr in America, he used electricity, massage, gymnastics, magnetism, hypnotism, herbal teas and homeopathic remedies. Homeopathy especially played an important role. At first he used it according to Hahnemann's strict principle of prescribing the single most similar remedy. However, he was disappointed with the results of single remedies in the treatment of chronic diseases. He concluded that a complex disease, which had evolved over years with layers of symptoms, had to be treated in a complex way.

> Instead of administering single remedies over a long period, he thought it better to prescribe a combination of different, carefully composed single remedies. Felke became, so to speak, the inventor of the combination remedies which are being offered in great numbers by many companies today (Schicke 1985, 12).

The "Felke Original Complex" remedies (abbreviated: Fcpl.) are still manufactured by Prof. Dr. Mauch in Göppingen. Classical homeopaths might scorn them, but Felke was a non-dogmatic eclectic who always tried to find the most suitable treatment for his patients. His eclecticism and versatility bring him in close kinship with modern naturopathic physicians, and the 8,000 German *Heilpraktikers* (naturopathic practitioners) identify more closely with Felke than any other great nature doctors. *Heilpraktikers* can't look back to a forebear like Benedict Lust who brought the classic nature cure tradition of Priessnitz, Schroth, Kneipp and Just to the United States. In Germany, this tradition was taken up by medical doctors, who became the successors of Priessnitz, Schroth, Kneipp and even Felke. These doctors now equip their nature cure sanitariums with the most modern facilities and direct them according to scientific principles to ensure national health insurance

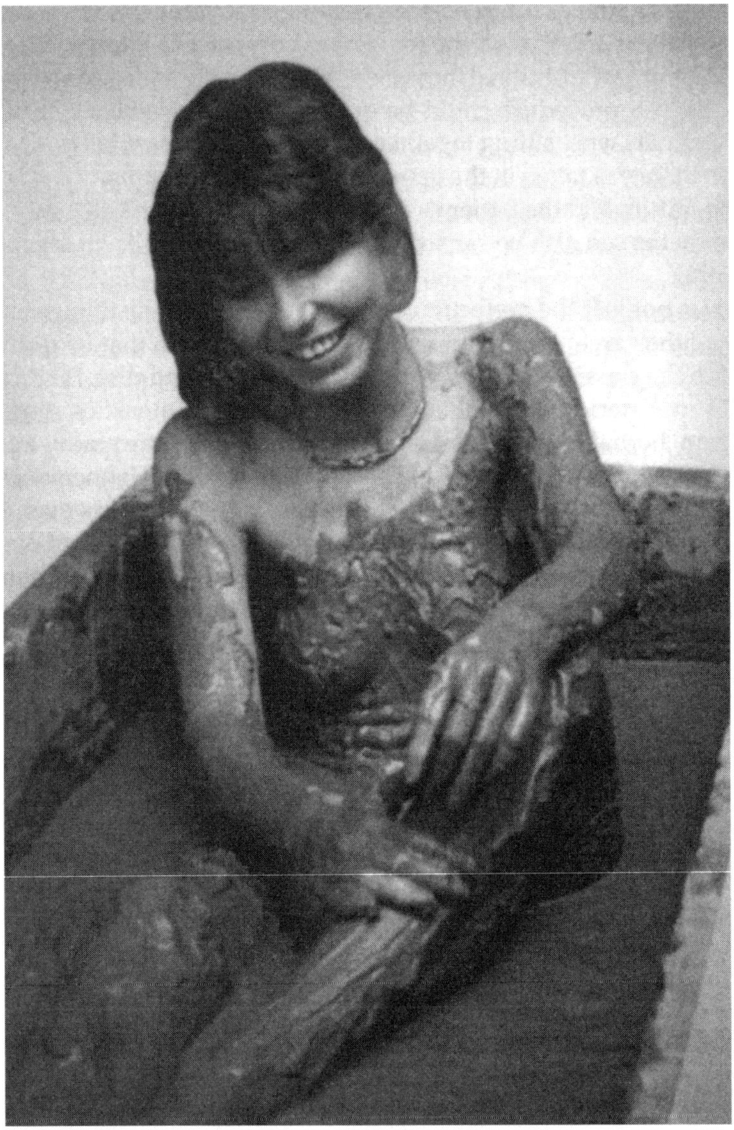

Loam Bath
(Prospectus Hotel Kurhaus am Maasberg, Sobernheim)

will pay for the patients' care. The German *Heipraktiker* is confined to a role as private alternative health practitioner.

Still it's heartening that Felke's legacy, like Schroth's and Kneipp's, is still alive. Besides the Felke Cure establishments in Sobernheim/Nahe and Diez/Lahn, a Felke Federation promotes his prescriptions for healthful living. A *Sobernheimer Kreis* or Sobernheim Circle, composed of *Heilpraktikers* and physicians, offers seminars on Felke's wholistic therapy. The Pastor Felke Institute for Iris Diagnosis and Wholistic Therapy in Heimsheim devotes itself to the training of qualified iridologists on a scientific basis. Finally, the Physicians' Study Group for Felke-Therapy, consisting of the directors of the Felke sanitariums, issues its own series of scientific publications about the effects of Felke Cure methods. Günther Schlau, the director of the Felke-Jungborn in Diez/Lahn wrote:

> The Felke Cure is not specifically directed towards a diseased organ or an isolated disturbance of bodily function, rather the body is put into a position, through the normalization of its regulatory system, to overcome the disease in its own individual way. We call this the strengthening of the nonspecific defense system or, in common language, the healing power of nature. (Schlau 1963, 15).

Schicke summarized Felke's creative achievement.

> Except for the loam baths, Felke did not invent the components of his wholistic therapy. His great accomplishment was to construct an ingenious edifice out of the different parts already in existence. The totality of all his measures and his powerful personality made it possible for him to be so immensely successful (Schicke 1985, 6).

Except for his loam therapies, Felke's approaches were duplicated by others in the United States, so he was of less consequence to the development of American naturopathy. But he deserves to be better known by the American naturopathic community, because he embodied its open-minded, eclectic approach more than any other great German nature doctor. He was a kindred spirit to Henry Lindlahr, with whom he shared a deep interest in iris diagnosis, homeopathy and the integration of other natural modalities.

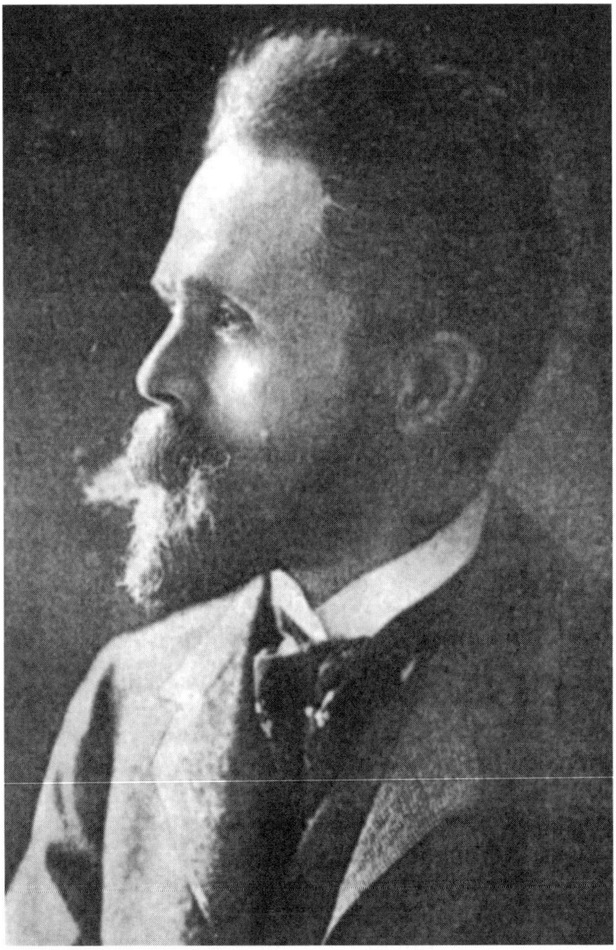

Heinrich Lahmann
(Brauchle 1933, 49)

The First Scientific Nature Doctor

Heinrich Lahmann

(1860-1905)

Heinrich Lahmann, "the first scientific nature doctor," is held in high esteem by lay nature doctors as well as medical doctors who specialize in natural therapeutics (Brauchle 1951, 228). Unlike other university-trained doctors who adopted nature cure, Lahmann never denied his indebtedness to the great lay healers such as Priessnitz, Rikli and Kneipp.

Heinrich Lahmann was born on March 30, 1860 in Bremen, a vital port city of northern Germany. His father was a hawser maker. When he was five years old, Lahmann suffered from laryngeal diphtheria which required a tracheotomy. From this time on he had a husky voice which gave the impression he was consumptive.

His parents were not wealthy, but rich relatives supported him through high school and college. He had a special talent for mechanical problems and started training as an engineer at the Technical University in Hanover. He found the courses on public health, building hygiene and sociology the most interesting so he switched to medicine after two years, first in Greifswald, then at the universities of Munich, Leipzig and finally Heidelberg where he obtained his doctor's degree in 1885. Benedict Lust wrote in his short sketch about Lahmann:

> When the University of Leipzig expelled H. Lahmann for spreading medical sedition among the students, it added a staunch advocate to Natural Healing. Dr. Lahmann finished his medical education in Switzerland and returned to Germany to refute in practice the false ideas of medical science (Lust 1918, 447).

Although Lahmann was outspoken, and such an occurrence is plausible, none of the German sources mentions this dramatic incident and it is not clear where Lust obtained this information.

Even as a student Lahmann's main interests were dietetics and disease prevention. Dissatisfied with the theories and results of scientific medicine, he delved deeply into the nature cure literature. He published articles on nutrition, adhered increasingly to a vegetarian diet and invented a plant milk which became so popular as a baby food that it was even imported by Benedict Lust. The display ad Lust ran in *The Naturopath* claimed that "Dr. Lahmann's Vegetable Milk" mixed with cow milk "is as palatable, as digestible, and as nutritive as mother's milk" (March 1905). He also offered other Lahmann products such as "Dr. Lahmann's Nutritive Salt Health Cocoa" and "Dr. Lahmanns Plant-Nutritive Salt-Extract" which "renders all foods more digestible by adding the parts lost in the preparation of the food." The chocolate factory of Hewel & Veithen in Cologne still manufactures "healthy" plant cocoa extract and chocolate bars according to Dr. Lahmann's original recipes with the slogan: "Eating chocolate without remorse and abdominal pain."

In 1885 Lahmann set up office as a general practitioner in Stuttgart, where he got involved in a controversy over the Jaeger system of dress reform then attracting many followers. The physician, Gustav Jaeger (1832-1917), had published several popular books recommending clothing from natural wool, without "poisonous dye," as a basic requirement for health. He himself had suffered from obesity, shortness of breath and colds for a long time.

> He finally found his salvation in the woolen clothing which became for him a basic element of any form of health care. It seemed to have helped him because he reached the 85th year in good health. Many followed his example (Rothschuh 1983, 123).

Although Lahmann was in favor of dress reform, he advised against the wearing of woolen underwear, "which excessively irritates the skin, and finally makes it flaccid" (Lahmann 1886, 98). He offered instead his own invention of the porous cotton underwear named after him.

In 1886, Von Zimmermann appointed Lahmann head of his nature cure institute in Chemnitz. Before taking up this new position, Lahmann went on a study tour to the most important nature cure establishments to learn the best methods and to determine the common denominator of these therapies which would yield a rational theory to explain them.

> Each one who practices the nature cure method uses it in a different way: one more complicated, one simpler; one fights a disease with low temperatures which another tries to master with higher temperatures, etc . . . It is impossible to point to the success of one method, in order to prove its absolute correctness, when the same success is achieved with a different method; if, for example, the different methods A, B and C all achieve the same

> goal, then this is proof that all three contain an unknown quantity X which guarantees that success; and that the rest of the procedure is redundant if not harmful. Our task in the future will be to find this quantity X; only then will we have a theory, only then a rational, scientific nature cure and only then the guarantee for the universal dissemination and continuation of a pure method (Lahmann 1886, 117).

Lahmann's scientifically trained mind brought a refreshing breeze of systematic thinking to the field of nature cure, previously chaotic with speculation on the reasons for the success of differing methods.

The Gräfenberg which Lahmann found on his study trip was no longer Priessnitz' Gräfenberg. He wrote:

> The conditions in Gräfenberg are not favorable because the Cure Commission is purely allopathic . . . .
>
> The explanation for all this is that great people usually have little sons. While Priessnitz' daughters became excellent women, the son inherited nothing from his father but his money which became an obstacle to his own development.
>
> When one examines the extensive library, many things appear in a different light and one becomes convinced that later authors, including Rausse and Hahn, wrote about Priessnitz without being sufficiently informed. Priessnitz constantly modified his system according to his experiences. He never proceeded, as he was often accused, in a stereotyped fashion.
>
> It is strange to be touched by the spirit of a man at the place where he was once active; by the spirit of a man who had the greatest influence on oneself—it is a feeling mixed with elevation, gratitude and enthusiasm (Lahmann 1886, 119-120).

Lahmann also visited the neighboring Lindewiese.

> Priessnitz followers often speak about Schroth with contempt and accuse him of ill motives; however, we as the representatives of the second generation, the representatives of the "combined" nature cure method, will not be distracted by questions of personalities but will stick to the facts, to the ideas. And we must admit in this respect, Schroth's idea is quite good. However, we understand it differently and modify Schroth's practice in exactly the same way that we change Priessnitz' while remaining truer to his original intentions than many of his fanatic followers (Lahmann 1886, 149).

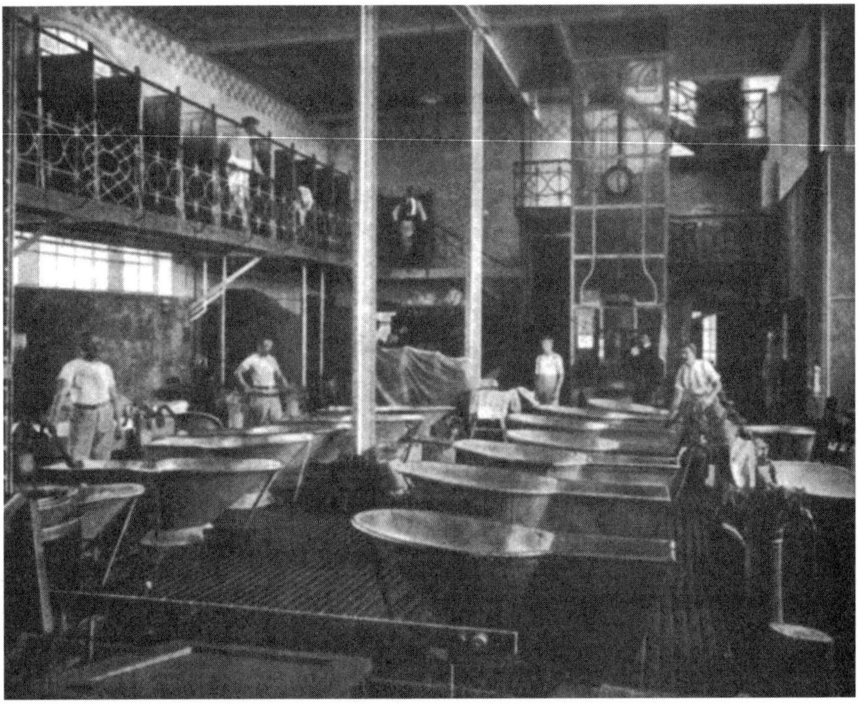

Inside view of the men's bath—Lahmann Sanatorium
(Prospectus of Dr. Lahmann's Sanatorium, Weisser Hirsch 1921/22
Archive of the Eden Foundation, Bad Soden)

In Veldes, Lahmann was deeply impressed by Rikli's light-and-air bath, later an essential part of his treatment program. He discussed its benefits in his book,*The Air Bath as a Curative and Hardening Agent* (1898), and quoted a letter by Benjamin Franklin, written to the French translator of his works in 1750:

> I rise very early each morning and remain sitting, without any clothes, for half or a full hour, according to the season, and read or write. This air bath is not unpleasant in the least, but on the contrary, pleasant; and when I crawl into bed again afterwards, as it sometimes happens, and I fall asleep for two hours, so to speak as a supplement to my night's rest, I enjoy a sleep which is the most peaceful imaginable. I cannot see any bad results from this custom and do not believe that it can harm my health, but on the contrary, it does much good (Brauchle 1951, 235-236).

Lahmann evaluated the dietary practices of several other nature cure establishments and concluded:

> The method of cooking is critical for the correct diet. As long as we leach out all vegetables, tubers, etc. in too much cooking water, we deprive them of their most important parts: the nutritive salts. It is the lack of nutritive salts which is responsible for deficient blood formation, deficient growth of bones, teeth and hair and for the nutritional disorders affecting the nervous system, etc. Further, the use of mild stimulants is necessary for many constitutions and the premature withdrawal of all stimulants downright harmful . . . . A rational diet is formulated in such a way that the fat one becomes thinner with it and the thin one stronger (Lahmann 1886, 164-165).

On a hiking tour Lahmann discovered the Weisser Hirsch (White Stag) near Dresden. He was taken by its beauty and its climatic advantages and decided to establish a sanatorium there according to his own principles. The site was a tiny village in the woods where people from Dresden, weary of city life, went for relaxation during the summer. The small spa hotel with the adjoining bath became successful only after Lahmann took it over, on January 1, 1888, and named it Dr. Lahmann's Sanatorium.

> The installments of the sanatorium were quite primitive in the beginning. The water supply functioned very poorly, and most of the time the bath water had to be brought in a hand-cart from the village well. However, Lahmann's personality soon attracted many patients. At the end of January, 1888, he had 20 patients, and in two more months he had to employ a medical assistant (Brauchle 1951, 229).

Lahmann gave public lectures on nature cure in Dresden to inform the public about his methods. His success was followed by bitter attacks from allopathic physicians, whom he answered in kind. Even homeopaths did not escape his criticism. He considered any artificial medicine a hindrance to nature's healing powers. But he accepted Schüssler's cell salts because they were similar to his own nutritive salts.

> The most advanced school of homeopathy . . . is the "Biochemic System" inaugurated by Schüssler which, like nature cure, regards nutritional deficiencies, especially the lack of certain mineral substances, as causes of most diseases . . . . Schüssler's ther-

> apy is the bridge which will hopefully lead homeopathy into the naturopathic camp (Lahmann 1885, 132-133).

Lahmann opened his sanatorium with two bathtubs and six attendants in 1888. In the same year he added three air huts. Additionally, he rented another house as the old spa hotel could no longer accommodate all his patients. In the fall of 1895 he established a biochemical laboratory to conduct scientific investigations into human metabolism and nutrition to establish a scientific basis for the nutritive salt preparations that he was marketing. This laboratory gained world-wide fame under the Swedish-born chemist, Ragnar Berg (1873- 1956), who headed it from 1909 to 1921. Berg's research focused on vitamins, trace elements and mineral metabolism, and he discovered the crucial importance of a low-protein, alkaline-rich diet as treatment for many conditions. He also suggested that the healthiest diet consisted primarily of potatoes, tubers, vegetables and fruits, preferably raw.

Lahmann's sanatorium never stopped growing. In 1900, it accommodated 2000 patients; in 1904, a year before his death, over 3500 patients received treatment there. By that time, twelve additional villas were attached to the sanatorium, and Lahmann headed a team of four senior physicians, three medical assistants and two auxiliary physicians.

After Lahmann's death the sanatorium continued to expand. The Prospectus and Annual Report of 1921/22 notes that over 5000 patients in 1908 and almost 7500 in 1913 visited to regain their health. In 1928 the sanatorium included 30 houses in addition to the main building and three estates supplying most of the fresh food for the special diets. It boasted a staff of 350 people. All patients were admitted except those suffering from hysteria, tuberculosis and acute infectious diseases and except "incurables, because our sanatorium is not a care institution, but a cure institution" (Prospectus, 9). A special birthing clinic, where young mothers could learn about dietetic care of their babies, was part of the sanatorium complex. Over a 40 years' period about 150,000 patients were guests at Lahmann's Sanatorium, among them such celebrities as the great poet Rainer Maria Rilke (1875-1926).

> Rilke married Clara Westhoff, a Protestant, in Bremen on April 28, 1901. They spent their honeymoon at the Weisser Hirsch, an exclusive sanatorium near Dresden and a most unusual place for newlyweds to stay. But in fact the groom was just recovering from scarlet fever, and at the time of the wedding he was "still very much a convalescent" . . . . Moreover, the Lahmann Method used at the sanatorium, which included therapeutic baths and a predominantly vegetarian diet, corresponded with his own ideas about healthy and natural living (Leppmann 1984, 136).

What is left of Dr. Lahmann's Sanatorium today? According to a newspaper reporter who visited Dresden-Bad Weisser Hirsch after Germany's reunification, the socialist regime had neglected the famous spa. He found it deserted and in decay. Only a few remnants of the famous sanatorium were visible behind a line of tall metallic palisades. The Red Army had turned it into a military hospital and ruined what had existed and otherwise been tended with loving care for almost 100 years (Hahn 1992, R 11). In May, 1992, these remnants were offered for sale at a price of 15 million German Marks.

Lahmann's death on June 1, 1905, at age 45, was due to overwork and exhaustion. He succumbed to a cardiac weakness which resulted from a neglected influenza. The nature cure world was shocked by his early death. A black-bordered obituary filling the front the page of Der Naturarzt read:

> Heinrich Lahmann was snatched from the world and the sick too early! Endowed with a weak constitution from his youth on, he was a victim of his restless productivity and phenomenal work load. It is simply and solely thanks to the strict practice of his hygienic teachings that this unique man even reached the age of 45 years in spite of his strenuous schedule. What the deceased has accomplished as a physician is demonstrated by the gratitude and unlimited love of his patients. Admirers from all levels of society, even from German princely houses, mourn at his grave. What Lahmann has achieved as a pioneer of science and as an advocate of nature cure can only be fully appreciated by later generations! (*Der Naturarzt* 33 (7) 1905,)

Another obituary noted that Lahmann's annual income was estimated to be 700,000 Marks, and that he left a fortune of 8 million Marks, bequeathing half of it for humanitarian and philanthropic causes (Schmidtbauer 1906, 126). His funeral made a deep impression.

> Lahmann was loved by all who really knew him . . . . I have never taken part in a funeral of a public figure where the sincerest mourning and love touched everyone's heart so deeply as during his funeral.
>
> The last wish of the deceased was not to be driven through the village to the graveyard but to be carried through the forest which he had loved so much. Accordingly, the solemn procession moved through the forest in its full spring-dress to the unique and beautiful location of the graveyard in silvan solitude, accompanied by the sounds of Chopin's funeral march and the loud warbling of thousands of feathered singers. Thus returned to

> nature what was mortal of Heinrich Lahmann (Ebert 1905, 304-305).

Despite his relatively short life Lahmann left a rich legacy of publications. In the polemical pamphlet, *Koch and the Kochians* (1890), he criticized Koch's overestimation of the role of bacteria as the cause of disease. In *Can Gynecologic Operations Be Prevented?* (1893) Lahmann advocated non-surgical treatments such as pelvic massage, gymnastics, sitz douches, alternating lavages, steam-applications and wet tampons for a variety of female disorders. His last publication,*The Disease-Producing Influence of Changes in Atmospheric Pressures* (1905), explored the negative impact of meteorological changes on nervous people. His two main works, *The Most Important Chapters of the Natural (Physical-Dietetic) Healing Method* and *The Dietetic Dysemia as the Fundamental Cause of All Diseases*, were published in 1890 and 1891 respectively. M. Schmidtbauer's claim that they "belong to the few immortal works of the healing arts for all time which will preserve their value in eternal youthfulness and truth" may be exaggerated (1905, 125). However, *Dietetic Dysemia* was translated into French and Russian and appeared in English under the title *Natural Hygiene or Healthy Blood* (1901). It was the first in a series of nutrition classics by Mikkel Hindhede, Robert McCarrisson, Max Bircher-Benner and Weston A. Price that established scientifically what had long been common knowledge for nature doctors, that poor dietary habits and denatured, adulterated foods contribute to degenerative diseases.

In *The Most Important Chapters of the Natural Healing Method*, a collection of articles from his early sanatorium years, he bitterly criticized the close-mindedness of official medicine towards other systems of healing.

> The behavior of orthodox medicine is wrong; it wants to be all-inclusive, yet it repels dissidents, thus causing deep splits among medical professionals as well as the public which slow the development of medicine . . . .
>
> Only the most independent-minded can prevail in such isolation and devote themselves to the ideas of reform . . . . It is not surprising, therefore, that the resulting void is filled by lay-healers . . . .
>
> These conflicts will not cease until orthodox medicine admits the free competition of divergent therapeutic systems by granting them a university department where they may either prove themselves or perish (Lahmann 1894, 3).

In this book Lahmann described his use of specific gravity as a simple measure for his patients' health condition. He determined the specific gravity by dividing the body weight by the volume of water displaced by the body. The specific gravity of a healthy person fluctuated between 1065 and 1072. Numbers below indicated adipose degeneration, higher numbers emaciation. A correct diet reduced a specific gravity which was too high and raised a specific gravity that was too low.

Lahmann had an astute diagnostic sense. The condition of the nails, skin, hair, eyes and teeth, the shape of the chest, the temperature of the hands as well as the odor of the body told him much about the diseases from which his patients suffered. He distinguished between alkaline and acid constitutions:

> Consumptives usually have good teeth and belong to the alkaline constitutions. The acid constitutions have bad teeth and are disposed to gout, diabetes, cancer, etc.
>
> Equipped with such knowledge, we can evaluate a person merely by looking at him as if he were made of glass. The sense-perception is sufficient for me in fifty of a hundred cases to know what is wrong with the patient; but I avoid passing judgment immediately to avoid gaining the reputation of a charlatan . . . . Certainly I would not like to do without the modern examination methods of percussion, auscultation, chemical and microscopic analysis, etc.; but I would not like to be a physician with only these methods. They are insufficient. There are countless persons who are not healthy; yet absolutely no findings of any illness can be detected on them with the common diagnostic methods (Lahmann 1894, 221-222).

It is interesting to note Lahmann's opinion about Louis Kuhne's face diagnosis:

> Some will say: But is there not the Master Kühne in Leipzig with his science of facial expression? Well, my answer is that he does not explain anything because his theories, lacking pertinent knowledge, are wrong. I concede that he developed the ability to detect certain diseases from the head and neck. But, as we have seen, that is not enough. I acknowledge that he achieves good results in numerous cases of disturbed metabolism or sluggish blood circulation, with sweat baths and friction sitz baths. But these cures don't make a wrong theory right . . . .
>
> A spark of truth is there; but the spark is smothered under nonsense; and there is no advantage for anyone; the least for the people as a whole. They can only be helped by teachings which

> have proven themselves in theory as well as in practice; for only what is theoretically correct, can we continue teaching (Lahmann 1894, 223-225).

In his second main work, *Natural Hygiene*, Lahmann contended that the principal cause of all disease was "dysemia," defined as "an imbalance of the food salts in the blood and especially a deficiency of those salts which are absolutely necessary to maintain us in good health" (Lahmann 1901, 28). Lahmann theorized how dysemia encouraged different diseases and how they could be prevented or cured by a diet rich in minerals from raw or sparingly cooked vegetable and fruits, but low in protein and without salt. Although Lahmann's nutritional theories, formulated when nutritional research on vitamins, minerals, enzymes and fibers was in its infancy, may have been replaced by scientific explanations, much dietary advice in his book is in accordance with modern naturopathic views. But he was not a fanatical purist.

> It is certainly good for the neurasthenic, and in fact for everybody, to deviate from his ordinary diet once every week or two; I even arrange for this in my sanatorium by giving stimulating dishes every now and then. This is not only harmless but even useful. The important point is, how we feed ourselves the other six days of the week (Lahmann 1901, 199).

The concluding chapter of *Natural Hygiene* outlined the future role of the physician in a way strikingly similar to Thomas A. Edison's often quoted statement, "The doctor of the future will give no medicine, but will interest his patients in the care of the human frame, in diet and in the cause and prevention of disease" (Werbach 1986, 178).

> As bodily misery and disease grow less, doctors will find less employment as physicians—they will have to become teachers of hygiene and protectors of health. Only then will the physician be able to develop the highest ideal of his art, the desire to help others to obtain perfect health. Today the main job of doctors is "mending work;" his patients merely use him to help them sin again against nature . . . .
>
> The day that hygiene is introduced as a subject into schools, the day physicians are appointed by the state as teachers of hygiene - that day will see the commencement of a new era, a time of progress unrivalled in the history of civilized nations (Lahmann 1901, 217-218).

Lust lists Lahmann as one of his "Great Pioneers."

> His work on diet is authoritative and his "nutritive salts theory" forms the basis of rational dietetic treatment. This work has but recently come to light in America and progressive dieticians are forsaking their old, worn-out, high protein, chemical and caloric theories for the "organic salts theory." Carque, Lindlahr, McCann and other wide awake Food Scientists have adopted it as the basis of their work. Dr. Lahmann was a medical nihilist. He denounced medicine as unscientific and entirely experimental in its practice and lived to prove the saneness of his ideas as evidenced by his thousands of cured patients (Lust 1918, 447).

Despite this praise, Lahmann enjoyed only name-recognition in America. The details of his work were hardly known. This is unfortunate for a doctor whom Brauchle called "the most comprehensive representative of nature cure of his time, the man with the most thorough scientific education, with the greatest gift for exact scientific research, achieving the most perfect harmony between intuitive insight and experimental proof" (Brauchle, 1951, 238).

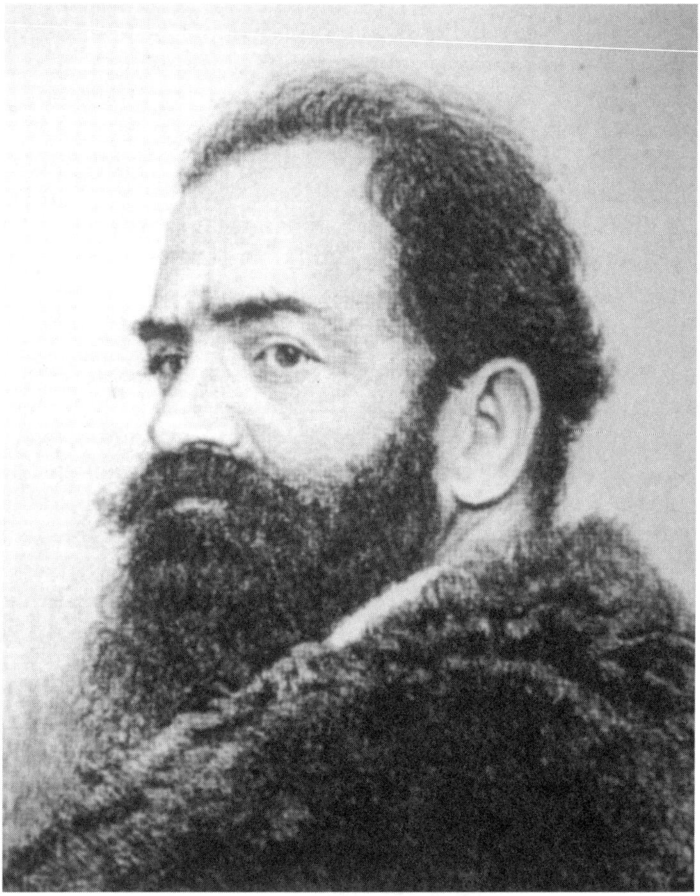

Ernst Schweninger
(Brauchle 1971, frontispiece)

The Physician Who Saved Bismarck and Established the First Nature Cure Hospital

Ernst Schweninger

(1850 - 1924)

Ernst Schweninger became famous as Otto von Bismarck's personal physician. He relieved the great German chancellor from excruciating pain and extended his life for years with pure nature cure methods.

Born June 15, 1850 in Freystadt, Schweninger was the son of a respected country doctor. He began his medical studies when he was sixteen years old and became a physician at the early age of twenty. He gained extensive surgical experience in military hospitals during the Franco-Prussian War in 1870-71. Later he became a lecturer at the Pathological Institute of the University of Munich and published several scientific papers.

Schweninger started out in the field of pathology, one of the strictest sciences in medicine, but his faith in allopathic practice was undermined at the dissection table. He saw its failures first hand, and became convinced that any cure was ultimately dependent on the healing power of nature. His interest in medical history led him to discover what such physicians as Hippocrates, Paracelsus and Hufeland thought about health and disease. "He did not select nature cure so much as arrived at it through his own evaluation of the processes of disease and cure" (Brauchle 1951, 313).

However, one physician in Munich influenced Schweninger. This was the laryngologist Max Joseph Oertel (1835-1897), who developed the famous Oertel cure, a special dietary withdrawal cure for the fatty degeneration of the heart. Oertel's two works,*The Dietetic-Physical Treatment of Myocardial Diseases* (1889) and *About Terrain-Spas for the Treatment of Patients with Cardio-vascular Disorders* (1904), contributed to the renewal of interest in physical-dietetic therapy among clinicians. The method included fluid intake, increased elimination through vigorous exercises, sweat-producing Roman-Irish baths and sun baths, small, frequent meals, separation of solid and liquid food, and increasing arterial blood pressure through a stay in a high altitude spa (Haberling 1932, 413). An American naturopathic textbook described the system of graded mountain-climbing which Oertel had used with good results on himself.

> The patient walks up an elevation slowly and until he is slightly fatigued but never to the point of dyspnea or palpitation. Gradually the speed and length of the walk are increased. The treatment is repeated every day or every other day for four, six or eight weeks or even longer. Massage is frequently added to Oertel's method. It acts as a splendid invigorator and has a specific value in as much as it helps to stimulate the venous flow (Juettner 1916, 478).

The advantage of the Oertel cure, which Schweninger modified and used on Bismarck successfully, was that it dispensed with all medicines (Griebel 1886, 54).

Schweninger became Bismarck's physician by first treating the Chancellor's son, who suffered from obesity, fatty degeneration of the heart and gout. Schweninger restored his health in a relatively short time by changing his diet and using simple nature cure methods. This "miraculous cure" won him the gratitude of the Bismarck family which immediately called the now 30 year-old physician from Munich to the bedside of the Iron Chancellor. In 1880, the overworked and overfed Bismarck was seriously ill. His unhealthy lifestyle had exhausted his once bullish energies, and his vigorous creative powers were paralyzed by a painful liver disease. He had consulted the most famous physicians of his time without benefit. The verdict of Professor Frerichs, the most prominent diagnostician of the University of Berlin, was that Bismarck suffered from stomach and liver cancer and at best had only a year to live.

> Then Schweninger entered this seemingly hopeless situation and saw it was very unlikely that Bismarck had cancer. Instead he found a misfed, over-strained, 250-pound man suffering from neuralgic pains who was being over-medicated with narcotics and sleeping pills. In consultation Schweninger told Prof. Frerichs that he did not want to treat "a diagnosis" but rather a sick man.
>
> No physician before Schweninger ever thought to help the heavy colossus with a simple natural weight-reducing cure. It was not easy to treat such a man as Bismarck, but Schweninger's strong personality allowed him to guide the domineering chancellor through the treatment program (Brauchle 1951, 307-308).

Erwin Liek (1878-1935), a respected surgeon and strong critic of contemporary medicine, wrote about this physician-patient relationship in his book, *The Doctor's Mission:*

> There are physicians who cringe before patients of wealth or high social standing. That attitude is deplorable. It gravely interferes with the effect of treatment. The faultiness of this attitude has been clearly pointed out by the wise saying of Bismarck: "My former doctors treated me as I directed them. They carried out my own ideas. I took them in hand, but my present man, Schweninger, treats me according to his own views." Bismarck had been treated "according to his own ideas" by no less than one hundred physicians, among them so great a celebrity as Professor Leyden (Liek 1930, 54).

Schweninger immediately restricted Bismarck's daily food portions, limited his intake of liquids, especially his beloved wines and champagnes, and did away with pain-killers and narcotics. He substituted hot compresses, warm baths, gentle massage and exercises.

> When Schweninger prescribed rest, even the great chancellor complied, and no emperor and no party leader could interfere. In the last sixteen years of his life Bismarck was under the naturopathic care of Schweninger (Brauchle 1951, 308).

Schweninger's success was not taken with good grace by the representatives of established medicine who had treated Bismarck. They looked down on this "Bavarian charlatan" who did not know how to use drugs but relied on "unscientific methods" of diet, packs and baths. The faculty of the University of Berlin under the leadership of the famous Rudolf Virchow did everything in its power to thwart his appointment as a professor there. But in 1884, after endless negotiations, Bismarck assigned Schweninger to the chair for dermatology without the consent of faculty. This did little to endear Schweninger to his colleagues who labelled him "the instant professor by the grace of Bismarck."

> When he met the faculty and presented them his card, the great Du Bois-Reymond returned it to him in a rage. Schweninger believed that he could only respond to this insult with a challenge to a duel. Fortunately, it never came about (Brauchle 1951, 311).

As a born physician, original thinker and eloquent speaker, Schweninger filled his new post with distinction. However, the limited position as professor and Director of the University Dermatology Clinic did not satisfy him professionally. He regarded it as a fortunate stroke of fate when, in 1900, he was offered the directorship of the newly constructed hospital of Gross-Lichterfelde near Berlin. Here he could prove on a grand scale the effectiveness of natural treatments. In his inaugural address he declared that "any difference between rich and poor was not compatible with the physician's mission, the purest of all endeavors to help others" (Asbeck 1977, 54). Schweninger had already shown his sense of social responsibility as Bismarck's adviser when he influenced the chancellor to put through universal health insurance, workmen's compensation, disability and old age insurance legislation fifty years before Franklin D. Roosevelt established similar programs in the United States.

Schweninger did not want to be the chief physician of a private sanatorium catering to rich, chronically ill patients. He wanted to treat poor patients suffering from acute diseases in a publicly funded hospital. When Schweninger was appointed head of the new hospital, his colleagues raised difficulties for him. The medical associations of the Berlin area boycotted him and refused to refer him patients. But the new hospital was soon so overcrowded that patients had to wait for months to be admitted. In his hospital, Schweninger avoided surgery and medicine as much as possible, focusing mainly on physical-dietetic treatment like sun, light, air, water, movement, rest, simple diet and psychological influences. The patients were made to feel at home in an atmosphere of light, fresh air and cleanliness which was completely different from the gloomy depressing fortresses which then passed for hospitals. The hospital rooms had access to gardens, air baths and a gymnasium. Until late November, patients, especially those suffering from tuberculosis, slept on open verandas:

> "The patients while being treated clinically should forget they are sick. Their stays should be made as pleasant as possible. . . . Rest and odorlessness in the hospital are the first requirements . . . . Strictest cleanliness, fresh air, hot water and marble soap are the best disinfectants. . . . One should not frighten the patient with a scientific diagnosis. . . . We try to give the rounds the character of a friendly visit which cheers up the patient, giving him comfort and advice so that he feels his problems are understood; the impression of a tiring inquisition must be avoided by all means."
> We can deduce from Schweninger's words how much he demanded from the physician not only to take care of the physical

> ills of his patient, but also of his psychic distress (Brauchle 1951, 314).

Schweninger advocated a generalized natural treatment not directed against a specific disease that had to be eliminated but towards the sick person's vital force. Schweninger was extremely conservative in using drugs and serums, which he considered merely "symptomatic medicines," cancelling the disease signs but not curing the patient. In his opinion the allopathic treatment often paralyzed the patient's best helper, the "inner physician." The doctor's task at the bedside was to awaken and strengthen the natural healing powers in the most natural way possible. He condemned "the misleading concept of diagnosis" that tempted doctors to treat diseases "instead of sick persons." "It is an error to believe that a treatment is only possible when a diagnosis is made .... No physician can cure! Only the confluence of all those forces which some call the vital force or the inner doctor ... can effect a cure. We can only unburden and support the organism; we can weaken or strengthen it, we can train it through exercise and make it fit through training" (cited in Brauchle 1951, 314).

He deplored blind faith in medicines:

> The patients stay away, unless they get their little bottle of magic drops. They don't want to be cheated. They believe that cure is impossible without medicine. We as physicians preached the power of drugs till they have come to believe in it. Every issue of a medical journal extols the virtues of new drugs, and doctors still read it without laughing! (cited in Bilz 1898, 991).

Schweninger was equally stringent in his criticism of stereotyped cures in spas, which were so fashionable:

> The method to live unreasonably during eleven months and then to look for the cure-all in a spa in the twelfth month always reminds me of the convenient but not always effective change of sinning and obtaining dispensation afterwards ....
>
> Whoever claims to eliminate diseases by so called "cures" without individualizing has no right to scoff at the nature doctors .... Nature does not permit anyone, however grandiose his title might be, to encroach on her domain .... Neither the baths nor fountains, neither the suggestive nor magnetic, neither the homeopathic nor the allopathic, neither the stale roll, fattening, slimming, meat, grape, iron, fruit, water nor the massage cure can

> be recognized as "cures" in the true sense of the word (Schweninger 1893, 215-21).
>
> Schweninger declared that in 1902 only 11 1/2 pennies per day were spent on medication for each patient in his hospital, including the surgical department; much less than in other hospitals (Brauchle 1951, 320-321).
>
> During the five-and-a-half years of his activity in Grosslichterfelde, he treated 8,359 patients with 262,118 days of hospitalization, among them 479 consumptives, 264 rheumatic cases, 219 patients with stomach diseases, 210 diphtheria cases, 165 scarlet fever cases, 155 heart patients, 141 syphilitics, 129 gonorrhea cases, 113 eczema cases, 104 patients with pneumonia .... Among the 129 gonorrhea patients admitted, 49 suffered from scrotitis and a number from suppurated inguinal glands. Schweninger treated all of them without injection into the urethra, only with hot sitz baths, hot compresses and diet (Brauchle 1951, 324-325).
>
> Schweninger treated 233 of the 264 rheumatic patients (almost 90%) druglessly with only physical-dietetic measures. Hot baths played a main role, followed by sweat packs and cotton packs with thermophore around the joints. After the fever subsided, he added sun baths, phototherapy, massage, exercise and showers. In the beginning he prescribed a liquid diet, then a meatless diet and later, after the fever was gone, a mixed diet with little meat (Brauchle 1951, 321).

Despite his documented successes, public lectures and case presentations, attacks from the allopathic community against Schweninger increased. He was denounced for wrong treatment of his patients, serious damage to their health and even accidental homicide. Although these accusations proved to be without substance and never came to trial, Schweninger was nevertheless forced to devote massive amounts of time and energy to refute them. This seemingly endless battle wore him down so much that he resigned his position as hospital director in 1906.

Schweninger's last work was the polemical manifesto *The Physician*. It is a powerful indictment of the physician as a soulless specialist who has completely lost sight of his true mission. It rings as true today as in 1906, when it was first published:

> Very well! Our physicians are scholars! But they hurt the patients by inserting tubes, lamps and cameras into every possible opening for the most trivial reason of finding out how it looks inside . . . .
>
> The scientist is a specialist who finds satisfaction in the dissection and analysis of objects and phenomena into the smallest parts. The physician deals with whole entities which he has to consider, evaluate and judge. He encounters them undivided in their living context as human beings. The scientific physician dissects this wholeness for the purpose of analyzing its minutest components. He does not see, examine and consider the person but only organs, cells, chemical transformations between biological entities . . . . The science of the physician destroys his humanity (Schweninger 1926, 43-46).

To Schweninger "being a physician is practicing an art, not exercising a science" (ibid., 38). He wanted a physician who combined "the courage of a warrior, the mildness of the philosopher, the decisiveness of the statesman, the aggressiveness of the conqueror, the familiarity with death of the priest, the tenderness of a mother, and the clear wisdom of the elder" (ibid., 96).

Schweninger wanted to see reform in the education of medical students so that they could be trained as physician-artists rather than physician-scientists. Today's medical schools could benefit from his advice:

> Take care that the students do not become scholars, bookworms and hair splitters; therefore check, too, whether they are physically qualified. No narrow-chested ones with broad buttocks! We need those with agile hands and eyes radiating from insatiable curiosity! Let among them be poets, painters, musicians! . . . with hearts from which a large and unobstructed road leads into nature, into the world.
>
> Let them experience a year of preparatory service. They shall learn the simple skills of nursing in a large hospital; to touch the patient, do jobs which look repulsive and overcome the aversion to wounded bodies . . . . Furnish them with the necessary portion of anatomy, physiology and biochemistry. But not too much of it!
>
> Whoever has proven his abilities after a year is permitted to enter the medical school which is nothing more than clinic - only observing, listening and taking part in the treatment of the sick, confirming by autopsy. Do not turn them into mere craftsmen who always cut from the same stencils; do not infuse them with

> disconnected scholastic material suitable only for memorizing! Teach them to see and judge, to absorb and assimilate the impression of a human physiognomy, posture, physical constitution. Sharpen their eagles' eyes and lions' paws! (Schweninger 1926, 43-46).

Like Lahmann, Schweninger wrote both for scientific journals and for the general public, on such topics as the "Corset and Woman's Future" and "Law Against Cholera." He discussed the cancer problem in the literary magazine, *Neue Rundschau*. He believed in the importance of "therapeutic touch:"

> The true physician knows about the power of his hands. He can sooth pain and spasms with them . . . . These hands cannot only relieve pain through laying on, stroking and grasping but can also produce demonstrable changes in superficial and even deep tissues (Schweninger 1926, 92).

Schweninger adhered strictly to his own natural health principles, but was troubled in his last years by the effects of a pelvic fracture he suffered in an elevator accident. He died at the age of seventy-four at his country estate near Munich, January 14, 1924.

Schweninger did not succeed in changing main stream medicine with his revolutionary views, but his students Franz Schönenberger, Emil Klein and Wilhelm Winsch became well known for their own attempts to introduce nature cure methods into medical training and practice. An obituary in *Der Naturarzt (The Nature Doctor)*, written by Schönenberger, praised Schweninger as "the pioneer who was the first to use nature cure in a hospital on a large scale."

> Although his detractors never dared belittle his medical skill and his philanthropy, they attacked his true greatness, his fight against the wrong path medicine had taken. He did not believe in the miracle of drug medicine . . . he did not bow down to the almighty power of surgeons; he did not have blind confidence in bacteriology . . . . He even dared to be skeptical of the blessings of vaccination and to testify in favor of some "so-called quacks." In short, he was the great heretic in medicine . . . .
>
> As Harden testified in the Zukunft, "I never saw him more concerned or more attentive in Bismarck's sickroom than at the

> bed of a day-laborer, factory girl or of a worker's child hospitalized at municipal costs."
>
> Thus Schweninger's dictum applies foremost to himself: "To be a physician is to be a humane artist" (Schönenberger 1924, 13-14).

P. Ziegelroth expressed the gratitude of all those physicians who knew Schweninger as a teacher:

> We will never forget the years during which Schweninger transformed the hospital into a training institution for true medical art. For all of us doctors who were there, these years were a great gift which fills us with gratitude. If there is any justice, the history of medicine will mark with golden letters the time when this gigantic experiment was made to reform medical education and hospital practice (cited in Asbeck 1977, 172).

Schweninger's achievements were original and substantial, but the history books did not mark them with golden letters. Only histories of naturopathic medicine can try to rectify this unjust omission. The saying ascribed to him, "A good physician can do more healing with a damp cloth than a poor one can do with an entire pharmacy," could grace the walls of the hydrotherapy department of any naturopathic clinic (Rauch 1991, 52). It embodies Schweninger's core belief that the true art of the physician is his skillful reliance upon nature.

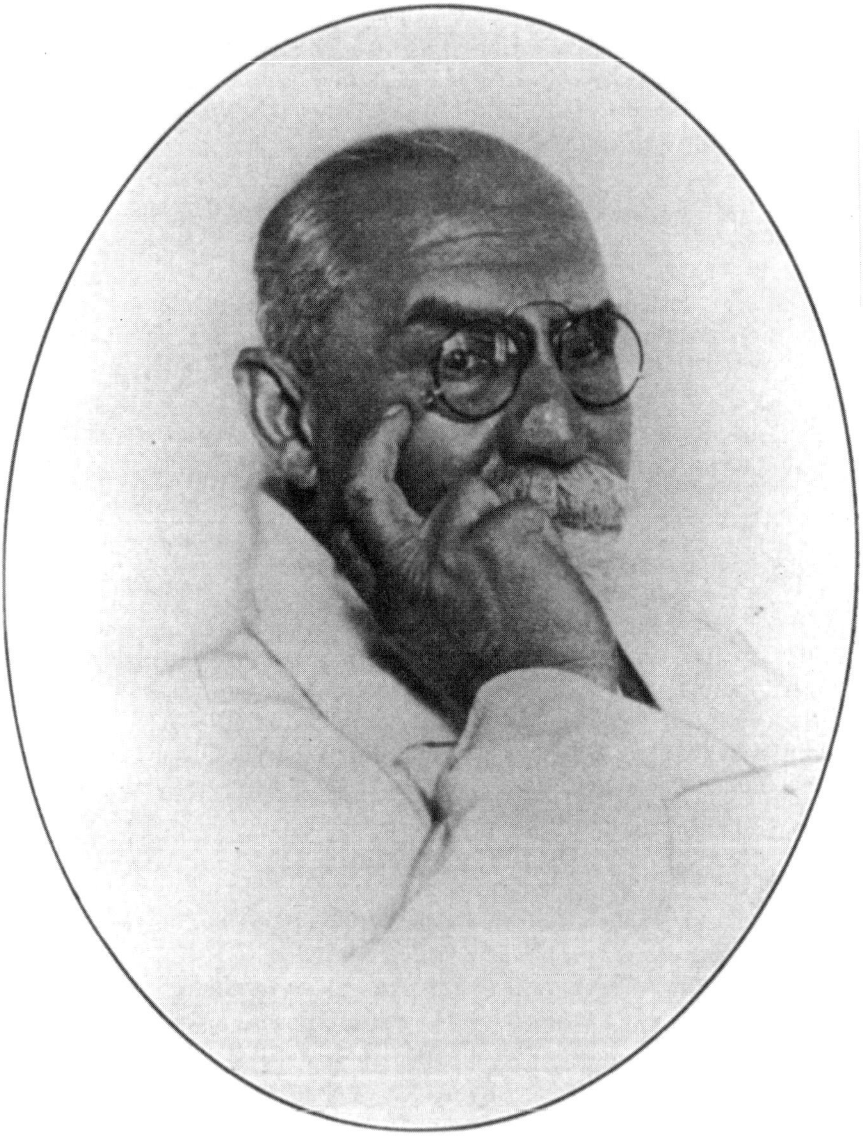

Franz Schönenberger
(Brauchle 1933)

The First University Professor for Nature Cure Methods: The Priessnitz-Hospital in Berlin

Franz Schönenberger

(1865-1933)

Ernst Schweninger was the first to introduce nature cure methods into a hospital near Berlin. This public hospital could not select its patients like a sanatorium but had to treat whomever walked through its door, including patients with acute diseases. The Priessnitz-Hospital in Mahlow, 20 kilometers south of Berlin, was established in 1907 under the directorship of Franz Schönenberger. Although privately funded, it also admitted patients with acute diseases, and was therefore the second nature cure hospital in existence.

A fund for the construction of a nature cure hospital in honor of Priessnitz' hundredth birthday had been established as early as 1898. But not until October 1, 1907, was the German Federation of Associations for Natural Living and Healing Methods, a union of Priessnitz-Associations founded in 1835, able to purchase a site of 100,000 square meters near Berlin. Due to World War I and inflation, almost another 20 years elapsed before sufficient funds were raised for construction to begin. On October 3, 1926, one day before Priessnitz' 127th birthday, the cornerstone was laid with the verse, "In honor of Priessnitz, as a bulwark against disease and as a lesson for the healthy (Priessnitz zur Ehr, der Krankheit zur Wehr, den Gesunden zur Lehr)." The cornerstone contained, among other documents, *Vincent Priessnitz: A Short Biography* by Philo vom Walde and Priessnitz' *Family Water-Book*. The following excerpt from one of the documents shows how proud the German nature cure movement was to have its own hospital at last:

> We call it Priessnitz-House in memory of the new discoverer of the water cure, Vincent Priessnitz, whose work became the impetus for the revolutionary nature cure movement. In the Priessnitz-House we want to put the innate healing power of nature into the physician's command for the benefit of the

> sick. . . .We hope to prove that natural methods are reliable and successful even in life-threatening diseases. We want the Priessnitz-House to become a place of recovery, an educational institution for the healing arts, a starting-point for a new way of life for everyone who is involved with it (Brauchle 1937, 394).

The inauguration of the new hospital took place on Pentecost, 1927. It had a modest beginning with 43 beds, but Paul Schirrmeister, President of the German Federation, expressed in his dedication speech his hopes for it.

> Natural healing methods can reduce much of the burgeoning costs which communities have to bear for their health care institutions . . . . The House shall be a research center for nature cure. Its staff will test and confirm scientifically what the ingenious instinct of our Priessnitz discovered many decades ago (Brauchle 1937, 396).

Professor Franz Schönenberger, M. D., appointed as the first medical director of the hospital, was singularly suited to such a challenge.

Schönenberger was born November 21, 1865 in Kiechlinsbergen on the edge of the Kaiserstuhl, a famous wine-district in Baden. His father managed the estate of the popular author of historical novels, Viktor von Scheffel, whose son was Schönenberger's playmate. Schönenberger became elementary school teacher in Karsau, a small village near Rheinfelden in Baden. Here a special talent for taking care of the sick soon came to light. He assisted the physician who came from Rheinfelden on horseback to look after the sick village folks. In the evening after their rounds they had a glass of wine together in the local tavern. One day Dr. Voigt, a nature doctor from Plauen, joined their conversations. He gave Schönenberger his writings and introduced him to nature cure.

Schönenberger described another early contact with nature cure as follows:

> My school house was located at the end of the village and was surrounded by meadows. During recess the young folks played with the usual frolic. When the rumpus got too loud, I investigated and found that the boys and girls had taken off their shoes and stockings and were gleefully jumping around in the grass which was wet from the rain. "Children, what are you doing there in the wet grass?" I asked with surprise. "Sir, we are playing

> Father Kneipp," answered one of the little rascals. This was the first time that I had heard the name "Kneipp."
>
> A year later Kneipp's book, *My Water Cure*, came out and was given to me by a pastor who was a water enthusiast . . . . I treated the sick with Priessnitz compresses; the youngsters hardened themselves through barefoot walking and playful splashing at the well. I was not drawn to Kneipp's herbal cures; I was always inclined more to Priessnitz' nature cure method (Schönenberger 1931, 172-173).

After Schönenberger had been converted to nature cure, he treated his sick school children and their parents with what he had learned and soon became convinced that he was born to be a physician, not a teacher. However, he had neither the academic prerequisites nor the money to study medicine. He attended some medical lectures at the nearby University of Basel, then he gave up his teaching job and trained with Dr. Voigt in Plauen as a bath attendant and nature curist. After completing his apprenticeship, he established a rural practice near Dresden. The black-bearded nature doctor, driving in a horse-drawn carriage to distant patients, was quickly in demand. But his desire for additional knowledge made him interrupt his nature cure practice to study medicine. This was not easy because he had to undergo the high school equivalency test when he was 28 years old. Thanks to the influence of his former neighbor, the writer, von Scheffel, he gained the personal protection of the Grand Duchess of Baden, who provided him with a scholarship:

> It was quite amusing to hear the white-bearded Schönenberger talk about that time: how he went into the examination with less than perfect knowledge of Latin and Greek, feeling intimidated by the stern examiners; when the examination did not go well, it was the Grand Duchess' personal inquiry which quickly dispersed all doubts of the examiners (Brauchle 1937, 406).

Entering the University of Berlin as a medical student in 1894, Schönenberger immediately established ties with nature cure associations. On Christmas, 1898, he took his examination in Kiel and subsequently received his medical doctor degree. The title of his dissertation,The Influence of Light on the Animal Organism including Investigations about the Changes of the Blood during the Removal of the Light, shows that even in an academic

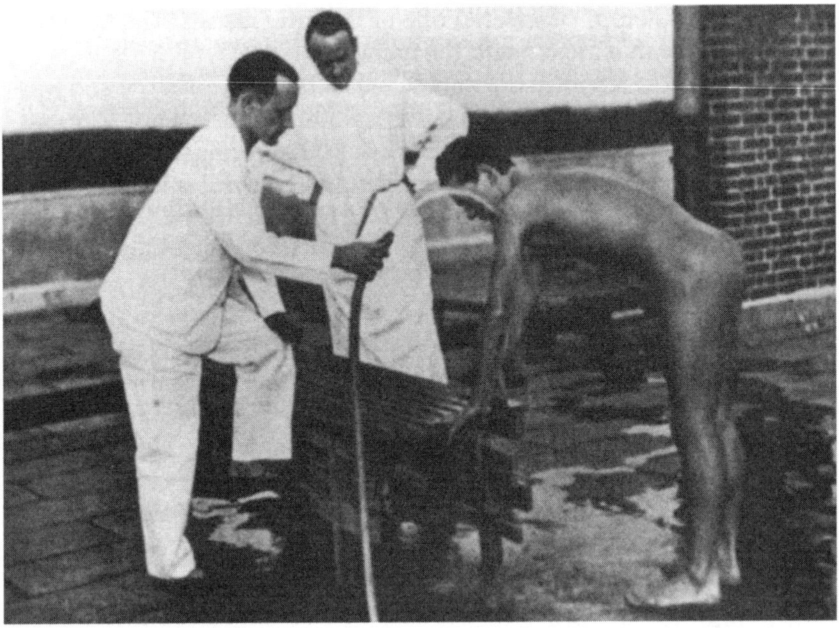

On the roof of the Priessnitz Hospital—The bathing attendant applies a cold arm spray in the physicians's presence. The roof is also used for sunbaths. The Patients enjoy a wide view over gardens and forests

setting Schönenberger focused his research on a subject relevant to nature cure.

He set up a general practice in Bremen. Although he had the same legitimate M.D. degree as his associates, they shunned the "water-doctor" like a leper.

> When I set up my practice as a so-called "nature doctor" in the nineties, all my medical colleagues boycotted me. At that time it was not considered professionally proper to appear at a patient's bedside with a colleague who used water treatments and gave lectures about natural health care any more than it was to greet him in the street.
>
> "Only chickens take a bath in the sun," they replied to me in 1900 when I sought the establishment of light and air baths. My advocacy of fasting days was also ridiculed.
>
> "Schönenberger cannot make us believe that it is possible to influence inflammations with baths, ablutions, packs, etc," was the comment of a court document about my treatment methods .

> . . . Meat and eggs were accepted as the only strengthening diet; vegetables, salad, etc. were regarded as goat food. Nutritional salts were considered worthless (Schönenberger 1930, 206-207).

Optimistic by nature, Schönenberger was not easily discouraged. He gave public lectures and wrote innumerable articles about nature cure which appeared in the magazine *Der Naturarzt (The Nature Doctor)*. In October, 1907, he was elected co-editor of this journal along with Wilhelm Siegert, a teacher, who would become his father-in-law. Looking back at the occasion of the journal's 60th anniversary in 1932, Schönenberger wrote:

> Since 1885 I have been a reader of this journal; I owe to it my first ideas about health. After I had become a physician, I also became a contributor to *Der Naturarzt*. For 25 years I have been co-editor and I have written approximately 500 articles in this journal (Groh 1968, 390).

He soon moved to Berlin where *Der Naturarzt* was published and where he practiced and lived for the remainder of his life. Siegert and he compiled the monumental two-volume work *Lebenskunst—Heilkunst (Art of Living—Art of Healing)* which was retitled in the 1930 edition as *Der Naturarzt (The Nature Doctor)*. This natural home medical adviser won a valued place on the bookshelves of many families. The book's preface showed Schönenberger's modest style, so different from the strident sermonizing of other nature doctors. He emphasized that the book didn't replace the physician or meddle with his work. It only removed obstacles and cleared the way for him. The treatment suggestions for specific diseases were not to be followed mechanically. They only pointed out the direction and goal, because among a hundred sick people not even two were the same:

> As the reader will soon discover, my position is on the side of the nature cure method. It has proved itself on me, my family and nearly 30,000 cases. However, it remains without effect where the natural healing power is gone. There is simply no remedy against death. Where there are still possibilities for the preservation of life, however, one will achieve the best results with the natural healing factors. 'Heilkräfte—nicht Heilsäfte (Healing powers —not healing potions)!' Whoever has struggled as a physician to reach this conclusion will never abandon it (Schönenberger 1906, v-vi).

In 1920 the Prussian Minister for Culture and Education, Konrad Haenisch, a Social Democrat and strong supporter of the nature cure movement, appointed Schönenberger Professor and Head of the Hydrotherapeutic University Institute. In the eyes of the medical establishment this was a scandalous act. Schönenberger's colleagues immediately made him feel unwelcome.

> It was not a happy beginning. They told me at the Ministry: "You will be thrown into a lion's den . . . ." The entire rage against nature cure was focused into attacks against me. My reply consisted in calmly taking-up my new task; in my spare time, however, I collected all the newspaper clippings devoted to my person and my new position. I had them pasted in a notebook very cleanly and tidily. Already I could see ahead to the value of this needlessly spluttered bile against me. Later these clippings would document how fast some scoffers could change their minds (Brauchle 1937, 408).

His inaugural lecture on May 10, 1920, where he invoked the teachings of Priessnitz, did little to dissuade the other professors that he was the "quack." Two chairs remained empty between him and the next professor during faculty meetings:

> When he prescribed a green salad for a patient as part of his cure, the kitchen complained because no professor had ever meddled in the affairs of the kitchen, and finally the chef crossed out the salad from the menu as too expensive for the winter-time . . . In his heart Schönenberger was not a fighter; he was only able to cope with these many serious conflicts thanks to his good humor (Groh 1968, 389).

In accordance with his new vision for the institute, Schönenberger changed its name to University Clinic for Natural Living and Healing. Its focus on prevention and nature cure methods was quite revolutionary, never seen before in a university setting. The clinic consisted of an ambulatory department with treatment rooms and a small in-patient ward with 20 beds. Alfred Brauchle, Schönenberger's assistant, wrote an account of the clinic's success.

> During nine years 25,000 patients, mostly from Berlin's poorest district in the North, received repeated counselling and treatment. Approximately 100 women and 50 men were treated daily in the baths. In those nine years 250,000 baths were administered, and 56,000 patients visited the electrotherapy department. The

> Department for Swedish therapeutic gymnastics and massage was established in 1921 and carried out 4,500 treatments within 8 years . . . .
>
> The enrollees for Schönenberger's lectures numbered 500 from 1921 to 1929. It must be pointed out that these were not required lectures and that it was very difficult for over-worked medical students to attend lectures which were not on obligatory examination subjects. Approximately 50 interns spent part of their practice year in the Clinic, and over 80 physicians worked there for various periods.
>
> Numerous scientific works originated from Schönenberger's Clinic, among them 25 dissertations. During my four years as Schönenberger's assistant I published the following articles in medical journals: "Chronically Cold Feet as a Cause of Disease," "Raw Food as a Therapeutic Diet," "Mass Suggestion as an Introduction into the Art of Influencing Oneself" (Brauchle 1937, 408).

When the Priessnitz Hospital opened in Berlin-Mahlow, there was no one better suited to be its chief physician than Schönenberger. Unfortunately he held this position for only two years, resigning in April, 1929, because it was too much of a burden for his advancing age. He did retain his university clinic position and continued as an editor of *Der Naturarzt* until his death on June 7, 1933. Lothar Strassburg, M.D., his successor at the university clinic from 1941-1951, noted that it was perhaps best that Schönenberger died in 1933 before the National Socialists seized power. This saved him from further humiliations, because a rigorous purge was conducted at the clinic, and one of the victims was his deputy, Dr. A. Würthle, whose Aryan genealogical certificate could not protect him from the suspicion of being a Jew (Strassburg 1979, 4).

Those who knew Schönenberger confirmed that he was not a fanatic, but rather an amiable, cheerful man who always had a joke on his lips. He tried to avoid conflicts, and if they occurred, he immediately arranged for compromise or reconciliation. This approach helped him to survive the hostile early years at the university before he gained the respect of his colleagues. Brauchle, his successor, wrote:

> Hundreds of students and dozens of physicians enjoyed this intelligent, ingenious and experienced teacher. When he stood at the bedside, he not only talked to his patients about their illnesses, but also about their origin, family and job. At these times it was evident that there was no corner of the country which was unfa-

> miliar to him and there was no field of human activity which had remained hidden from his alert mind. And when he talked with us assistants outside the ward about the present and the past, we felt we were listening to someone who turned over the leaves of world history. Many people—writers, artists, scholars, politicians—had passed through his consulting room, and he had established personal relations with many of them beyond their diseases (Brauchle 1937, 407).

Schönenberger's last contribution to *Der Naturarzt* were comments of Priessnitz' contemporaries about Priessnitz, and he arrived at the often quoted conclusion: "We are still far from surpassing Priessnitz; we can only try harder and harder to live up to him" (cited in Groh 1968, 390).

Cooperation Between Natural and Orthodox Medicine: The Great Nature Cure Experiment in the Dresden Hospital

Alfred Brauchle

(1898-1964)

Alfred Brauchle, M.D., who assisted Franz Schönenberger at the Priessnitz-Hospital in Mahlow, followed him as director from 1929 to 1934. Brauchle had a more forceful personality than the mild-mannered Schönenberger, but like him was an outstanding clinician, teacher and writer. He was also the first historian of the nature cure movement, and his work, *Nature Cure in Biographies* (1937), later re-issued in abbreviated editions under different titles, remains the most comprehensive standard work on the subject.

Brauchle was born in Schopfheim (Baden) on March 22, 1898. He completed his medical studies at Freiburg after an interruption due to World War I. The promising young doctor spent his internship at the University Hospital of Berlin, making a name for himself as the author of a much used textbook, *Fundamentals of Normal Histological and Microscopic Anatomy* (1925). It was also there that he met Schönenberger, who introduced him to nature cure methods.

> In 1924 I became an intern at his clinic. The original arrangement was that I should stay for only three months. During this brief time Schönenberger succeeded in completely winning me over to nature cure which had been foreign to me until that time. Since then I have never thought for even a single moment of abandoning it (Brauchle 1957, 134).

Indeed, Brauchle became one of nature cure's most ardent, talented and eloquent defenders among the medical doctors who converted to nature cure.

After his internship he studied with Emile Coué in France from whom he learned the method of autosuggestion.

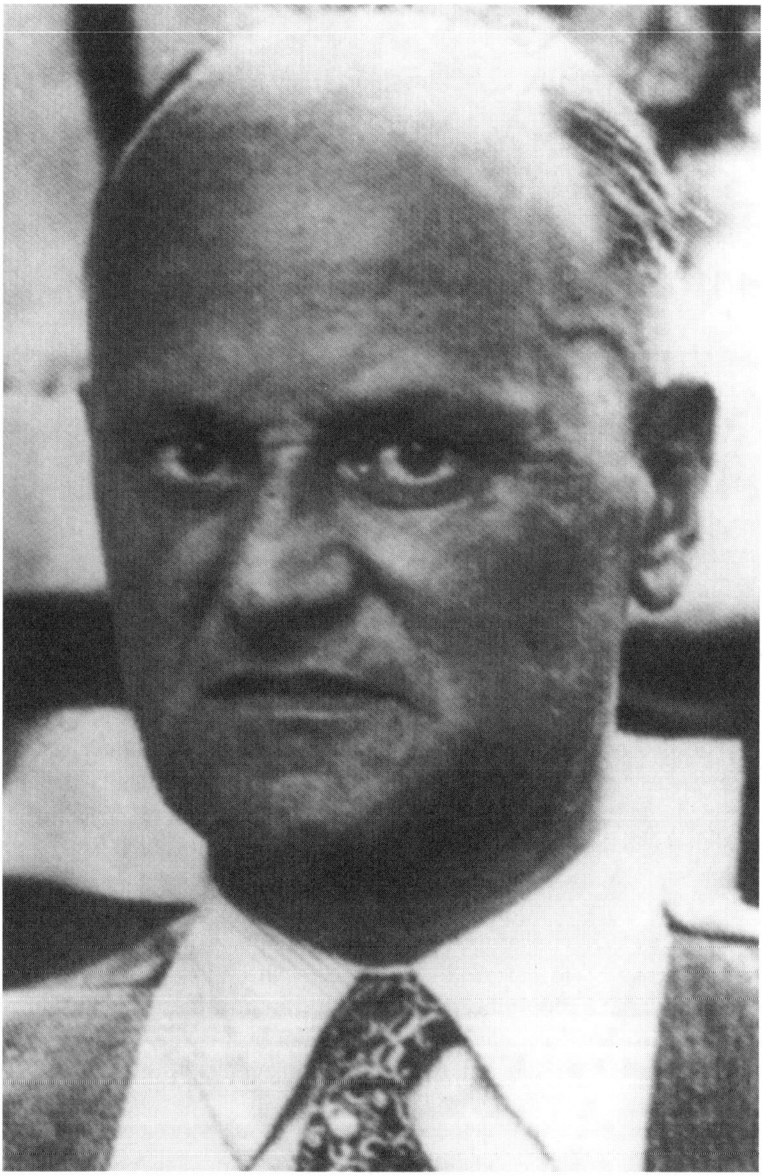

Alfred Brauchle
(Rothschuh 1983, 32)

> I discovered Coué's work after I had suffered for fifteen years from stomach and intestinal disturbances which were not relieved by the removal of the gallbladder and the appendix. After reading his small book, *Self-mastery through Conscious Auto-Suggestion,* I was seized by such a swell of hope that I was able by my own efforts to become healthy within a short time and I have remained free from all stomach and intestinal ills until this day. Then I visited Coué myself in Nancy in March 1925 (Brauchle 1951, 362-363).

Brauchle was deeply impressed by the success of Coué's methods, and came to believe that hypnotic suggestion could help unlock the inner healing power and speed recovery in all kinds of illnesses. The Frenchman's lucidity and modest, unassuming appearance convinced Brauchle that he was not a charlatan. Later he used Coué's methods on his patients as an adjunct to his nature cure treatments with excellent results.

> I introduced the mass suggestions which I had seen at Coué's into the University Clinic for Hydrotherapy in Berlin. Once every week approximately 100 patients who were pre-screened took part in the sessions . . . . Gradually I gave a personal touch to the method . . . . For six years I conducted mass suggestions as the chief physician of the Priessnitz-Hospital in Berlin-Mahlow. At the Dresden Hospital from 1934-43, I treated approximately 500 patients weekly with mass suggestions. I concluded from these extraordinary experiences that such psychological group therapies are a valuable and effective instrument to multiply the effect of a physical treatment so long as it is in the hands of an experienced physician who believes in the power of the mind (Brauchle 1951, 366).

> I consider nature cure without psychological guidance incomplete. Therefore, I always placed a special emphasis on the development of a "psychological nature cure" or "naturopathic psychotherapy" (ibid., 341-342).

Brauchle concluded his book, *History of Nature Cure in Biographies,* with a chapter entitled "Psychological Nature Cure," devoted to the three great hypnotherapists, Franz Anton Mesmer (1734-1815), Emile Coué (1857-1926) and the Swedish physician Otto Wetterstrand (1845-1907). The scientifically-trained Brauchle remained open-minded even towards Mesmer and his "animal magnetism," when many considered Mesmer to be a charlatan.

> Relaxation, gentle massage and emotional impression alone can explain the success of the magnetic treatment. It is not necessary to assume a transference of magnetic forces from person to person. We have not yet been able to prove such a transference scientifically. However, I believe that it is quite within the realm of possibility. Only the future will bring us clarity in this respect. In any case, I acknowledge that the magnetic treatment, if freed from all unnecessary hocus-pocus, is a valuable method of influence, impression and mild treatment (Brauchle 1951, 361).

As Schönenberger's successor at the Priessnitz-Hospital in Berlin-Mahlow, Brauchle implemented nature cure methods in a pure way. Even herbal, homeopathic and vitamin preparations, popular among many naturopathic physicians, played no role in his program.

> Until 1935 I was the medical director of the Priessnitz-Hospital in Mahlow and tried to be a physician in the spirit of Schweninger and Schönenberger. Soon the influx of patients was so great that the 75 beds were constantly occupied, and patients had to wait for months to be admitted. I introduced the raw food diet according to Bircher Benner, practiced the cold water treatment according to Priessnitz and Kneipp, the heat treatment according to Schweninger and Winsch, air and sun baths according to Rikli and Lahmann and practiced the principles of natural treatment as elaborated by Theodor Hahn. Even Schroth-Cures were carried out in limited numbers. In addition, fasting, massage and gymnastics played a major role (Brauchle 1951, 341).

One of the fruits of his work during six years at the Priessnitz Hospital was the *Handbook of Nature Cure on a Scientific Basis* (1933), one of the first nature cure textbooks written specifically for physicians. It was divided into two parts. The first part dealt with nature cure in general, its theory, methods and history. The second, larger, clinical section covered the etiology and natural treatment of various diseases, including nervous and mental disorders. Detailed case histories enlivened the second part, including one of a 66-year old man, referred to the hospital with pneumonia.

> When examined, the patient was very pale. He had difficulty breathing, and his lips were slightly bluish. The lower lobes of the lungs showed signs of inflammation—dullness and diminished bronchial respiration—on both sides. The pulse was greatly accelerated (120 per minute) and his temperature measured 39.5 C. The case was further complicated by the advanced age of the patient, by the chronic bronchial catarrh he had suffered from for years and the fact that he was a heavy smoker. Three days after his admission an embolus developed on his left wrist.
>
> The treatment emphasized complete bed rest. Even during the warm whole body ablutions the patient was hardly allowed to move. Leg packs, steam compresses and Priessnitz wraps around the chest were given daily. The windows were kept wide open day and night. During the first five days, while the patient was feverish, he was given only fruit juice and honey water. From the sixth day on his temperature was completely normal, and two weeks after his admission the patient got out of bed for the first time. After another six days he was discharged as completely cured (Brauchle 1933, 310-311).

Like other nature doctors Brauchle was also a teacher who tried to reach the masses through a number of popular books on natural healing. *The Great Book of Nature Cure* (1957), a worthy successor of the encyclopedic nature cure books for the home by Theodor Hahn, Kneipp/Reile and Schönenberger, differed from theirs in that it contained extensive chapters on the history and theory of nature cure. Brauchle also showed his awareness of the great spiritual influence which the physician can exert on the patient years before this topic was addressed by Norman Cousins and Bernie S. Siegel in their best-selling books.

> It is through the soul that the inner doctor can be enlivened, encouraged or inhibited. Therefore the success of many nature cures depends on the physician who carries them out. After all, the physician has a strong impact on his patient's soul and can inspire it with hope and confidence which in turn can enliven the central regulatory mechanism. In other words, the inner and the external physician must cooperate on the basis of friendship and mutual understanding in order to achieve a complete curative success (Brauchle 1957, 142).

In 1934, Brauchle was appointed head of the Department for Nature Cure Methods at the 1,200-bed Johannstädter Hospital in Dresden. For the first time in its history nature cure was given the chance to prove itself in a large hospital setting under the watchful eye of official medicine. Brauchle and his counterpart, Professor Louis R. Grote (1886-1960), made this historical experiment a success. Although Grote, the Director of the Department for Internal Medicine, represented orthodox medicine, he was not prejudiced against nature cure. Early in his career he was chief physician of Dr. Lahmann's Sanatorium, where he saw firsthand the effectiveness of nature cure methods. Grote was a man of high culture, great charm, sparkling wit and extraordinary intelligence. He was also a talented pianist and had difficulty choosing between a musical or medical career. Grote was in a delicate position. The followers of nature cure hoped that he would open wide the doors of official medicine for their methods, while his orthodox colleagues expected "that he would soon put an end to this spook" (Strassburg 1979, 4). Grote considered it his task to observe the methods of nature cure with "constructive criticism" and to integrate them as much as possible into orthodox medicine. Brauchle described the playing field for "the contest between orthodox medicine and nature cure" as follows:

> The real struggle for mutual understanding occurred in a ward of 30 beds shared by both departments which was occupied by patients without any prior selection. I or one of my interns was responsible for the treatment there while Grote or one of his interns saw to it that all diagnostic requirements were meticulously observed. Once or twice a week Grote and I made our grand rounds there together (Brauchle 1951, 346-347).

The results of this great experiment, lasting from 1934 to 1943, were manifold and found their expression in numerous articles by Grote and Brauchle, and in the dissertations of their students, which were published in many respected allopathic medical journals. From 1935 to 1939 the Dresden Hospital, now renamed Rudolf Hess Hospital by the Nazis, regularly offered continuing education seminars titled "Nature Cure within the Scope of Medicine as a Whole." Approximately 1,000 physicians took part in thirty-seven courses (Brauchle/Groh 1971, 161). But the greatest triumph of cooperation came at a 1936 conference on internal medicine in Wiesbaden.

> Grote acknowledged in public for the first time the success of nature cure methods in the treatment of pneumonia, bronchial asthma, heart diseases, gastric ulcers, cirrhosis of the liver and

> rheumatism and demonstrated them to the allopathically oriented audience with the help of his charts and precise technical data (Brauchle 1951, 347).

In America, Benedict Lust was aware of these events, and described them as "a sweeping vindication of Naturopathy" (Lust 1936, 99):

> Naturopathy and Allopathy are shaking hands and promise to respect each other . . . . But this is in Europe. When will America wake up? When will the people of the United States realize that again they are limping behind the old world? Let us hope that the American public will show their common sense if the medical world fails to do so (ibid., 114).

The most impressive testimony of Brauchle's and Grote's successful partnership were their books, *Results from the Cooperation between Nature Cure and Orthodox Medicine* (3 volumes, 1938-40) and *Conversations about Orthodox Medicine and Nature Cure* (1935). The latter was an intelligent and conciliatory dialogue between the two representatives of different schools of medicine.

> **Brauchle:** The natural stimuli, such as air, light, water, movement, breathing, diet, fasting, etc. are capable of much greater healing than orthodox medicine wants to believe. I concede, however, that nature cure cannot do completely without surgical intervention or medicine if it has to treat patients without prior selection. Where we can no longer cure, we must bring relief; but for the real business of curing, the natural stimuli are very far-reaching (Grote 1935, 14-15).

> **Grote:** I believe I am quite familiar with the nature cure literature. At least I read Lahmann very carefully and some of Bircher-Benner's writings. I was always disappointed by the contrast between the grand theoretical statements and the meagerness of their documented proofs. I might also observe: the leading figures of nature cure did not enjoy stable health. I only have to remind you at what early age the great Lahmann died, now just 30 years ago. You know yourself that Schroth and Priessnitz did not get old, and, in fact, only Kneipp reached a patriarchal age. Perhaps one psychological root for nature cure can be found in this fact; persons with poor constitutions have an immanent drive

> to that health which is embodied by a life in untouched nature far from the city (Grote 1935, 30).
>
> **Brauchle:** If there is a conflict between a theory and a practical success, the nature doctor doesn't hesitate to take the side of the success and leave the theory to itself. There is a basic ability in the human heart which perceives and knows a priori what is right. This ability can be paralyzed or inhibited by an academic education . . . . I make it my interns' duty to spend part of their day in the air bath, to go swimming and hiking and give themselves to Nature. If there is a conflict with their paper work or chemical analyses, I decide in favor of Nature, for the physician himself must embody something of living nature if he wants to re-connect the sick patient to the power of Nature again (Grote 1935, 63-64).
>
> **Grote:** Each therapeutic action by a physician must be evaluated as to whether it can equally live up to the knowledge of orthodox medicine and the skill of nature cure (Grote 1935, 117).

Conversations was dedicated to Rudolf Hess, Adolf Hitler's deputy, and had a preface by Gerhard Wagner, M.D., the Reich Physicians' Leader, who wanted to create a new German medicine, a "synthesis of the so far one-sided orthodox medicine with the nature cure method" (Brauchle, 1937, 411). There can be no doubt that the nature cure experiment at Dresden hospital would have never taken place without the support of the Nazi top brass. Brauchle begins his chapter on the Rudolf Hess Hospital in the first edition of his history of nature cure with a quote from Hess:

> I have experienced the effects of nature cure on my own body. I also know many astonishing successful cures with natural healing methods experienced by friends and acquaintances. I would be a coward if I did not acknowledge this in public and draw practical consequences from it. It would be a crime against my people if I did not do everything in my power so that the nature cure is given the position which it deserves (Brauchle 1937, 411).

A number of prominent figures in the nature cure movement were attracted to National Socialism. Nature cure's rallying cry, "Return to Nature," and its condemnation of the ills of civilization could easily be distorted to fit the infamous "blood and soil" ideology of the Nazis, just as nature cure's cultivation of strong, healthy bodies could be perverted in support of the eugenic breeding of the Aryan superman, with its inhuman consequences. Lothar Strassburg, who was an intern under him, maintained that Brauchle despised the Nazis, but Brauchle's writings from this time were not without kowtows to National Socialism (1979, 5). Brauchle's lip-service to the regime might have been given in the interest of nature cure, but it casts a shadow on him. Interestingly, in the 1951 edition of his *History of Nature Cure in Biographies* the Rudolf Hess Hospital is once again the Dresden Hospital, and the Hess quote is purged from the text.

World War II called most of the hospital staff to arms and overshadowed the last years of the Dresden experiment. Brauchle abandoned it in 1943, and retreated to his native Black Forest, taking over the Sanatorium Glottertal near Freiburg (1943-1946), and later the Park Sanatorium Schönau (1949-1960). Brauchle and Grote remained friends for the rest of their lives. Strassburg drew an amiable picture of Brauchle's personality.

> Despite all his writing and teaching, Brauchle's main interest was the bedside care of the sick. Here in long, intensive visits he tried to understand the patient in his totality. He analyzed all discernible harmful factors of the patient's inner and external life with great understanding. Such individual investigations then determined the focus of his therapy. With relatively simple means he was able to improve or cure the patient . . . .
>
> In no way a bookworm, Brauchle was a true child of nature who found relaxation in outdoor athletics . . . . As a young man he had won the Southwest German championship throwing the discus . . . . In later years he had a special passion for horseback riding, even writing a small book about it. Until shortly before his death, already ailing and half blind, he let himself be carried on his loyal horse through his beloved Black Forest mountains. In Dresden I was sometimes allowed to accompany him on his rides into the beautiful Dresden Heath. Then, free from all professional burdens, he seemed to be transformed. He could not be bothered with any conversation about the medical questions of the day. Completely turned inwards, he was only interested in timeless, metaphysical subjects.
>
> On the whole, the constant public engagements and professional challenges didn't agree with his true nature. He was also not as robust as his imposing appearance suggested. His own body was not spared the suffering of illness. His often quoted

> saying: "Only those whose lives are threatened take up nature cure," seemed to be applicable to himself (1979, 4).

On February 11, 1951, the Central Association of Physicians for Nature Cure Methods *(Zentralverband der Ärzte für Naturheilverfahren)* was formed with Brauchle as its first president. He maintained his private practice in Schönenberg near Schönau in the Black Forest from 1960 until his death on November 21, 1964. Brauchle had been a member of the Research Council of the Emerson University, Los Angeles; Honorary Member of the American Balneological Society; and holder of the Swiss Rikli Honor Medal (Brauchle/Groh 1971,164). In 1964, Brauchle was one of the first recipients of the prestigious Hufeland Medal, still awarded by the Central Association of Physicians for Nature Cure Methods to eminent physicians "who contribute to an all-encompassing wholistic concept of medicine" (Schimmel 1983, 470). Grote summarized Brauchle's achievements.

> Modern nature cure physicians owe much to him; we can almost say: everything . . . . When nature cure therapies are no longer regarded as methods for outsiders only, when fasting, a raw vegetarian diet and hydrotherapy have become legitimate tools of the clinician and found their appropriate places in medical texts, then it was Professor Brauchle's indefatigable work which not only opened the path but also paved it (Brauchle/Groh 1971, 164).

After the war a few municipal hospitals established nature cure departments, foremost among them the Hospital on the Kreuzberg in Berlin, which gained special reputation under Dr. Lothar Strassburg (1904-1983), a Brauchle disciple and strong advocate of the classical nature cure methods (Podszus 1992, 864). A well-known private 120-bed Hospital for Nature Cure Methods, headed by nature cure physician Walther Zimmermann, M.D., exists in Munich-Harlaching. However, these institutions have never reached the same status as the Dresden Hospital, especially in terms of cooperation between orthodox medicine and nature cure. Despite the early promise of Schönenberger's and Brauchle's accomplishments, the dream of a nature cure hospital in every large city or of a nature cure department in every large hospital still awaits fulfillment in Germany as well as in the rest of the world.

Part II

Pioneers of Naturopathy in North America and Great Britain

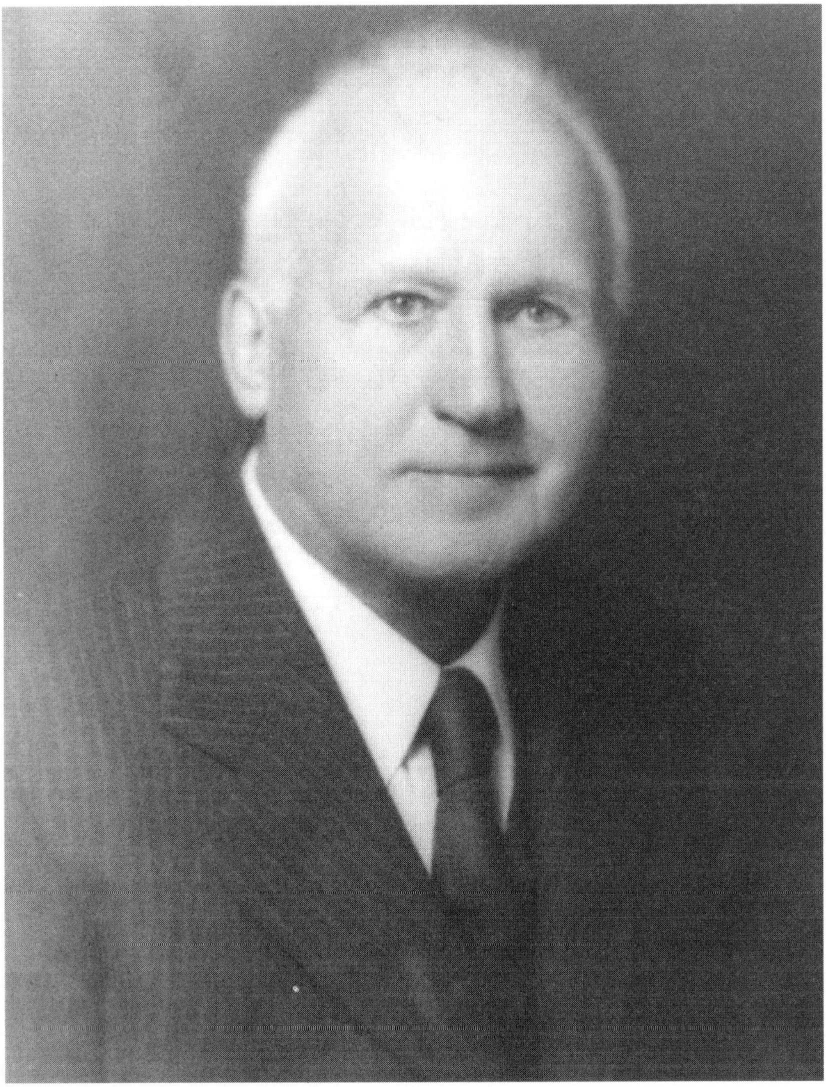

Benedict Lust
(National College of Naturopathic Medicine—Gift of John B. Lust)

The Father of Naturopathy

Benedict Lust

(1872 - 1945)

Nature cure, consisting of hydrotherapy, air and light baths, a vegetarian diet, and herbal remedies, originated in Europe with the work of Priessnitz, Rikli, Kneipp and others. Naturopathy, combining nature cure with homeopathy, massage, spinal manipulation, and therapeutic electricity was developed in America largely through the efforts of Benedict Lust.

Lust (pronounced Loost, meaning "joy" in German) was born in Michelbach near Gaggenau (Baden), Germany on February 3, 1872, and came to America in 1892. Weakened by several operations and "six vaccinations enforced upon me in different parts of the world" (1919, 438), he developed a serious case of tuberculosis. Despite the best efforts of homeopathy and allopathy he wasted away to 104 pounds and was given up to die by American doctors who made out a death certificate in his presence. He decided to return to Germany to die in his homeland and managed to travel to Wörishofen to see Sebastian Kneipp. The good father examined him, listened to his story and at the end of the interview said, "I don't know whether I can put you together again or not, but I will see what we can do" (1904, 145).

Immediately upon starting the Kneipp cure, Lust's health began to improve, and in eight months he had completely regained his health. This was the turning point in his life. Having experienced the value of Father Kneipp's treatments firsthand, he was determined to share the benefits of the system of healing with others.

In 1896, after his successful recovery, Lust had an audience with Kneipp during which he was authorized by the prelate to carry the Kneipp methods to America. Some historians mistakenly lump together Lust's 1892 and 1896 moves to America and incorrectly state that he undertook Kneipp's work in 1892 (Cody 1983, 1; Wardwell 1992, 37). Lust came to America in 1892 to seek his fortune; after becoming ill and returning to Germany and being healed by Kneipp, he came back to America in 1896 to be Kneipp's official representative. This was the start of naturopathy in America.

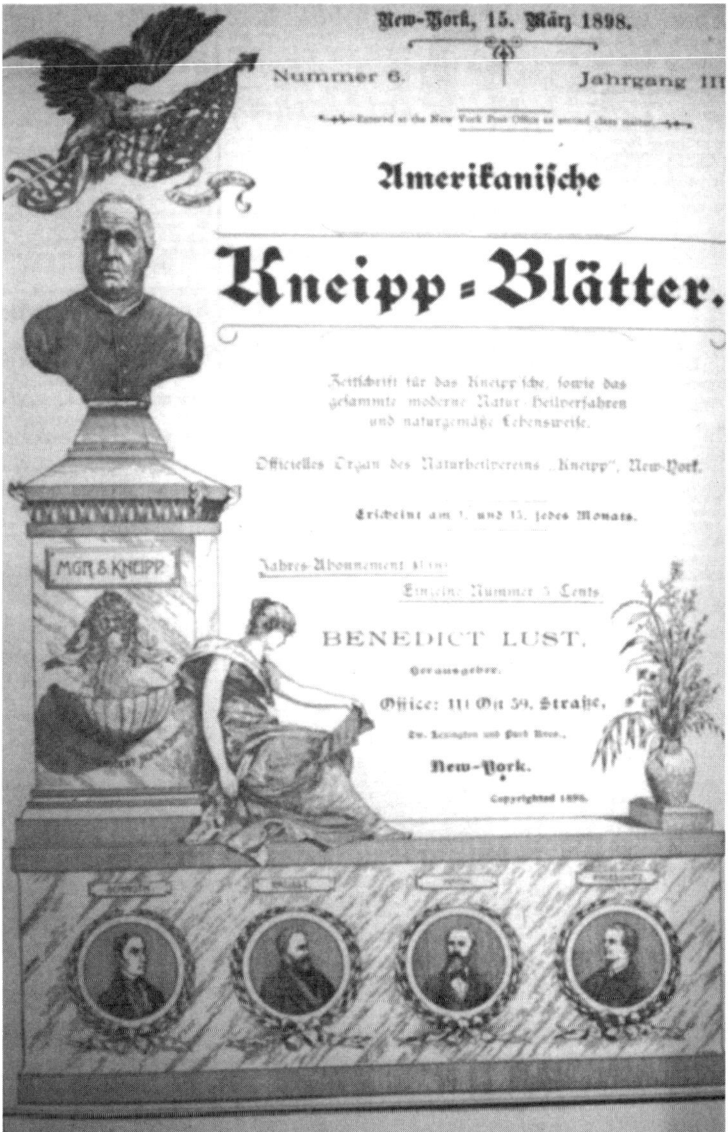

Cover of *Amerikanische Kneipp-Blätter*
published in New York by Benedict Lust

Lust was not the first to bring Kneipp's methods to these shores. A number of Kneipp institutions were already in existence throughout the country, including the German-speaking immigrant communities in New York where Lust settled. But he was the first to be commissioned by Kneipp as well as the first to sense the need to Americanize Kneippism and make it acceptable to the population at large.

From the start he intended to combine Kneippism with other nature cure practices. Indeed, after his recovery he visited other German sanatoriums and broadened his perspective beyond that of Kneipp. When he discovered that the percentage of cures at other nature cure establishments to be even greater than that of Wörishofen, he undertook to study the systems of Kuhne, Lahmann, Just and other European nature doctors. Later he wrote:

> The Kneipp Cure had no dietetics to speak of, nor did it give due place to sun-air baths, massage, electrotherapy, mechanotherapy, physical culture, and suggestive therapeutics (1903, 36).

When Lust arrived back in America in 1896 he was "a raw German youth" with a "small sum in his grasp, and a large purpose in his heart" (1902, 168). The sum was small because a road trickster relieved him of most of his savings. But he was still able to establish a school, a clinic and a magazine. Soon he was shocked to find his message of natural health opposed by medical authorities and Kneipp purists, stolen by "polite plagiarists" who hyped it for profit, and completely ignored by the majority of the population. Hampered at first by the language barrier, he soon mastered English, and rapidly became wise in the rough-and-tumble ways of New York City.

Lust always gave honor and credit to Father Kneipp but didn't hesitate to distance himself from Kneippism when he realized the limits of its appeal to Americans. While the Kneipp purists decried Lust's mixing of Kneippism with other methods, Lust found their insistence on public performance of dew walking barefoot in Central Park stupid and self-defeating. It made Kneippism an easy target for ethnic ridicule. He cherished many of Kneipp's methods but often belittled the Kneippists as "hose-[ap]pliers and compress wringers" and took special measures to keep them out of his naturopathic organizations (1903, 37). He didn't repudiate the Kneipp Cure but went beyond it. Five years after Kneipp's death he wrote:

> The Kneipp Cure was largely prescriptive—naturopathy is first instruction, then inspiration, and ultimately growth. And the cleavage line is increasingly distinct (1902, 485).

As a new generation was emerging in America which was not familiar with Father Kneipp's name, Lust felt it was time to change the name of his successful magazine from *Kneipp Water Cure Monthly* to *The Naturopath* (1902, 14). He continued for some years to have a German-language section in each issue.

By this time Lust was heading a naturopathic sanatorium with scores of faithful patients, a naturopathic college with a growing number of students, a naturopathic magazine with thousands of readers, and a Kneipp store with many eager customers. His success did not escape the attention of the New York medical authorities. He wrote:

> From the very outset I was hounded and persecuted by emissaries, sleuths, detectives, stool-pigeons, and spittle-lickers of the New York County Medical Association (1939, 438).

As early as 1899, he was arrested for the practice of medicine and surgery without a license, for giving a bath and massage to an agent of the County Medical Association. This secret agent, Mrs. Frances Benzecry, made a career of bringing charges against naturopaths, chiropractors and even Christian Scientists. She was responsible for the arrests of over 800 naturopathic doctors during a twelve-year period (*New York Times* July 14, 1914, 4). Although found not guilty, Lust paid $800 in fines and fees.

When Lust complained editorially in *The Naturopath* and called Mrs. Benzecry, "a disgrace to American womanhood and to the free soil of America on which she treads," he was arrested, handcuffed and "carried to the Tombs as if I had committed murder" (1919, 439). Subsequently indicted for criminal libel and released under a $10,000 bond, he was under this bond for 18 months until the trial was set. In open court Lust's attorneys made a motion that the County Medical Association "show their charter to the jury and prove their rights to exercise police power." This forced the Medical Association to offer a retraction and the libel case was dropped (1921, 480).

Thereafter, prosecutions trailed off. At a 1907 New York County Medical Association meeting, one member is reported to have said:

> Our Association cannot take a second chance as it did in the Lust case. We had better give up the prosecutions (1934, 298).

But before the prosecutions ended, Lust had been arrested 16 times by New York authorities and 3 times by federal authorities. One newspaper headline simply read: "They Have Lust Again." This was a shock to the "simple-hearted" young man inspired to come to this country by the American idealism of Washington, Franklin and Lincoln. He even found himself mocked in the German-American newspapers which said that the letters N.D. after Lust's name stood for "Narren Doktor" or "Fool's Doctor" (ibid., 297). When he was not being arrested himself, Lust was frequently called in to bail out other naturopaths who had been jailed. Lust described a typical experience.

> One judge scolded me for calling Carl Newmann a doctor, and he scolded me for contempt of court, because I asked whether a murder had been committed. When I got the particulars of the case, the charge was that he had given a bath to a stool pigeon and that he sold a pound of clay for mud pack to a sleuth who worked for this stool pigeon. Think of it, being arrested for giving a bath and selling a pound of clay for health (1934, 37).

Lust took it as a point of honor never to accept the terms offered by the prosecutors.

> Many Chiropractors pleaded guilty in those days rather than pay the lawyer's fee and go to trial. But we are proud to say not one Naturopath ever pleaded guilty (1921, 480).

It is interesting to note that when she retired as an undercover agent for the Medical Association, Mrs. Benzecry took advantage of her celebrity status to write her life story for publication in the *New York Times.* She stated that although she was variously vibrated, stretched, rubbed, steamed, and prayed over, she came to no harm. "I am unhurt," she wrote. "Nothing happened to me." As Lust pointed out, "What if she had gone around to all the regular doctors for 12 years and underwent their treatments—would anything be left of her if she had submitted to their operations?" (1934, 298)

Looking back, he wrote:

> It is all over now but not forgotten. Some of our members served a year in jail; a woman drugless doctor committed suicide on the Island in despair, several died of broken hearts in the struggle, and many happy homes were ruined (1921, 480).

Lust sought to defuse some of the hostility by studying medicine, but it didn't work. "When he entered medical college, he was a pariah." The other students "badgered him, taunted him and even drenched him in water" (Anonymous 1925, 945) because of his advocacy of water cure. When his publishing office burned down, his fellow students asked him why he hadn't cured the flames with hydrotherapy.

This period of persecution was the crucible in which the fighting spirit of Lust and the other early American naturopaths was forged. It also gave rise to the adoption of the term "naturopathy" to designate the emerging science of natural healing in America, a term originally coined in 1892 by the Drs. Scheel who combined the terms "nature cure" and "homeopathy"

(Faulkner 1934, 102). Dr. John Scheel was a water curist whose wife, Sophie, was a homeopath and Lust's preceptor in medical school. The Scheels had opened one of the first water cure institutions in New York, called the "Badekur," and in 1896 they gave Lust the right to use the name in association with his ventures (Lust 1921, 479). Their term, naturopathy, came to Lust's attention during a competition. "It was chosen out of some 150 submitted as the most comprehensive and endearing" (1902, 33). A conflicting and probably inaccurate version of the term's evolution given by George Cody states that it was coined in 1895 by Dr. Scheel and purchased by Lust in 1902 (1985, 1). A third version is offered by Herbert Shelton, the leader of Natural Hygienists, who began as one of Lust's students but later became a critic.

> One morning in the year 1901 a young man, flushed with enthusiasm, rushed into the establishment of Dr. August F. Reinhold, of New York City, and exclaimed, "We now have a name for our work!" That young man was Benedict Lust, just then becoming a figure in the field of Kneippism. Besides giving baths, he had a supply store where he sold Kneipp pills, undershirts, sandals and other Kneipp supplies. The new word that had given rise to such enthusiasm was NATUROPATHY, a word that had just been coined by Sophie Scheel, an instructor in the local homeopathic college. The word naturepathy appeared in an editorial by R. T. Trall in the *Water Cure Journal* during the Civil War. It may well be that Dr. Scheel had read this editorial and had merely modified the term used by Trall. On the other hand, it may be that she coined the term out of whole cloth.

Shelton added, sarcastically, that other system builders had to find other terms for similar systems since the word "naturopathy" was copyrighted. "Thus Macfadden called his system Physcultopathy; Lindlahr called his Natural Therapeutics; a man in the Northwest called his system Sanipractic, etc." (1949, 88).

Whatever the exact truth about its origin, Lust credited the term "naturopathy" with the successful squelching of the Benzecry libel suit and with helping bring an end to the persecution.

> The prosecution became so intense that we could not use the words cure, healing, therapy, therapist, physician, doctor, or any other similar title. We were all in despair. Finally we decided to use the word 'Naturopath' as being the only safe term by which we could designate ourselves as having to do with nature cure and disease. By this term we did not hold ourselves out as practi-

> tioners. In one year we had more than fifty arrests. The word "Naturopath" was the magic word that set us free. Although being a misnomer, it covered the subject. It has come to stay as a living protest against the autocracy, coercion, imposition, intolerance, and persecution of the New York Medical Society Trust in particular, and the American Medical Association Trust in general (1921, 479).

The term "naturopathy" has been criticized on two grounds. First, it is a misnomer, translating from its roots to "natural disease" rather than "natural healing," its intended meaning. It might be for this reason that Henry Lindlahr never used this term in his writings and preferred "nature cure" and "natural therapeutics," the equivalent of the German "Naturheilkunde." Second, the term is considered poor coinage because it combines a Latin root (nature) with a Greek root (pathos). Lust defended its "bastard Graeco-Latin birth" (1903, 206) by making a virtue of its fault:

> Naturopathy is a hybrid word. It is purposely so. No single tongue could distinguish a system whose origin, scope, and purpose is universal-broad as the world, deep as love, high as heaven (1902, 32).

In 1948, Harry Riley Spitler, Dean of the Central College of Physiatrics in Eaton, Ohio, still deplored the choice of the term in *Basic Naturopathy*, a textbook published by the American Naturopathic Association. He preferred the more correct term "physiatrics," but admitted: "It is now too late for the profession to change its name because long usage — fifty-five years — makes it to be an impossibility."

Lust was a skillful practitioner, and it was said that he could apply water in a thousand different ways. The early volumes of his journal are filled with articles on hydrotherapy, many from his own pen; others were translations from the writings of Kneipp and his successors. No other water application captured Lust's fancy more than "the blood-washing method," a shower bath constructed and patented by a Dr. Christos Parasco. This sophisticated detoxifying shower was taken in eight hour units for 20 to 30 days. Parasco and Lust promoted this "Ultimate Bath" in the pamphlet with the ponderous title *The Apocalypsis of Physical Immortality* in which Lust testified to its effects:

> I have had personal experience with practically every form of water cure known to mankind; and I can say without qualification that there is nothing in any way comparable to this treatment. I am not exaggerating a bit when I say that it made me, a man of sixty, feel twenty-five years younger by the time I had

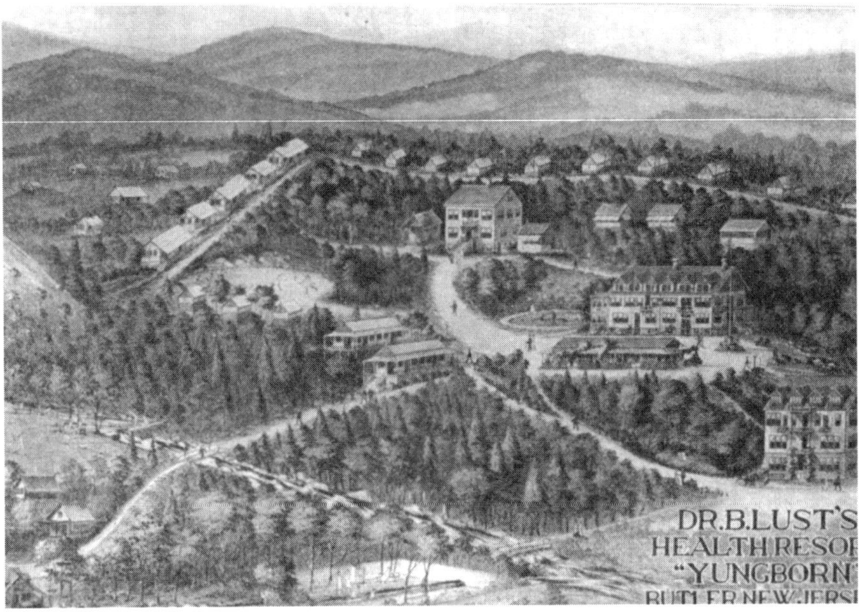

Yungborn, Butler, New Jersey
(Lust 1918, 795 *Universal Naturopathic Encyclopedia*)

taken three of those eight hour units which Parasco recommended (1923,18).

This reveals an important characteristic of Lust as a chief spokesman for naturopathy. His exuberant enthusiasm for a new healing method or fad sometimes interfered with his ability to evaluate something critically and to sift the wheat from the chaff.

One of Lust's first accomplishments upon arrival in America was to cure his brother, Louis, of typhoid fever. He did so in a matter of two weeks, "chiefly by means of a watering-can and his knowledge of the Kneipp cure."

> It is no easy matter to cure one's own brother of anything—and this brother had been given up to die by all the local doctors (Purinton 1914, 279).

Louis, under the influence of Benedict, opened a health food bakery, and with a fleet of trucks he delivered fresh-baked whole-grain products all over New York City.

It was not as a practitioner, however, but as an educator, promoter and organizer of naturopathy that Lust had his greatest impact. He believed that "the human body was created to be perfect—to be well at all times," and that within each person was "a certain mysterious power which regulates his health and strength" (1944,8). Lust seems not to have been familiar with the term *vis medicatrix maturae*, or the healing power of nature, as he referred to this force as "natural power." Echoing Kneipp, he wrote:

> Naturopathy, with all its various methods of treatments, has always one end in view and one only: to increase the vital force (1903, 195).

At one point in his career, apparently under the influence of various "New Thought" and theosophical movements, Lust injected a religious dimension into his philosophy.

> Naturopathy agrees with Mental Science, Christian Science, New Thought and other mental pathologies in that all disease is originally thought, but with Physical Culture, Sex Specialism, Dietotherapy, Hydropathy, et al. in that the manifestation is distinctly material . . .
>
> Naturopathy comes from the heart of Nature through the heart of man to the heart of God. Deopathy would perhaps be a truer name, save that Nature is, and must be, the starting-point for the weary, weak, diseased, discouraged, chronic invalid (1903, 165-166).

Lust was sincerely idealistic and his youthful enthusiasm often went to over-exuberance. He originally named his college "The Naturopathic School of Regeneration" and gave it the motto: "We Stand for Humanity." (1902, 33). He once referred to the "Naturopathic gospel of love" in describing his efforts to promote altruism in daily life. However, the sound core of his philosophy survived the comings and goings of these excesses and kept him and the profession in good stead.

One zealous aspect of Lust's philosophy which remained constant throughout his career was his insistence on the necessity of changing people's lives through naturopathy. "It depends on the revolution of one's daily life," he wrote, "and the regeneration of his thought habits" (1903, 165). He believed naturopathy's purpose was "to reach and transform and transfigure everyday lives" (1905, 319).

In 1903, he stated, "Naturopathy believes in Pathological Monism and Therapeutic Universalism" (165). By this he meant that all diseases arose from violation of nature's laws and that all of nature's agents could be used to correct disease. He insisted on a multilateral approach to natural healing. He was the "sole official representative for America of all the great Naturist movements in Europe-such as those of Kneipp, Bilz, Lahmann, Rikli, Just" (Purinton 1905, 253).

From first-hand experience he understood the merits and limits of each approach. "Each factor," he wrote, "was one-sided—ever exclusive—in its development" (1905, 97). His contribution was to combine these one-sided approaches into a single coherent system. He defined naturopathy as "a distinct school of healing, employing the beneficent agency of Nature's forces, of water, air, sunlight, earthpower, electricity, magnetism, exercise, rest, proper diet, various kinds of mechanical treatments, such as massage, osteopathy, and chiropractic, mental and moral science." This was not just to claim as much territory as possible, but rather to offer a more efficacious system. "As none of these agents of rejuvenation can cure every disease," he wrote, "the Naturopath rightly employs the combination that is best adapted to each individual case" (1918, 1175). "If he really understands how to individualize and administer the nature cure methods in every case . . . " he promised, "then cures are the result and the practitioner has no competition, especially not from the medical cult nor from other single track practitioners" (1925, 368). It was Lust's genius to assemble these various methods and promote them as a single naturopathic package. He proclaimed:

> Naturopathy is the mother, all-inclusive, of natural therapy. It is the basic platform for all methods of healing; without it any healing art will be a failure (ibid.)

Lust's "therapeutic universalism" also had its disadvantages. The student of naturopathy was burdened with the demanding task of becoming a jack of all healing methods with the possible result that he did not become a true master in any one. This universalism could have caused naturopathy to perish with Lust's death, due to the impression that it was his charisma, and not a special method, that was the unifying principle behind the profession. Chiropractic didn't suffer the same decline after its founder's death because his method was so easily identifiable to the public's eye. Homeopaths, acupuncturists, herbalists or nutritionists can practice under the "universalist" label ND (Naturopathic Doctor), so the public has difficulty forming a distinct picture of the naturopathic profession.

Nowhere was Lust's commitment to an eclectic integrated practice of naturopathic methods more evident than in the health sanatoriums he established in New Jersey and Florida. One of his first acts upon returning to America in 1896, under Father Kneipp's commission, was the founding of a natural health retreat in the Ramapo Mountains near Butler, New Jersey. He eventually called this the Yungborn in honor of Just's sanatorium in Germany, one of his models. He considered the Butler Yungborn to be "the

American reproduction of, and improvement on, the original Kneipp Cure in Germany" (Purinton 1914, 279). Lust started out modestly but made gradual improvements over the years. The first building was a crude hut of live tree branches with a roof made of store boxes. By 1908 he announced the opening of an elaborate new building "fitted up with a large sun parlor so that sun and air baths can be indulged in even in the coldest weather" (Lust 1908, 288).

Lust was not the only naturopathic physician who established a German-style nature cure institution. Around the turn of the century, other pioneers, most of them also of German origin, founded similar institutions. While the earliest institutions used mainly German nature cure methods, the later ones broadened their scope and added massage, Swedish movements, osteopathy, chiropractic, electrotherapy, physical culture and other naturopathic modalities. None of these establishments, however, gained the same fame and endured as did Lust's Yungborn.

The Butler Yungborn was jointly owned by Lust and his wife Louisa, a naturopathic physician practicing in Butler when she met him. A one-hour train ride from New York City, the spa was situated on "sixty acres of forest and fruit, of hill and dale, of glorious foliage" (Shaw 1911, 145). It accommodated 100 guests at a time and often operated at full capacity. Some locals opposed the Yungborn. Half a century later one old-timer reminisced about how, as a boy, he peeked through the fence of the Yungborn to watch nude women bathing in the brook (O'Brien 1978, 1).

Descriptions of the Butler Yungborn are invariably given in idyllic superlatives. Austin Shaw considered it the best of the American health homes and described it as an "Eden Spot" where one would "let Dame Nature make you new again." Guests who lived in air cottages or tent colonies would rise at 5 in the morning for a day of walks, sports, lectures, mud baths, vegetarian meals, health naps, stream plunges and sun bathing, garbed in nature's apparel only. They retired at 9 p.m. Men's and women's sections were separate. No meat, tobacco, or contagious diseases were allowed. One guest wrote that after a week or two of this regimen, "You feel so comfortable that you want to shout in your ecstasy" (Shaw 1911, 146).

Even allowing for the probable exaggeration in these exuberant accounts, the Butler Yungborn was no doubt an exceptional health retreat. Thousands of early twentieth-century city dwellers chose to spend their "health" vacations there. Charges were $2.50 per day, $16 per week, and $60 per month. The patients received good natural health care but were not pampered. Lust retained no nurses at the Yungborn and didn't allow wealthy guests to bring their own.

> A nurse adds to your sense of weakness, helplessness, and irresponsibility. And the whole idea of the Nature Cure is to make the invalid responsible to himself for every thought, act, and emotion of his life (Purinton 1914, 282).

In 1908 Lust scored something of a national public-relations coup when the Chinese Imperial ambassador to Washington, Wu Ting Fang, who cured his own sciatica by giving up meat, liquor, tea, and coffee, expressed "a great desire to come and look over" the Butler Yungborn. The ambassador was received at the sanatorium with due pomp. As an anonymous writer recorded with a simple, almost poetic expression.

> Great was the interest of Wu Ting Fang when the technique and application of the clay baths were demonstrated. Several of the patients were introduced to him, and in a charming way, full of sympathy and appreciation, the conversation was briskly kept up (Anonymous 1908, 288).

At the end of his stay, the ambassador said he felt 20 years younger and expressed his expectation to live to be 200.

Lust, licensed to practice in Florida in 1914, also conducted a Yungborn at Tangerine, Florida called Qui-si-sana. He established it in 1913 after an expensive search for the ideal location in the ideal climate. Located in Western Orange County at 300 feet above sea level, it sat at the highest point in the state "amidst beautiful pine woods, orange groves, and fine voids, lakes, and springs." Described as a "commodious caravansary on the shores of Lake Ola," it contained two solaria, one for men and one for women, and Its motto was "In the sun, life is won" (Bradshaw 1918, 884-890). Fire destroyed it in April, 1943, marking the beginning of the end of Lust's career and life. Lust also established a Natural Life Colony at Palm City near Nuevitas in Cuba.

Just as Lust's local successes drew the unwelcome attention of the New York County medical authorities, so invited his national successes the scrutiny of the American Medical Association. Morris Fishbein, editor of the prestigious *Journal of the American Medical Association* attacked Lust and his methods with alacrity. Fishbein was a formidable polemicist who liked to refer to Lust as a "minor prophet of healing" and "one of the kingpins of the naturopathic cult" (Fishbein 1932, 122, 133). His favored characterizations of naturopathy were that it was crazy, having "embraced every strange system of healing that has come across the American horizon," and greedy, representing the "capitalization for purposes of financial gain of the old advice that outdoor life, good diet, enough exercise, and rest are conducive to health and longevity" (121, 126). He liked to portray Lust and Lindlahr as gold-digging frauds who bastardized an otherwise worthy tradition, and invoked the memory of the movement's founders, long-since dead and safely buried on another continent.

The real naturopaths were, of course, such healers as Father Kneipp, Priessnitz, and others who advocated natural healing and healed by the use of sunlight, baths, fresh air and cold water.

This sounded like a ringing endorsement of naturopathic principles by the AMA, but then Fishbein continued:

> But there is little money to be made by these methods. Hence the modern naturopath embraces every form of healing that offers opportunity for exploitation. Thus, there have grown from naturopathy a myriad of peculiar doctrines which run the gamut from aeropathy to zonotherapy (125).

Lust proved a worthy antagonist to Fishbein, being himself a natural polemicist and an eager fighter who thrived on conflict. After four decades of struggle against the medical establishment he would write:

> As long as I can fight, I will fight and stay younger and younger. After each fight I have better health (1935, 250).

He responded to the attacks from Fishbein and the medical authorities in two basic ways. First, he readily acknowledged that there were quacks in the naturopathic movement. He liked to call them "Pseudo-Naturopaths."

> New York City is this moment at the mercy of some of the worst abortioners of Naturopathy that ever disgraced a mushroom by a likeness to its growth (1902, 169-171).

He railed against the "outright fakers and cheats masking as Naturopaths" and added woefully:

> That is the fate of any science—any profession—which the unjust laws have placed beyond the pale. Where there is no official recognition and regulation, you will find the plotters, the thieves, the charlatans operating on the same basis as the conscientious practitioners. And these riff-raff opportunists bring the whole art into disrepute. Frankly such conditions cannot be remedied until suitable safeguards are erected by law, or by the profession itself, around the practice of Naturopathy (Wendel 1951, 41)

He fought a dual battle against orthodox medicine on one hand and illegitimate naturopathy on the other. "The worst enemy of Naturopathy," he wrote toward the end of his career, "is the Naturopath—those without character, dedication, fairness" (1935, 251). To him the ideal naturopathic doctor was not a sectarian but rather an eclectic who studied "every new philosophy and practice that appears, whether he finds it in the confines of Naturopathic teachings or otherwise" (1938, 291). He was "intuitionally a physician" who devoted his life "to teaching ideal living more than curing needless ills" (1902, 171), and he considered the ideal naturopaths on a mission of service as "ministers of God, of nature and of man" (1937, 303). For this the naturopath must be endowed with two things "in large measure—knowledge and love." While Lust's description of the purpose of the naturopath as "not the wrenching of a paltry fee from a trembling patient, but the loving into wholeness of a triumphant brother" may be a little excessive, it's a sufficient answer to Fishbein's charges of unbridled greed (1902, 170).

Lust's second response to assaults against him by organized medicine was the counter-attack, at which he excelled. Before aiming his barbs, Lust always took care to distinguish between "the regular, clean medical man, especially the old-time family doctor who was a friend to all" and "the devilish, hellish political doctor" for whom "we sharpen our axe" (1938, 266).

With this qualification established, Lust was ready to do battle. An energetic writer, he was in his element when stringing together a series of epithets against the orthodox medical "trust" which he held in undisguised contempt:

> There never was a cult, a religion, a political party, a government, a king, a soviet or an institution so narrow, so egotistic, criminal, materialistic and selfish as the medical trust. All the other cults, such as homeopaths, eclectics, osteopaths, chiropractic, etc., are absolutely harmless and should all be left severely alone. Naturopathy is the only system of healing that is not a cult, not a fanatical narrow creed, nor a system of control by one man, one school or group; it is the science of nature . . . . All the cults, even the regular medical cult, are off-shoots from the old nature cure that started in the Garden of Eden. In the future we will have only MDs and NDs. All the other systems, if they are biologically correct, must belong to naturopathy or nature cure; and if contrary to nature, superstitious, dangerous, criminal in their practices and results, they are sure to belong to regular medicine—regular licensed quackery (1925, 366).

One writer claimed Lust had a thick German accent which made him hard to understand (O'Brien 1979, 12), but this is warmly disputed by Lust's niece, who as a young girl enjoyed weekly visits from her "Uncle Ben" (Proctor 1991). Whatever the case, Lust appears to have been an effective public speaker. At public lectures he was often challenged by orthodox medical doctors, and he relished the hot debates which ensued. In one case a Dr. Apfil, who claimed syphilis was harmless and perfectly curable by mercury, was driven from the hall by Lust's pointed rejoinders.

Lust cast his counter-attacks in terms of medical freedom, which was as big an issue during his time as it is today. In June 1920, he nominated his long-time ally Dr. Frederick W. Collins for President of the United States on a platform adopted by the Constitutional Liberty League of Philadelphia. Its libertarian platform denounced the increasing curtailment of citizens' rights by the federal government and opposed "compulsory vaccination and all similar assaults upon the health and privacy of person."

Lust was a populist whose views were sometimes suffused with radical perceptions. "Medical laws are all class laws and unconstitutional," he wrote.

> Without free competition in the art of healing, the American people will be deprived of their unalienable rights under the constitution to select the method and the doctor of their choice and to have the best in the prevention and cure of disease (1919, 440).

He was not above injecting patriotism into his arguments. Indeed, he sincerely believed that the "medical trust" was subverting the health and strength of the nation. He labeled it "un-American" a decade before that term became a watchword of American politics (1938, 33).

> The medical machine in this country is the greatest curse ever visited on America. It is interested in keeping the people sick by undermining their health by vaccination and other medical superstitions and crimes. Eventually the plans of the medical trust will cause widespread damage to the American people if they are not checked. Only nature cure can bring health, happiness, and long life (1935, 322).

Lust was ahead of his time in his concern for patient rights. He criticized the hospitals of his day "where the feelings of the patient are never considered," and the attitude at the teaching hospital which was "lie down and die that we may observe the process." His prediction that "a century from now, the 'regular' therapeutic methods of today will be seen as barbarous as blood-letting and Voodoo-craft appear to us," may prove to be hauntingly true (1909, 87-88). Lust's "new conception of health" was embodied in three terms: "People's health, People's doctors, People's health institutions." The naturopathic doctor would practice in a "modern people's hospital" where patients would be free from harmful medicines and unnecessary operations. Lust anticipated by decades the growing importance of prevention in health care. "The hospital of the future," would be a place where "the inmates will not only increase their power of life and come back to normal but where they will also learn how they can regulate their lives in the future so as not to become ill again" (1938, 266).

Although Lust remained a lifelong enemy of what he regarded as the medical trust, he never became personally embittered by the relentless persecution which cost him tens of thousands of dollars in fines and bail and countless hours in court and jail suffered at its hands. He accepted it quite matter-of-factly, "The prosecution and persecution is part of our life as naturopaths" (1935, 227).

Besides establishing and popularizing naturopathy in the United States, Lust must be credited with four other accomplishments. On March 1, 1901, he founded the American School of Naturopathy. Located at 124 East 59th Street in New York City, it was the first institution in America to offer personal instruction in naturopathy. The school taught every branch of Nature Cure in a two-year general course. Advanced and Post Graduate courses were also offered along with special summer instruction at the Yungborn sanatorium in New Jersey. When the school acquired a charter in 1905, it conferred the degree of Doctor of Naturopathy on Lust. Lust had already graduated from the Universal Osteopathic College in 1898, received his medical degree at the New York Homeopathic College in 1902, and garnered an Eclectic Medical degree from the Eclectic Medical College in New York in 1913. He was licensed as an M.D. in Florida in 1914. When the school later moved to West 76th Street, it was sued by a New York State Senator who lived nearby because it attracted persons "undesirable to the exclusive residential district." It was also the source of "unseemly noises" (Anonymous 1924, 8).

At first, Lust used only Kneipp's books as texts. Later the school's program would be expanded to four years. Its curriculum was modernized to include basic sciences, physiotherapy, phytotherapy, geotherapy, electrotherapy, mechanotherapy. Degrees in naturopathy and chiropractic were granted. At least one source claimed that the school held high academic standards and counted PhDs from Columbia University on its faculty (O'Brien 1978, 19). One source claimed that Lust helped train 8,000 practicing naturopaths by 1924 (Anonymous 1924, 766). In 1927, investigators of the Council on Medical Education and Hospitals of the American Medical Association inspected "Schools of Chiropractic and of Naturopathy in the

United States," among them the American School of Naturopathy and the American School of Chiropractic.

> This school, known by the two names given above, is the famous (?) institution founded by Benedict Lust, N.D., D. O., D.C., M.D., and is now a night school only. It is located in an old apartment house at 236 East Thirty-Fifth Street, New York, where it makes use of two floors and a portion of the third. It has two small lecture rooms each containing about a dozen chairs, a very small demonstration room containing a McMannis osteopathic table, a small clinic room into which five chiropractic adjusting tables have been crowded, and a little chemical laboratory with one table (offering room for two or three students) . . . . Quite a number of chiropractic adjusting tables were said to be stored—evidence of the balmier days that once were known.
>
> There were said to be twenty students at present. Fifteen were graduated last year. The school does not publish a catalogue: it is too expensive. A four-year course is offered, covering nine months of the year, the classes being in session from 7 to 10:30 p.m. . . .
>
> The tuition is $250 annually. Textbooks and other supplies are offered to students at discounts; Lust has a book store at his business and publishing office, 124 East Forty-First Street.
>
> Benedict Lust is the great national organizer of naturopathy. He is now in Florida and the inspector did not meet him personally, but his school is a very sorry looking affair. Aside from the giving of chiropractic adjustments the instruction must be almost altogether didactic. The dean, whose name is Sinai Gershanek, is deaf, nervous and thick-headed (1928, 1738).

The *Journal of the American Medical Association* had to retract the statement that the Dean is thick-headed.

> Mr. Gershanek properly takes exception to that portion of the statement which says that he is thick-headed. *The Journal* wishes to apologize for the publication of this statement (JAMA 91 (Sept.1928:654).

The school was closed in 1942. However, Lust had established the New York School of Massage and Training School for Physiotherapy, which he operated until his death. He also offered naturopathic home study and post-graduate courses through his journal.

Lust seemed to understand that his school was at best of regional importance. One of his unrealized goals was a nationally recognized college of naturopathy. "Naturopathy will never meet the American people on a fair footing," he wrote, "until there is a great college organized and legalized, whose diploma will distinguish its possessor from the crowd of copyists now imposing on the ignorance of the public" (1902, 171). A decade after his death such a school was founded but it was decades more before it would achieve the status he envisioned.

Lust's second important accomplishment was the founding of the American Naturopathic Association (ANA). Although Lust liked to date the start of this and most of his other endeavors from 1896, the ANA came into existence in 1902 as the Naturopathic Society of America after Lust had achieved sufficient distance from the Kneipp Societies. It was reorganized due to insolvency on December, 1919, as the ANA, and eventually incorporated 18 additional constituent state organizations.

The ANA was the first professional organization of naturopathic physicians. It played a vital role in unifying the profession in the face of many difficult circumstances. Its annual conventions held variously in New York, Cleveland, Philadelphia, Chicago, Minneapolis, Denver, Portland (Oregon) and Milwaukee grew to become impressive affairs. The 1922 convention was held in Washington, D.C., where Lust was permitted to lay a wreath at the tomb of George Washington in Mt. Vernon, "an honor extended only to great dignitaries" (Mock 1923, 442). As Lust recalled years later:

> The officers and delegates of the ANA were received by President Harding. Mrs. Harding was cured, at that time, by a Naturopath after the medical doctors had given her up. At that time the medical persecution went wild (Lust 1942).

The U.S. Post Office withdrew second class mail privileges for Lust's naturopathic publications, ruling that they were "a danger to the public health" and were of "no educational value." Outraged, Lust threatened to "go straight to the White House," and the postal service quickly reversed itself (1942, 199).

The ANA was primarily a vehicle for Lust's prodigious organizational energies to advance the profession. Wardwell states that Lust was its "president until 1921" (1992, 37), but in that year he was elected president-for-life and continued to head the organization for the next twenty-four years. As he could say in an address to the members of the ANA without self-righteousness or self-importance, "For thirty years I have personally carried the naturopathic movement on my shoulders" (1925, 673). However, a number of capable doctors assumed responsible positions in the state and national associations, greatly strengthening the organization. Their efforts, combined with Lust's and the general membership gave the early profession a valuable sense of identity as well as the political wherewithal to establish legal protection for their practice of naturopathic medicine.

The ANA foundered after Lust's death in 1945 due to regional factionalism. The introduction and popularity of "miracle drugs" and technological medicine after World War II are often cited as the main reason for the decline of naturopathy. But these unfavorable conditions were made worse by the in-fighting within the profession which accelerated its decline. The following report in one of the naturopathic journals shows how difficult it was to unite the profession:

> Dr. Henry Schlichting reports that the Unification Convention held in St. Louis, Mo. by the two ANA's resulted in amalgamation of both groups . . . . Dr. Paul Wendel, President of the Eastern ANA has just informed us that amalgamation did not take place in St. Louis . . . . Previous to the St. Louis convention, Dr. J. Gehmann issued a folder addressed to the profession at large stating, among other things, that he was still President of the ANA (Parent Body), and that the "Parent Body" was not holding their convention in St. Louis.
>
> All this is very confusing, to say the least. According to our summation, it seems that we still have three ANA's (*Journal of Naturopathic Medicine* Sept. 1950, 20).

At one time there were six naturopathic associations which claimed to represent the profession. According to George Floden, President of the Sierra States University College of Naturopathy in Los Angeles, the split did not come about suddenly but had begun during Lust's lifetime. He gave the following account of the events which led to the demise of the organization which Lust had founded 40 years earlier:

> It was not a quarrel over principles but rather between personalities. The constitution and by-laws of the ANA were filed in Washington, D.C. 1919, and in 1935 Dr. Robert V. Carroll, asked by Dr. Lust, wrote a new constitution and by-laws which were duly signed and accepted by the ANA board of directors at an annual convention in Omaha, Nebraska. But here is where various individuals' lust for power took such proportions that in the year 1942 an open split occurred. The "rebels," later known as the "Western Group," and headed by Drs. Dugdale, Carroll and Schlichting held their convention in Chicago, while the original

> ANA met in Atlantic City, N.J., headed by Drs. Lust and Schippell. It is indeed strange to note that both parties claimed to be "the original ANA" Shameful attacks and accusations did much to destroy the faith in Naturopathy which Dr. Lust had built to great proportions, not only as a profession but also in public esteem. The fight over who could lay claim to "the original" was carried into the courts, but finally a disgusted judge threw it out of court. Efforts were made to mend the breach, and would perhaps have been fruitful, but after the passing of Dr. Lust it became obvious that amalgamation was an impossibility. There were good naturopaths in both camps, but each had its "hot-heads" and sheer stubbornness without acceptable reasoning ended the efforts for some time to come (1964, 2).

Floden was not entirely correct when he stated that "it was not a quarrel about principles but rather between personalities." It was also a conflict between traditionalists and modernists which still flares up in the corridors of the naturopathic colleges today when some students criticize their training as too medically oriented. Dr. Jesse Mercer Gehmann, Lust's successor as the president of the Eastern ANA, expressed the anti-medical view at the Golden Jubilee Congress in New York, July 27 to August 2, 1947.

> We need standards and we need more, to stand by them, once they are established . . . . These standards should insist upon a thorough training in basic Nature Cure. All students should be required to be thoroughly competent in applying the methods of the old Masters and should be taught the fundamental principles and discoveries of Drs. Bechamp and Powell, Trall and Lindlahr, as opposed to the dangerous semi-acceptance of the germ disease theory advanced by Pasteur and the theory of Phagocytosis which fits into it and was advanced by Eli Metchnikoff. Neither Pasteur or the Metchnikoff theory can be accepted by the true understanding naturopath.
>
> Our standards should include thorough training through study of Kneipp, Priessnitz, Just, Kuhne, Rikli, Trall, Schroth, Graham, Jennings, Lust and Macfadden.
>
> We need adequate standards for entrance upon training for a Doctorate in Naturopathy, but these standards need NOT be, nor should they be patterned after the medical requirements. Our work is not based on a warped and decadent pathology, bacteriology, or biology (cited in Freibott 1990, 7).

Gehmann and his entourage liked to refer to the Western group, which tried to raise naturopathic standards by imitating conventional medicine in education and research, as "pseudo-group" or "pseudo-medical group." Dr. Robert V. Carroll, the President of the Western group, expressed his opposite view in a 1948 editorial.

> The writer recently received a letter from a good Naturopath in which he suggested our type of Naturopathy was not desired by good Naturopaths. We appreciated that criticism and began to take stock of ourselves. Lindlahr laid down some good rules to the approach to disease. One of them was hereditary soil, which is difficult to observe. The many "wonder" drugs that have come and gone have left their marks in the human body. The old "water cure" upsets the patient pretty badly in a healing crisis in unloading these suppressive drugs. So it is to prove the old unstable and find new ways, Naturopathically, to remove the bad effects of Preventative medicine as well as suppressive drugs, that we work towards.
>
> We say this because we want to eliminate any *fads* and *fancies*, if there be such, from Naturopathy and prove same to the entire field through Scientific Naturopathic Research . . . . We must quit bickering over "penny-ante" matters and learn to respect each other in one progressive, co-operative organization for Naturopathy (Carroll 1948, 3).

The two camps developed their own textbooks which showed their different point of view: Paul Wendel's *Standardized Naturopathy* (1951) and Harry Riley Spitler's *Basic Naturopathy* (1948). An echo of this conflict could still be heard thirty years later when Dr. William A. Turska condemned the "narrow-path and simplistic" approach of Wendel and others that defined naturopathy as "a therapeutic system which does not use drugs but employs natural forces such as light, heat, air, water and massage," a definition still found in the 1989 edition of *Taber's Cyclopedic Medical Dictionary.* Turska argued, "all therapeutic agents are drugs, good drugs can become bad drugs and bad, good, it's all in how you use them" (Jayne 1990, 3). In his opinion "drugless" did not properly describe the philosophy of the practitioners of constitutional therapy.

> At the turn of the century, Henry Lindlahr, M. D., established a school in Chicago patterned after Dr. Benedict Lust's naturopathic institution founded in New York in 1896. The curricula and disciplines of these were truly constitutional therapy. Lindlahr

> was looking for a distinctive rather than a descriptive name for constitutional therapy. He stumbled on "National College of Drugless Physicians" and the fiction was started. However, general acceptance of the term "drugless" was never achieved, not even among constitutional practitioners. To the average citizen, "drugless physician" has an unprofessional connotation, conjuring up images of herbalists, health farms, nudist camps, Swedish massage, the towel and bucket brigade, colonic houses, bathhouse rubbers and the like. Almost never does he equate the term with a Doctor of Medicine . . . .
>
> Our conclusion is this: No practitioner of constitutional medicine or any of its branches, who uses biological substances and procedures in the restoration and maintenance of normal body chemistry is a "drugless" physician. If he prescribes only orange juice and/or water, he is not a "drugless" physician because both contain drugs within the broadest definition of the word (Turska, 1976, 5).

Turska insisted on including the word "medicine," which had a bad connotation for the old-school naturopaths, to describe the naturopathic profession. Dr. Turska's view prevailed in Oregon when in March, 1993, the Senate there passed a bill that changed the term "naturopathy" to "Naturopathic medicine," and removed the word "drugless" from the practice act (Campbell 1993, 4). Although the "pseudo-medical" naturopaths seemed to have won the battle, the great naturopathic physicians like Lust, Lindlahr, Turska and Bastyr have always been above such ideological controversies. They were neither narrow-minded dogmatists who only looked back to the past nor did they uncritically embrace every new fad in medical science and nutrition. They used the best from the past and the present and from different schools of medicine; whatever would enhance the patient's own natural healing power.

The split within the ANA darkened Lust's last two years of life. He expressed his distress in a moving letter, written to Dr. Paul Wendel, author of *Father Kneipp's Health Teachings* (1947), on February 16th, 1945, six months before his death (Freibott 1990, exhibit F). This letter also shows how much Lust still felt that he was Kneipp's heir.

> My dear Dr. Wendel:
>
> Thank you for your letter of February 8th.
>
> Charlie wrote me that the lectures were well attended and everybody was pleased. I always said you were a natural born Naturopath. Regarding our talk, I want you to undertake to write

Father Kneipp's Health Teachings and books on Naturopathy, as you are the only one I know that was raised on Father Kneipp's teachings and natural healing. Your father was my friend and fellow Naturopath. We both fought for natural healing.

Dr. Wendel: I hereby give you full permission and authority to copy and use any of my books on Father Kneipp or any articles in *Naturopath, Nature Path Magazines* or *Kneipp Blatters,* without payment and I hereby give you the same commission Father Kneipp gave me in 1892 to spread his teachings and water cure, which I began in 1896. This is my right and I give it to you to take effect after my death. You are to pass it along to some worthy Naturopath when you lay down your work.

I do not know if I will live to see the 50th Golden Jubilee Congress (which I hope I will do) but if I do not, I want you to ask the Congress to elect Dr. Frederick Collins of Newark, N.J. as he fought for Naturopathy and stood side by side when trouble came.

If Dr. Collins declines then I would like to see you take my place as you know the ups and downs in Naturopathy. I also want you to stand by Dr. Schippell, as you know she spent her time and money and did much for Naturopathy and deserves consideration at the 50th Golden Jubilee.

I hope you will be able to get all groups together into one Naturopathic Association, as I cannot understand why the group wants to cause a split as my struggles and sacrifices have been great, and my efforts in establishing a profession for the Nature doctors has been a sad disappointment to me. I hope and pray you succeed in your efforts. May the spirit of Father Kneipp guide you in your work to which you have my blessing and good wishes.

Sincerely yours,
Dr. B. Lust

Paul Wendel's father was Dr. Hugo Wendel (1857-1929) who taught Kneipp water cure for Dr. Lust. Paul Wendel became President of the Eastern ANA, but neither he nor Theresa M. Schippell nor Otis C. Carroll, who strived for the amalgamation of the two groups, succeeded in their efforts to fulfill Dr. Lust's last will to keep the profession unified. When Dr. Wendel died on December 21, 1956, he was hailed as "the clarion of Naturopathy."

"With his passing, Naturopathy, in both its spiritual as well as material sense, lost one of its most gallant warriors—for its

> cause, for its principles, yes, for its very survival" (*Journal of Naturopathy*, January 1957, 27).

The editorials of the naturopathic journals in the years after Lust's death were filled with urgent pleas for unity. In 1949, the President of the Western ANA, Dr. Henry Schlichting, Jr., sent out the following appeal:

> I am convinced that the leaders and thinkers in the profession realize that this is a *must* for our survival and progress. Naturopathy has truly reached the crossroads. The crisis is here. It is *now* or *never*—*do* or *die*—one for *all* and *all* for *one*. In Unity is strength! Too long have we as a profession been rugged individualists. We must learn to become ORGANIZED and work through organized channels (1949 (7), 5).

And Mario T. Campanella, the President of the International Society of Naturopathic Physicians, echoed the same when he wrote in 1952:

> The bigotry, intolerance and general rivalry that has increasingly manifested itself in recent years should be exploded once and for all—leaving no hatred or obstacles to progress . . . .
>
> The greatest danger to naturopathy lies in ourselves—not in the opposition. The profession has been aroused to the ever-increasing necessity for unity of purpose. Until we do just that we will not accomplish anything to speak of (4).

Not until 1980 when the American Association of Naturopathic Physicians was founded was the profession unified enough to start an organization like Lust's ANA which could speak for the large majority of naturopathic physicians.

It is difficult to separate the success of Lust's organizations from that of his publications. The Kneipp Societies were served by the *Kneipp Water Cure Monthly*; and the Naturopathic Societies were served by *The Naturopath and Herald of Health*, which became the official publication of the American Naturopathic Association. Later *Nature's Path*, a popular magazine for the lay population, was also published. For the most part Lust was the editor and chief writer of these magazines, although he did turn the editorship of *The Naturopath and Herald of Health* over to Edwin Earle Purinton temporarily in 1902 so that he could pursue a medical degree. These journals articulated Lust's philosophy, educated readers about naturopathy, gave instructions about treatment methods for various conditions, exhorted members to renewed dedication of action, and gave state-by-state news on legal developments concerning naturopathy. The magazines also promoted Lust's school, practice, and books. They did much to keep the naturopathic profession before the American public and constituted one of Lust's major accomplishments. They provide the best records we have on the naturopathic movement for the first half of this century.

Lust was successful in his publishing just as he was in most of his endeavors. The first issue of *Nature's Path* in 1925 sold 50,000 copies. Later he extended his media success into the airwaves with his "Dr. Benedict Lust's Radio Health Talks" on WLT, otherwise known as "The Air School of Naturopathy." But just as important as these media successes were Lust's contributions of translating, publishing, and promoting the works of Kneipp, Kuhne, Just and Bilz. One work which he could not advertise enough in his magazines was Bilz' *The Natural Method of Healing* (1898), an encyclopedic nature cure compendium the author had published in several languages. Little biographical information is available about F. E. Bilz (1842-1922). One source claimed that he directed the largest sanitarium in the world (Cordingley 1938, 308). The Bilz Sanitarium occupied a great castle in the village of Radebeul near Dresden. The estate of over 300 acres and the spectacular Victorian castle was the gift of a titled patient Bilz cured. Although Lust ranked Bilz on the same level with Kneipp, Kuhne, Just and other naturopathic pioneers, he is not mentioned by German nature cure historians, possibly because his book is mainly a compilation of cases and treatments taken from other nature doctors' writings without his own original methods and thoughts.

In 1918, Lust published the monumental *Universal Naturopathic Encyclopedia, Directory and Buyers' Guide: Yearbook of Drugless Therapy for 1918-19,* a colorful historical record of the state of drugless healing after World War I. This included pictures, manifestos, advertisements, and biographies and directories of drugless physicians, schools and sanatoriums. It listed several hundred publications, including titles in German, which could be mail-ordered from Lust's own Nature Cure Publishing Co. in Butler, New Jersey. Representatives of every kind of drugless school were allowed to present their specialty in the *Yearbook.* There were departments on electro-medicine, neuropathy, dietology, chiropractic, mechanotherapy, osteopathy, phytotherapy, apyrtrophy, physiculture, natural divine healing, astroscopy and phrenology. In Lust's universalist concept the strangest healing systems were admitted as long as they were drugless. Only homeopathy, which plays such an important role in modern naturopathic medicine, was left out. He must not have considered it a drugless therapy. Lust wanted his *Yearbook* to be truly universal with "every Naturopathic practitioner, from the Arctic Circle to the furthest limits of Patagonia, represented" (12). A larger edition was planned for 1920, but the 1918-1919 *Yearbook* has remained the only one of its kind.

The most tangible of Lust's accomplishments was the legal status naturopathy attained as a result of his efforts. The statement that during his career as many as twenty-five to thirty states plus Hawaii accorded naturopathy complete or partial legal recognition is inflated to include such limited provisions as massage laws. But many of the solid naturopathic statutes which endure today in such states as Oregon, Washington and Connecticut can properly be "attributed to the vision and dogged perseverance of one man, Dr. Benedict Lust, who traveled the length and breadth of the land lecturing and organizing state societies, branches" (*Naturopath* 1944, 1).

Given the medico-political climate of America in the twentieth century, licensure for naturopathy was its only hope for survival. Lust was quick to perceive that the medical freedom he and his cohorts sought could only be guaranteed by laws specifically legalizing their practice. Currently only a handful of jurisdictions protect the full practice of naturopathic medicine, and most of them do so with laws passed under Lust's influence. While the legal protection of naturopathic medicine was almost snuffed out in the Eastern U.S. after Lust's death, it survived in the favorable legal climate of the Northwest and is now being transplanted to new jurisdictions. Without Lust's efforts there would be no licensure of naturopathy and without licensure there would be no naturopathic medicine as we know it today in the U.S.

Lust's success in establishing naturopathic medicine in the United States was remarkable, but not all of his goals were realized. Lust recognized the need for a national examining board for naturopathic physicians, but despite his best efforts none was formed before his death.

Like many naturopathic doctors since him, Lust also dreamed of establishing a naturopathic hospital. In 1909 he wrote:

> What this country needs most is a practical demonstration of Naturopathy on a large scale—an institution corresponding to that of Bilz, Kneipp, Lahmann, or Just, where the great masses of people may come and be healed, then go forth and tell their friends. Every large city could easily support a wisely directed Home of Natural Healing.

A skilled fundraiser, Lust pledged $1,000 toward the hospital and exhorted his readers to send in even the most meager contributions:

> We would rather have a hundred $1.00 subscriptions than a single $1,000 offer; because the moral support and mental encouragement of a hundred individuals will advance the work more than anybody's lump of gold possibly could (1909, 88-89).

Nonetheless, this goal remains unrealized to this day.

Lust was a widely-known figure of his day. The impact of his work and fame was confined neither to America nor naturopathy. When air travel was in its infancy, Lust became famous as one of the original "frequent fliers" because of his many trips between New York and Florida to oversee his far-flung interests. Outside the United States, the German government recognized him early in his career with a gold medal "for distinguished services rendered to mankind," transplanting nature cure and drugless methods to the U.S. (1919, 438). The most prestigious German nature cure magazine, *Der Naturarzt,* praised "the organizational talent of the German Dr. B. Lust, a student of Kneipp, who succeeded in unifying the principal groups of drugless practitioners in their fight against their common enemy, the medical trust" (Sommer 1925, 817). Later he was honored by the Nature Cure Association of Great Britain and Ireland for his pioneer work in America (1927, 143).

In the summer of 1926, Lust travelled to Europe to visit his birthplace and the birthplaces of nature cure, Kneipp's Wörishofen, Priessnitz' Gräfenberg and Schroth's Lindewiese. He reported about "Our Trip to the Fatherland" in a delightful series of articles in *The Naturopath* which began with the description of his triumphal welcome as guest of honor in his home town:

> Although I have been away from home for forty years, we never forgot the place of our birth, and the indebtedness to our parents, our village and our fellow citizens . . . .
>
> During the war the people in our home town suffered much distress and destitution was great. We did all we could and so did my departed wife, Mrs. Louisa Lust, by helping the institutions, the orphans, the church, and especially by replacing the chimes of the church steeple which were removed during the war for making cannons. After leaving the R. R. Station which is two miles from the village, the auto stopped about two thirds of the way and we saw a big crowd of people along the road in the meadows. The President of one of the village societies came up and presented us with a beautiful bouquet of flowers and made a fine speech of welcome to the "Heimat." When he stopped speaking, the chimes

> of the church steeple began ringing, the music band played, and the parade began to move. With the different societies in front of the car and all the school children of the town behind the car, it was a joy to see all the children barefooted, clean and happy. Our reception in the old town was certainly a great surprise. The natives threw flowers in the auto from every side. We were received by authorities such as the mayor, the Board of Aldermen, the teachers, the priest, the Sisters of the Mercy and the rest of the town (Lust 1916, 580).

Lust was not alone in his struggle to establish naturopathy as a recognized branch of drugless healing. He gained allies and friends and forged alliances with other camps such as chiropractic, physical culture and diet reformers. He was a tireless traveler, criss-crossed the United States several times on speaking tours and in defense of beleaguered colleagues in courts or legislative battles. One of his important allies in the West was Carl Schultz, the "Benedict Lust" of the West and the "Father of Naturopathy" in California.

Dr. Carl Schultz (1849-1935) studied medicine, homeopathy and nature cure in Germany before he came to California in 1885 after losing his wife and fortune in Germany. In 1901, Schultz organized the Association of Naturopathic Physicians of California which was incorporated on August 8, 1904. He was its secretary and president for many years. In 1905, he opened the Naturopathic Institute and Sanitarium of California at 1319 South Grand Avenue, Los Angeles, and later organized the Naturopathic College of California at 556-560 South Hope Street, Los Angeles (Keating 1994, 94). Nearly every naturopath in California and many in Oregon and Washington were graduates of his institution (Lust 1918, 901-902). He was one of the first naturopaths who studied osteopathy and chiropractic. His success challenged California's medical establishment which declared war on Dr. Schultz and other naturopaths in the state. For over six years, he fought the allopaths almost single-handed at a cost of thousands of dollars. He studied law at night for three years in order to better help himself and other similar practitioners. "His crowning triumph as naturopath and lawyer" was the passage of a bill in 1909 that licensed all those who were accepted for membership in the Association of Naturopathic Physicians of California. "Yet with all these activities he was able to keep his office practice and to attend to approximately sixty patients a day" (*Yearbook* 1945, 12). On May 18, 1914, Schultz obtained a charter for the "California University of Liberal Physicians" which he ran as owner and president conjointly with his Naturopathic Institute of California. In June 1936, the charter was taken over by Dr. Clarence William

Tyndal, who changed the name to "Emerson University." A naturopathic department headed by Dr. Arthur Schramm, who became the founder and president of the International Society of Naturopathic Physicians, was maintained at the university and a standard course of 4500 hours in a four year program was being taught until January 1944 (*Yearbook* 1945, 29).

Having founded the American School of Chiropractic and having acquired a D.C. degree, Lust was well-known to the chiropractic profession. In 1915, he was invited to the Mecca College of Chiropractic in Newark, N.J., founded by Dr. Frederick W. Collins (1873-1948). His lecture was so enthusiastically received that the students gave him three rousing cheers and presented him with a bouquet of chrysanthemums so gigantic that "it completely covered Dr. Lust." Later Lust visited the chiropractic college in Davenport, Iowa, run by B. J. Palmer, son of D. D. Palmer, the founder of chiropractic. Palmer was furious with Lust and "jumped all over him" for his association with F. W. Collins, a rival whom he regarded as a "mountebank." Lust "gave Palmer one good Nature Cure adjustment" and told him that Collins and he were friends and worked closely together for medical freedom. "B. J. immediately cooled down" and ordered his assistant to show Lust the greatest hospitality (Collins 1916, 21).

Collins graduated in June, 1907, from the American School of Naturopathy, "claimed degrees in chiropractic from half a dozen institutions, including one signed by both Palmers, and also used every other degree known in that period when academic mills were a small cottage industry" (Gibbons 1989, 41). The authors of the *Yearbook of the International Society of Naturopathic Physicians* were more positive in their appraisal of Collins' credentials and wrote that "he, like Dr. Carl Schultz of California, has the happy faculty of abstracting all that is good in Naturopathy, Osteopathy and Chiropractic" and "attended the founders' schools in these three fields—Lust's, Still's and Palmer's—believing in the fountain heads as the true source of knowledge" (1945, 17). The same AMA report about "Schools of Chiropractic and of Naturopathy in the U.S.," that had nothing positive to say about Lust's American School of Naturopathy, was not more flattering about Collins' First National University of Naturopathy in Newark, New Jersey.

> The First National University of Naturopathy is supposedly the result of a merging of the Mecca College of Chiropractic, the New Jersey College of Osteopathy, and the United States Schools of Naturopathy, a year or more ago. The fact seems to be that these three are creations of F. W. Collins, who also chartered the United States School of Physiotherapy, the American Academy of Medicine and Surgery, and about fifteen other similar paper colleges .

> . . . The twenty or more institutions are all crowded into the one building, and there are now said to be twenty-six students . . . .
>
> Two or three diplomas are given each graduate, from as many different "schools." The tuition is $600. In short, for this price a student may get all the diplomas the walls of one small office will offer space for, and have them with no great effort on his part, with no preliminary education insisted on, and with the school frankly cooperating in the faking of everything that can be conveniently faked in this preparation to fool the public (1928, 1738).

According to the *Yearbook,* over four thousand World War I veterans graduated from this University under the sponsorship of the United States Government. Collins was also the first physician in America to establish a free clinic for infantile paralysis where he treated polio victims with methods developed by Sister Elizabeth Kenny (1886-1952). The Australian nurse revolutionized the treatment of polio and became world-famous using methods which can only be called naturopathic, including stimulation and reeducation of the paralyzed muscles through gentle movement and hydrotherapy. Dr. Collins was a popular speaker on iridology at ANA conventions. The congress brochure of 1943 praised him as "one of the most colorful and most dynamic individuals in his profession."

Another chiropractic ally was Dr. Joe Shelby Riley (1889-1946). Riley was Dean of the New England and Washington, D.C. Schools of Chiropractic. According to Harry Runge, he was not a Palmer man, but "a mixer who included everything possible under chiropractic: lamp, vibrator, medical diagnostic instruments like the stethoscope, osteopathic manipulation, and urinalysis; he was an osteopath, a lawyer, and a preacher, so we didn't know what he really was" (Wardwell 1992, 122). On Lust's 60th birthday, he wrote a poem celebrating Lust as the "Leader of the Drugless World" (1921, 525) which began, "Of the men I have met and the men I would trust, There are none to excel Dr. Benedict Lust." It was thanks to the influence of Riley and his wife, Dr. Elizabeth Riley, the organizers of the 1922 Naturopathic Convention at Washington, D.C., that President Harding received the delegates at the White House. In 1928 Lust published a little book on zone therapy, and it was Riley who had awakened his interest in this early forerunner of reflexotherapy and acupressure. Riley became an untiring developer and practitioner of this therapy, originated by William Fitzgerald (1872-1942), a medical doctor of Hartford, Connecticut. During the early 1930s, Eunice Ingham (1879-1974), known as the "Mother of Modern Reflexology," worked with Dr. Riley as his therapist in St. Petersburg, Florida.

Among the diet reformers Lust featured in his magazines, such as Dr. John Harvey Kellogg, George J. Drews, Otto Carqué, Eugene Christian and V. G. Rocine, German-born Arnold Ehret (1866-1922) had the greatest influence. Ehret cured himself from Bright's disease after he had been given up by medical doctors, and after nature cure could only bring him temporary relief. He travelled all over Europe and North Africa searching for health, discovering that fasting and a diet "free of mucus and albumin" consisting mainly of fruits cured not only his own illness but other chronic diseases (1970, ii).

> Disease is internal uncleanliness acquired over all ages by wrong food. My revelation of diseases and their healing through corrective diet is based on proof and backed by experiments on my own body as well as on thousands of patients at Dr. Benedict Lust's Yungborn Sanitarium during a period of over five years (Ehret 1980, 15).

Ehret became a much sought-after lecturer and settled in Los Angeles. Lust published his books on fasting and the Mucusless Diet Healing System which still has followers today. He wrote: "Cures have been made by Prof. Ehret all over the world, and his diet seems to be far superior to any other diet so far known in the world" (1922, 557). Ehret's life ended in a tragicomic accident. Returning home from a lecture on a poorly-lit street in Los Angeles, and wearing a new pair of shoes, he stepped off the curb, lost his balance, fell and fractured his skull on the curb stone (Hirsch 1923, 11-12). Lust praised Ehret as "one of the pillars on which the drugless movement stands today in America" (1922, 557).

Finally, Bernarr Macfadden (1868-1955) cannot be omitted; the father of physical culture and author, editor, manager of a publishing empire, and director of several sanitariums. Although called a "sensationalist," a "crank of the worst type" (Day 1979, 92) and a "monomaniacal campaigner for better health for all" (Whorton 1986, 296), he was immensely successful in popularizing nature cure principles such as diet, fasting, fresh air, exercise, hydrotherapy and nudism to a prudish Victorian society. He wrote: "Health means vim, vigor, snap, energy. Health means clarity and strength of mind, purity and beauty of soul" (Macfadden 1914, 1). Practicing what he preached and performing extraordinary athletic feats, he himself was a superb male specimen. He was the celebrated guest speaker at many naturopathic conventions and graduation ceremonies of the American School of Naturopathy. Lust had great respect for Macfadden and considered him an important ally.

> The nature cure movement, Naturopathy, with the fundamental basis of a healing art, *Naturology*, natural living, and with

> its sister, the great physical culture movement, launched and championed by our big brother, Bernarr Macfadden, constitute a great revolutionary movement for rational medicine and true prevention of disease. Combined with medical freedom, which we must and will get, it will usher in the new day of better health, more happiness and liberty for our bodies and souls. The nature cure and physical culture movements are the only popular movements for a broad education for the people on the prevention of disease (1921, 480).

Lust was even influential in the introduction of Yoga to America. Yogendra Mastamini visited the U.S. from 1919-1922 and met Lust during this time. A recent writer noted:

> This was a watershed meeting because in the next decades hatha yoga would be introduced to America largely as an adjunct to the multiplicity of alternative healing techniques advocated by naturopathy (Leviton 1990, 44).

Herbert M. Shelton (1895-1985), the leading force in the natural hygiene movement, was a 1922 graduate of Lust's American School of Naturopathy. Shelton taught evening courses in dietetics there to pay for his education. He was disappointed in his education which was marked by "endless disagreements about which treatment was important" (Oswald 1989, 25). Shelton was an independent and outspoken thinker. For a time he contributed a regular column to Lust's *Naturopath*, but when his articles began criticizing some of the founders of naturopathy such as Kneipp, Lust verbally "spanked" Shelton for insulting the "parents and progenitors in the movement" (Lust 1924, 569), and they went their separate ways.

After overcoming his early medical problems, Lust's own personal health was always good. Blessed with a strong constitution and following the nature cure principles he advocated, Lust kept up with his demanding schedule of writing, teaching, speaking, and administering his practice and business interests. He remained a formidable gymnasium wrestler well into his sixties.

However, in 1943 a fire of undetermined origin swept through the Yungborn in Tangerine, Florida. During the blaze Lust was severely burned. The sanatorium had been "packed to capacity," his nephew wrote. "Twice Dr. Lust's clothes and hair caught fire and it was necessary to beat out the flames" (John Lust 1953, 4). He was treated by medical doctors at the scene with sulfa drugs. His health went steadily downhill for the next two years and although he was living alone during this time and not taking care of himself, many of his friends felt the sulfa more than anything contributed to his decline. He died September 5, 1945. The official cause of death was listed as coronary thrombosis.

Lust was buried at the Mt. Calvary cemetery in Butler, New Jersey, next to his wife, Louisa Lust, just a few miles from the Butler Yungborn. Jesse Mercer Gehmann, a close associate in his last years, gave a slightly florid description of the funeral.

> The sun never shined more brightly nor was the sky ever clearer then when we bore the mortal remains of Nature's son, Naturopathy's Father from the Yungborn through Grace Valley and the portals of St. Anthony's Church and thence to Mount Calvary. There was scarcely a whisp of a breeze as we made our grievous way from the Yungborn to the Church and thence to Cemetery . . . . The spirit of Benedict Lust will ever live even as does that of those great pioneers he has joined in the realm from which no mortal returns. He is now communing with the old Masters of Nature Cure whose shrines he visited in years gone by. With him are Vincent Priessnitz, Louis Kuhne, Adolph Just, Arnold Rikli, Father Kneipp, Schroth, Trall, D. D. Palmer and Still, Lindlahr and Bechamp, whose works he correlated to formulate the basic systems of Nature Cure of Naturopathy (1947, 12-13)

A recent writer gave the following account of his visit to Lust's grave:

> When I visited his gravesite in Butler, I was enveloped by a great sense of humility. It was a humility that seemed to say Lust knew that he was a competent man, but he knew his place in the universe. It seemed to me at the time that a man of his stature should have been buried in some pretentious manner, but I can now see it would have been inappropriate. I could sense how hard he tried, how important his efforts were, especially in comparison to what most of us today consider to be important (O'Brien 1978, 28).

Lust's friends, family and associates immediately set in motion plans to construct a "Light of Naturopathy" monument at the Butler Yungborn to memorialize the life and work of their hero. Their "Benedict Lust Permanent Memorial" received enthusiastic responses and contributions from many naturopathic doctors. An architect's drawing was completed and the cornerstone was laid on September 5, 1946, one year after Lust's death, but the project was never completed. Dr. Jesse Gehmann, President of the American Naturopathic Association, inserted a number of documents important to the history into the cornerstone, among them the first issue of the *Kneipp Water*

Cure Monthly, a copy of the incorporation papers of the ANA, the Dr. Louise Lust memorial issue of the *Naturopath*, a photo of Dr. Lust and Kneipp together and the definition of Naturopathy as given in the *Congressional Record*. The finished monument would have been a tower visible from New York with the sculpture of a man on top, arms outstretched to a sun made of lucite or glass containing a perpetual light, "'The Light of Naturopathy'—a promise of hope to suffering humanity" (*Nature's Path* 1946, 643, 663).

Lust always put the naturopathic movement before himself and had no interest in money except as it advanced the profession. He contributed over $200,000 of his personal funds to the ANA. He was prideful only in the dents he could put in the facade of orthodox medicine. He believed his greatest honor, besides being commissioned by Kneipp to bring his methods to America, was in being considered the worst enemy of orthodox medicine. He took it as a compliment when arrested along with other naturopaths that his bond was set at six hundred dollars, twice that of the others. Except by his enemies, Lust was universally admired. George Floden found it "befitting Naturopathy that Dr. Benedict be placed among our National Heroes. In his field he rates with George Washington and Abraham Lincoln—liberators of mankind!" (Gehmann 1947, 19).

Lust remained militant to the end in his battles with official medicine but softened later in his career concerning treatment methods. "We don't want iconoclasts and extremists," he wrote. "We want to give the patient the best." In a passage which would prove to be prophetic he wrote:

> The naturopath of the future will be a regular doctor. He will have changed his methods and adjusted his system to give complete service. Our schools must advance and our schools must teach what is right in surgery and obstetrics. There are times even when drugs are necessary. Don't be so radical (1935, 251).

Lust lost his life the way he had lived it—trying to save other people. He may have sensed that the naturopathic movement would falter after he was gone, but he remained confident of his earlier vision.

> The rising sun of the nature cure movement will come into its full glory, will light the darkest corners of official quackery and future generations will exonerate the naturopaths from the superstition of the dark age of our present day (1921, 480).

On August 30th 1945, a few days before his death, he dictated the following for the 49th Annual Congress of the ANA:

> The increasing lack of confidence in the infallibility of Modern Medicine will eventually make itself felt to such an extent that

the man on the street will turn upon these self-constituted oppressors and not only demand but force a change. I may not be here to witness this revolution but I believe with all my soul that it is coming. Yes, the future of Naturopathy is indeed bright. It merely requires that each and every true Naturopath carry on—carry on—to the best of his and her abilities (cited in Wendel 1951, 41).

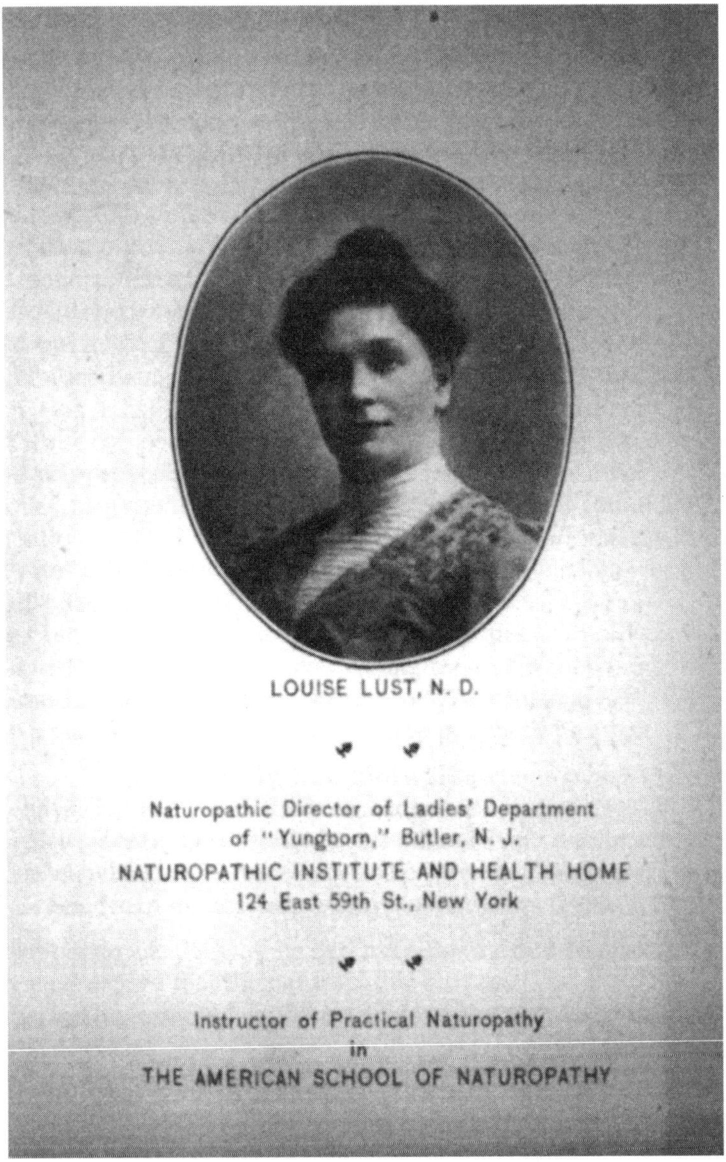
LOUISE LUST, N. D.
Naturopathic Director of Ladies' Department
of "Yungborn," Butler, N. J.
NATUROPATHIC INSTITUTE AND HEALTH HOME
124 East 59th St., New York
Instructor of Practical Naturopathy
in
THE AMERICAN SCHOOL OF NATUROPATHY

Louisa Lust
(L. Lust 1907, frontispiece)

The Matriarch of Naturopathy

Louisa Lust

(1868 - 1925)

Louisa Lust is one of the unsung heroines of naturopathic medicine. Born Aloysia Stroebele, daughter of the mayor of Sigmaringen, Germany, she immigrated to America and became an accomplished naturopathic physician specializing in the treatment of women. During the early 1890s she was doctor-in-charge of Bellevue Sanitarium, a nature cure retreat in Butler, New Jersey. Later she headed the women's department at the "Yungborn" retreats in New Jersey and Florida, modeled after the European nature cure institutions. In her practice she employed the time-honored nature cure methods of hydrotherapy, vegetarian diet, air-and-light baths and rational life style with great skill and success.

Aloysia Stroebele met Benedict Lust in 1896, after he returned to America to establish Father Kneipp's methods on this side of the Atlantic. A devout Catholic, Benedict Lust made regular religious pilgrimages from his base in New York City to the beautiful countryside of Butler, New Jersey. These pilgrimages, known as the "Procession through Grace Valley," were conducted by Rev. Albert Stroebele, the priest at St. Anthony's Church in Butler, and Louisa's only brother (Proctor 1991). It is probable that Benedict would have met Louisa on these pilgrimages in any case, but that likelihood was enhanced by the fact that she was already a successful practitioner in the field to which he aspired.

Shortly after they met, Louisa and Benedict, with the help of her brother, Father Albert, established the Butler "Yungborn," which was closely modeled after the Hartz Mountain namesake founded by Adolph Just. Louisa was the leading financial partner in this enterprise. Benedict once said that she "owned the health resort at Butler long before we were married" (Collins 1924, 659). She promoted it as "an ideal summer resort for lovers of nature" and compared it to the Swiss Alps. She touted its advantage of being "only thirty miles from New York" as compared to the popular but more distant Catskill Mountain retreats. (L. Stroebele 1899, 141).

Louisa studied the nature cure methods of Rikli and Kuhne in London before coming to America. After establishing her practice in this country, she continued her studies at the Columbia Institute, where she was taught hydrotherapeutics, presumably Kneipp's method, by Benedict Lust. Their marriage in 1901 was a cause for celebration by the naturopathic community, which feted them with a wedding breakfast of "refreshments and dainties . . . not in strict keeping with the 'doctrines of Kneipp'" (Anonymous 1901, 163). After overcoming an inauspicious beginning (they both suffered food poisoning on their Niagara Falls honeymoon), they embarked on a twenty-five-year partnership that established naturopathy as a medical force to be contended with in the United States.

Besides being "the greatest woman doctor in the whole history of the naturopathic movement," (B. Lust 1937, 175) Louisa Lust was also an accomplished preparer of healthful foods. She saw to it that the patients' meals at the Yungborn sanitariums were as tasty and enjoyable as they were nutritious. After fifteen years in practice she "found the need of a simple, wholesome vegetarian cookery book." (L. Lust 1907, 9) Her *Practical Naturopathic-Vegetarian Cook Book,* the first strictly naturopathic guide for food preparation, was popular and influential. This book showed her knowledge of dietetics, much of which has been validated today:

> A large part of food among Americans is composed of white flour, sugar, and butter. People who try to live on such stuff gradually starve to death (L. Lust 1907, 40).

She was influenced by the writings of Luigi Cornaro who improved his health and prolonged his life by a frugal diet. "We can lengthen our life," she wrote, "or shorten it by eating." In sickness she recommended the lightest possible diet. "One of the greatest evils to be avoided by those who are nursing the sick," she wrote, "is that of overfeeding" (L. Lust 1907, 11). In health she recommended a sparse, simple diet for the prevention of disease:

> Minimum of food means a minimum of digestive work. Nervous breakdowns can more often be traced to overwork of the digestive, than the mental apparatus (L. Lust 1924, 812).

Her advice to her patients was always simple, clear and to the point:

> Do not under any circumstances, shut the air and sunshine from your home. Do not mind if the furniture, curtains, draperies, etc. will fade. It is better to let them fade than you should (L. Lust 1911, 99).

This revealed a practicality often lacking in her more idealistic male counterparts. What good was it to be cured at a naturopathic sanatorium if one returned to a bad diet and unhealthy home, only to become sick again? Time and again she emphasized the importance of homemaking skills for maintaining family health:

> Good housekeeping is the science of combining perfect cleanliness with economy and comfort; of giving the inmates of the house healthy bodies through the preparation of wholesome and palatable food, careful and intelligent attention to sanitation and the laws of hygiene (L. Lust 1907, 9).

She considered these skills to have revolutionary potential:

> If mothers would learn how to live . . . to prepare simple healthy food and by example teach their children the all-important lessons of how and what to feed the body, sickness would be out-grown and forgotten in one generation. (L. Lust, 1911, 99).

The issue was not that these were women's tasks of low prestige but rather indispensable elements of a healthy life, transcending any menial connotations society placed on them.

Her common-sense approach to naturopathy involved all aspects of her practice. She believed firmly in "the life force within" as the "great healing agent," but was not doctrinaire in her approach. "General principles may be laid down," she wrote, "but it is better to leave details to the individual's own experience" (L. Lust 1907, 10). For her the successful practice of naturopathy rested on three factors:

> Freedom from fear, mastery of hygiene, and to never forget to treat the individual . . . to modify and adjust treatments to the individual case (L. Lust 1923, 437).

She did not thrust radical changes upon her patients. She advocated the "nut and fruit diet" as the ideal. However, "knowing through experience the difficulty we meet with most people in suddenly adapting themselves to such a simple style of living as nature would dictate, a step at a time, slowly but surely, is the wisest in the end." She even pointed out a rarely appreciated implication of the simple, naturopathic lifestyle she advocated. "Raw food or a fruitarian diet," she wrote, "will also solve the servant question considerably" (L. Lust 1907, 12).

Louisa Lust was a staunch advocate of hydrotherapy. "If all people understood how to use water," she wrote, "one half of all the afflictions from disease would be removed." The other half would be taken care of by understanding "how and when to eat, how to breathe and the necessity of daily exercise" (L. Lust, 1911, 231). She believed there was no better treatment for acute or chronic disease than the steam bath, especially in pneumonias, flus and severe colds. For preventing disease she recommended that "the daily cool natural bath should be as regularly taken as meals." Like Kneipp, she was a firm believer in the value of order. "Do nothing in a careless manner," she wrote. "Order is law, and to be happy we must obey all of nature's laws" (L. Lust, 1911, 99)

Her belief in the benevolence of fever typified her clinical approach:

> When there is fever of any kind, the vital force is trying to get rid of the poisons . . . . Give the patient an enema of lukewarm water and a tea of rhubarb powder once a day. No solid food whatsoever . . . . Give the patient an ablution of cool water every hour . . . . Normal function of the organs will take place and the fever will stop. It is the poison and the toxins in the system and the foolish medicines which kill, not the fever. Fever should never be suppressed (L. Lust 1923, 437).

The achievements of Louisa Lust and Benedict Lust are difficult to separate. She was a great inspiration to him, his prime counsellor, co-worker, and financial backer. They worked as partners and their accomplishments were mutual successes. She helped him start the Yungborn. In fact, she had already started it under a different concept and name and directed its "Ladies Department." She lived a spartan existence to make her "hard earned savings" available for the promotion of the naturopathic profession (Posner 1925, 708). She helped provide the financial wherewithal for the establishment of the first naturopathic college, the American College of Naturopathy in New York, where she served as "Instructor of Practical Naturopathy." She helped fund the publication of the *Naturopath*, the magazine which her husband edited and to which she regularly contributed. This widely distributed journal brought naturopathic principles before the public, provided an important forum for discussion of health issues, and was the instrument which united the early profession in this country. She helped pay for the legal defense of naturopathy in at least seventeen legal actions taken against it (B. Lust 1937, 175). She kept herself and Benedict Lust going through many dark, discouraging days of persecution. On several occasions she prevented him from giving up the whole naturopathic enterprise in despair. She was said to have "brought out the captainship of Dr. Benedict Lust" (Posner, 1925 708). Although she studiously avoided the limelight, she was a powerful presence behind the scene.

Negative comments about Louisa Lust are difficult to find. Her low profile did not invite attacks from the allopathic enemies of naturopathy. Those who did know her were won over by her modesty, conscientiousness, erudition, dedication, wisdom and selflessness. Her motto, which inspired and re-inspired the profession, was "Don't give up your enthusiasm" (Posner 1925, 708).

But like many naturopathic doctors, Louisa Lust worked herself to death on behalf of her profession. One writer described her as "racked by the rigors" of thirty years of self-sacrifice (Kern 1925, 709). She knew secretly for months she was dying but remained devoted to the care of her patients up to the last hours of her life. She was frequently referred to as the "Clara Barton of Naturopathy." Her unexpected death in 1925 at the age of 57—her death certificate listed the cause as "chronic endocarditis"—was a devastating blow to the profession from which it recovered only slowly.

The shock to her husband, Benedict, was the greatest of all, not only because her death represented "the loss of a great general in the ranks of Naturopathy" (B. Lust 1925, 759), but also because she died intestate, i.e., without a will, thus depriving him of financial resources which he and the profession had relied upon for decades. He seriously considered abandoning naturopathy after her death and only relented because he knew "in a land beyond this mortal state, he must render unto her an accounting of his stewardship" (Kern 1925, 708). One writer said:

> Dr. Louisa Lust could not tolerate the whimperings of a coward; she loved the fighting spirit in him (Benedict), and he is conscious of her feeling (Anonymous 1925, 944).

The naturopathic profession owes an unacknowledged debt to Louisa Lust. Throughout this century, thousands of naturopaths unaware of the influence she wielded, have been able to practice naturopathic medicine because of her efforts. As one admirer put it:

> Dr. Louisa Lust was original, because she was "natural"—that is, she was herself; she learned early in life the secret of happiness: helping others to help themselves. The praise of her work echoes from the four corners of the globe (Posner 1925, 708).

And Louisa Lust is not the only female nature doctor who deserves more recognition in naturopathic history. One of them, Susanna Way Dodds, M.D. (1830-1911), a student of Russell T. Trall, practiced nature cure in the water cure and hygienist tradition going back to Priessnitz. She founded a college in St. Louis, Missouri, in 1897, which taught hygiene, obstetrics and surgery. Unfortunately, it only lasted a few years. She published the magazine, *The Sanitarian,* and the outstanding textbook *Drugless Medicine: Hygeiotherapy* (1915) with the motto, "Nature is the True Physician, Hygiene is Her Handmaid."

Benedict Lust's right hand in his later years was Dr. Theresa M. Schippell, Secretary/Treasurer of the American Naturopathic Association. Sometime after Lust's death she served as a President of the ANA and resumed the publication of the *Naturopath* as a professional journal. Dr. Paul Wendel credited her with having "fought practically alone to have Naturopathy recognized in the District of Columbia." He paid the same tribute to a Dr. Louisa of Salt Lake City who achieved the legalization of Naturopathy in Utah, because "the Governor of Utah at that time was her patient" (Wendel 1951, 134).

For the last fifteen years, more than half of the graduates from naturopathic colleges have been women, and naturopathic history will be as much a history of women as of men.

Founder of Scientific Naturopathy

Henry Lindlahr

(1862-1924)

In 1893, Henry Lindlahr was a prosperous business man, banker, mayor, and leading citizen of Kalispell, Montana. He had made his fortune in land speculation, buying cheap land ahead of the railroads, then selling it to them at high prices for their transcontinental line. He was 5'6" and weighed over 250 pounds, and considered a brace of ducks a fitting appetizer to a full course dinner. At this pinnacle of success, he was diagnosed with sugar diabetes and advised by the ablest doctors to set his affairs in order. Ten years later, in 1903, he was one year away from graduation from medical school and had already started a successful nature cure practice in Chicago as a licensed Drugless Practitioner. Eating a modified vegetarian diet, he no longer had diabetes; indeed, he was enjoying unprecedented health. Over the next twenty years he became the foremost practitioner of scientific naturopathy in America.

Lindlahr's transition from business tycoon to scientific nature doctor is an absorbing tale. He was born in Germany on March 1, 1862, and spent the first twenty years of his life there. He was educated as a brewing and baking chemist, but after emigrating to America he followed his fortune west and entered the world of business. Having achieved his highest goals, ready to enjoy the fruits of his labor, he was informed that he had a fatal disease for which there was no cure. He later summed up his situation in this way:

> At the age of thirty-five I found myself a physical and mental wreck without faith in God, in Nature or in myself. Many times the desire to end my miserable existence threatened to overwhelm me. The terror of it all was my utter ignorance and helplessness. I failed to see the causes of my troubles, much less the way out of them (H. Lindlahr 1923, 439).

A sympathetic friend gave him a copy of Louis Kuhne's *The New Science of Healing*, which introduced him to the concept of disease being caused by violations of nature's laws. As Lindlahr read the book, "it was as though a

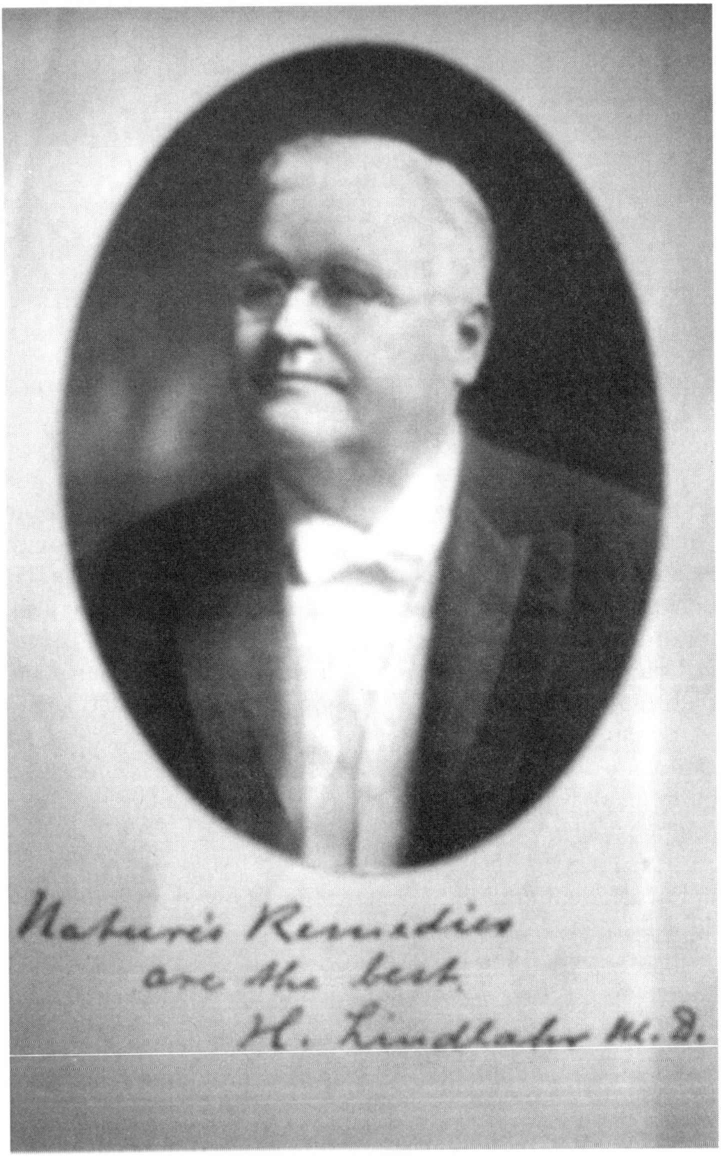

Henry Lindlahr
(Lindlahr 1922, frontispiece)

great light were arising before me and illuminating my darkened consciousness." He began to realize that health was regulated by natural laws just as immutable as those governing gravitation. He immediately began to practice the Kuhne's regimen on himself and found the results "most gratifying" (ibid.).

While Lindlahr's condition improved under his makeshift home care, his diabetes and the threat it posed to his life remained. Having exhausted the possibilities for help from the best of America's doctors, he undertook a journey to Vienna to seek out the most noted physicians of Europe, where he received the same diagnosis and hopeless prognosis. Then Lindlahr was prevailed upon by a companion to visit Wörishofen in Bavaria where Father Kneipp practiced his natural healing. His interview with the priest was short and to the point.

> The priest smelled his breath, surveyed his 250-odd pounds, and said bluntly: 'You have the sugar disease. You are a pig (glutton). You will take sitz baths, live on fruits and greens and vegetables alone. You shall have no breads, no cereals, no meats (V. Lindlahr 1973, 14).

By the next spring, Lindlahr was free of sugar and within a few more months he had lost 43 pounds and fully regained his health. Lindlahr stayed in Europe several additional months to travel to other natural healing centers. What he observed and experienced there and at Wörishofen changed his health and revolutionized his whole outlook on life. Having been saved himself by natural health methods, he began to wonder about his friends and family members who had died before him at early ages from similar conditions.

> In our halcyon days of youthful vigor, we are apt to look upon health culture, mind culture and higher philosophy with contempt and derision, but suffering is the great awakener, revealer and teacher . . . .
>
> In my youth I had learned the Ten Commandments, but neither in church, school nor college had I been taught that there is a decalogue and a morality of the physical as well as the spiritual . . . .
>
> I accepted the popular belief that life and death, health and disease are largely matters of chance or dependent upon drafts, wet feet, germs and bacteria or upon the will of a capricious Providence. My friends of the medical profession assured me that

> eating and drinking and the use of liquor and tobacco had little to do with physical condition . . . . (H. Lindlahr 1923, 438-439)

Lindlahr felt betrayed by official medicine. He believed his doctors should have warned him and his loved ones of the mistakes of eating and living which could lead to unnecessary disease and early death. He never forgot that his health was saved by laymen such as Kuhne and Kneipp whom most medical doctors considered quacks. Having completed his cure in Europe, Lindlahr returned to America, moved to Texas and re-entered the world of business. However, he found himself strangely discontent. He wrote:

> I realized that commercial pursuits, no matter how remunerative, could never again satisfy me. Money making had lost its charm. Higher and finer ideals had taken its place . . . . I had grasped the law of service which ordains that we achieve contentment and happiness only as we make others happy. "Freely ye have received, freely give." In compliance with this injunction of the Master, I decided to make Nature Cure my life work (H. Lindlahr 1923, 440).
>
> The wonderful results I witnessed in others, and experienced myself, filled me with such enthusiasm for the work that I was not able to think or plan anything else (H. Lindlahr 1914, 251).

Although he was nearly forty, Lindlahr decided, "for the peace of my soul," to study medicine. He thought that as a medical doctor he could help correct the wrong thinking which had kept American medicine ignorant of the natural health principles that saved his life. Undecided where to study, he chose Chicago over San Francisco on the flip of a coin.

Lindlahr was an eager student both inside and outside of class. In every free moment he haunted the John Crear library to study diet and nutrition. He also hired a doctor to give him private instruction in osteopathy. By 1902, he had qualified to sit for the Illinois Drugless Practitioner Examination, which he passed. With this license he started a nutritional practice which grew to such proportions that it threatened his regular medical studies.

In 1904, he graduated from medical school, received his medical license and began to practice full-time. His first patient was a waiter at a prominent Chicago restaurant with a nasty varicose leg ulcer. The referrals which came from the rapid cure of this patient got Lindlahr's practice off to a fast start.

Another early case was not so successful. A noted businessman with gallbladder disease did not improve as expected despite Lindlahr's most strenuous efforts and most careful instructions. When he stopped at a nearby

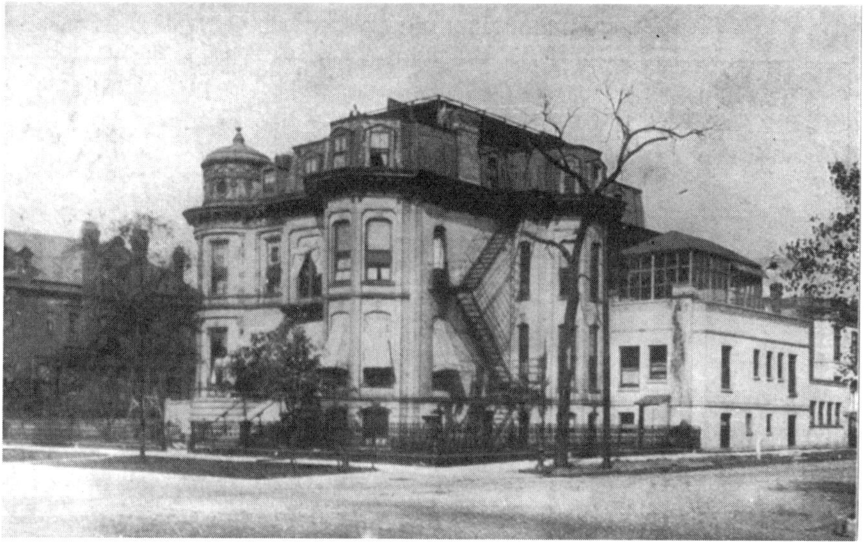

Dr. Lindlahr's Sanitarium for Nature Cure and Osteopathy
(Lindlahr 1913, back page)

restaurant to buy a loaf of pumpernickel bread, he happened to see his gallbladder patient feasting on roast duck and dressing. He realized that his chances for a successful nature cure practice were limited unless he could find a way to supervise his patients' activities and meals. Two months later he purchased a large property on Chicago's Ashland Boulevard, which he converted to a sanitarium.

This property, located on 515-529 South Ashland Blvd., was known as the Mike McDonald homestead, "the former residence of the well known millionaire, politician and gambler." By January, 1906, the conversion of the mansion to a sanitarium was complete. Lindlahr started the sanitarium from scratch with "not a single friend or acquaintance to aid him in the propaganda of the new gospel of living and healing" (Davidson 1923, 454). He entered into this venture against the advice of his friends and family, because he "wanted to demonstrate to suffering humanity and to the medical profession the possibility of curing chronic disease" (H. Lindlahr 1918, 123). During his training in medical school he was fully exposed to the therapeutic nihilism regarding chronic disease which he had first encountered when his doctors had told him there was nothing to be done for his diabetes except to go home and prepare to die. His European nature cure experiences had opened his eyes to a radically different concept of disease which allowed for the cure of chronic conditions.

Lindlahr believed, like the early nature doctors before him, that chronic disease was "due to the accumulation of waste matter and poisons" and that "every so-called acute disease is the result of a cleansing and healing effort of Nature" (H. Lindlahr 1922, 19). He felt that all diseases were acute before they became chronic, that chronic disease was the result of suppression of acute disease. "If acute diseases are treated in the natural way," he wrote, "there are no chronic diseases to cure."

> Such chronic supposed-to-be-incurable diseases as tuberculosis, cancer, locomotor ataxia, paresis, paralysis agitans, infantile paralysis, secondary and tertiary syphilis, etc., yield to the natural treatment, provided there is enough vitality in the system to respond to treatment and the destruction of vital parts and organs has not too far advanced (H. Lindlahr 1914, 252).

He was fond of using secondary and tertiary syphilis as examples of chronic diseases which were the result of neglect or suppressive drug treatment of the primary, acute stage, and he claimed to have cured hundreds of cases, many "far advanced." Like Lust, he was a staunch enemy of the mercurial treatment of this disease.

> Be not deceived: neither this nor any other disease can be cured by putting poisons into the human bodies. The only possibility of cure lies in taking the old poisons out of the system, and this can be accomplished solely by natural methods of treatment (H. Lindlahr 1913, 16).

In his experience, adding drug poisons to the body's poisons only made matters worse. To Lindlahr, nothing was more harmful in medicine than the suppression of disease. He believed that disease was nature's effort to eliminate morbid matter from the body and restore normal function. "What the Old School of Medicine calls the disease," he said, "we look upon as the Cure" (H. Lindlahr 1922, 221).Therefore to suppress disease was to suppress its cure. He deplored orthodox medical reliance on "fighting" disease.

> The combative method fights disease with disease, poison with poison, and germs with germs and germ products. In the language of the Good Book, it is 'Beelzebub against the Devil' (ibid., 16).

This view necessarily held that germs were not the causes of infectious diseases but rather secondary manifestations of a disturbed metabolic environment. To Lindlahr, the common cold was "vicarious elimination," where the mucus lining of the respiratory tract was taking up the slack for sluggish skin, intestines, liver and kidneys (ibid., 86). His early training as a brewery and bakery chemist introduced him to the concept that not all germs were bad. Indeed, the brewer's and baker's art depended on beneficial strains of microbes. He felt that fear instilled by the bacterial theory of disease often did more harm than the organisms themselves. His approach was not to kill the germs but rather to remove the morbid matter, or "cell feces," upon which they thrived. Lindlahr believed that health came from nature, not that disease came from germs. "Every moment," he wrote, "there are enacted in our bodies innumerable mechanical, chemical and psychological miracles. Who or what performs these miracles? We call it Nature" (V. Lindlahr 1973, 229).

Since health came from nature, then nature must be given free reign. Lindlahr regarded the *vis medicatrix naturae*, or the healing power of nature, as the true physician which pervades every body cell and repairs and heals from within. He was highly critical of the allopathic approach of fighting nature. "When nature pulls right," he wrote, "the doctor pulls left. Every serious problem is counteracted" (H. Lindlahr 1919, 39). He felt the physician's job was to remove obstructions and establish normal conditions so that the healing power of nature could work to best advantage. Avoiding the suppression of disease was to Lindlahr the medical equivalent to the biblical injunction, "Resist not Evil" (H. Lindlahr 1922, 229).

Thus Lindlahr, with his patients securely in a controlled environment, embarked on his mission to demonstrate the curability of chronic disease. His methods were those of the nature cure doctors in the old country adapted to twentieth-century Chicago and integrated with the manipulative therapies emerging in America. Like Lust, he saw the one-sidedness of many of the European nature cures, and strove to integrate the best of all of them; in eclectic fashion. While one admirer's assessment of Lindlahr's work as "the first effort ever made to combine in one system all that is good in the various methods of treating human ailments" may be too exuberant, Lindlahr was an effective combiner of the various natural methods because he thoroughly understood their underlying principles (H. Lindlahr 1923, 441).

In his *Catechism of Nature Cure* Lindlahr recognized five categories of natural therapy: 1) Return to nature, 2) Elementary remedies, 3) Chemical remedies, 4) Mechanical remedies, and 5) Mental/spiritual remedies (H. Lindlahr 1922, 22-23). The first category, Return to nature, played the biggest role in the therapies practiced and taught at the Lindlahr Sanitarium, and especially meant a return to a more natural diet. Lindlahr believed strongly in nutrition and kept up-to-date on all the latest findings in that field. He understood and used the action of foods as medicines, long before vitamins were discovered. When he said, "Our head cook is the chief pharmacist," he was earnest (V. Lindlahr 1973, 41). He used fruits, now known to contain vitamin C, to cure scurvy; brown rice, now known to contain thiamine, to cure beriberi; green leafy vegetables, now known to contain iron, to cure anemia; and Irish moss, now known to contain iodine, to cure goiter. Indeed, he sometimes filled his doctor's bag with oranges, a rare commodity in those days, when going on house calls for sick children.

> Within the plants lie vital life principles . . . which defy description and are not discoverable by chemical analysis. These act specifically in different ailments . . . Time will undoubtedly disclose these mysteries which explain vitality and life itself, but now we must content ourselves with the secure knowledge that certain foods and plants are medicines (ibid., 45).

Lindlahr had studied nutrition in Europe with the famous Swiss doctor and "living food" advocate Max Bircher-Benner (1867-1939), and so became a sworn enemy of the rich American diet in which he had so freely indulged as a younger man. He believed that strong blood did not need large quantities of fats and proteins from meat and dairy products but rather "positive mineral salts" from fruits and vegetables (H. Lindlahr 1981, 55). He felt that overeating created morbid toxins which taxed these vital mineral salts and could actually lead to nutritional deficiencies. Lindlahr emphasized a vegetarian diet at the sanitarium, and his wife, Anna, wrote *The Vegetarian Kitchen,* a masterfully concise and accurate explanation of the relationship between diet and health. However, Lindlahr did not "intend to make a fetish of vegetarianism" (H. Lindlahr 1910, 290). He often incurred the wrath of militant vegetarians by suggesting that properly prepared and combined vegetables and meats could be more wholesome than certain bad vegetarian combinations.

> It is not wise to be too finicky about food selection. Constant slavish fear of eating this, and eating that; of eating too much and eating too little is just about as bad as the other extreme of priggish promiscuousness. A hypochondriac mind will sour and poison the best of viands, and too great a monotony in food selection will destroy the wholesome zest and enjoyment of foods which is the best stimulus for the secretion of digestive juices (ibid., 289)

Lindlahr liked to point out that the "narrow fanaticism of Simon pure vegetarianism" repels rather than attracts intelligent converts and was the biggest factor preventing the wider adoption of a rational vegetarian diet. "We would eat a piece of meat once in a while ourselves," he wrote, "just to save us from that unfortunate frame of mind." A keynote for Lindlahr in diet and all therapies was, "It is good to be natural but by all means let us be rational" (ibid., 290).

Lindlahr was one of the earliest practitioners to recognize that some patients had bad reactions to certain foods. His "foundation diet," which restricted foods he found to be the most commonly offending, was a precursor to the "elimination diets" used by many allergy doctors today.

Lindlahr also practiced therapeutic fasting on his patients in a cautious, limited way during acute phases of their conditions such as in healing crises. With some patients Lindlahr even used his own version of the "dry diet," a modification of the Schroth Cure. He substituted dried fruit for the dry white bread and found that he could forego the wine, which he felt was only necessary in the Schroth plan to counteract the morbid effects of the bread.

Return to nature also meant adopting a rational lifestyle. This frequently meant making changes in occupation or working conditions. Lindlahr attracted patients from coal mines and quarries throughout the Midwest. "You don't need a doctor," he often told them, "you need a new job" (V. Lindlahr 1973, 84). He was very concerned about occupational health. Some of his most difficult cases were those which were under the constant stress of a noxious working environment. He believed that dangerous industries such as mining and quarrying should be taken under government control to ensure healthy working conditions. For voicing these sentiments Lindlahr was branded by some as a socialist. This may have been what attracted Eugene B. Debs, the famous socialist and labor leader, to become a patient at the sanitarium. Debs was sixty-six and an ill and wary man when President Harding ordered his release from prison in 1921. Nevertheless, as historian Arthur M. Schlesinger, Jr., noted, "Gene pressed ahead in his work, writing on the need for prison reform, working for the party, till fatigue would overtake him and send him, ashen-gray and trembling, to his bed or to Lindlahr, the Socialist sanitarium in Chicago" (Debs 1948, xii). Debs entered the Lindlahr Sanitarium in mid-July 1922, and was well enough by September that "he ran foot races with a young tuberculosis patient" (Ginger 1949, 434). He also brought excitement to the sanitarium with the many prominent visitors who came to see him, among them Sinclair Lewis, the famous author of *Main Street* (1920), and Carl Sandburg:

> Sinclair Lewis arrived at Lindlahr in August for a brief rest, and he was quickly recruited for the discussions held by Debs and Sandburg. One Saturday night Sandburg even brought his guitar and gave the patients "a most charming entertainment in folk lore, etc. It was a complete conquest," Debs wrote David Karsner, "and they all love him. Lewis will also entertain them and the patients

> here feel big with importance. No 'Main Streeters' here" (ibid., 436).

When Lindlahr had difficulty getting a patient well with natural methods, he went to the patient's home or workplace to inspect environmental conditions which might be inhibiting the cure. In one instance, he cured a successful bakery owner of his hypertension and obesity by ordering him to give up his sedentary managerial style and go back into the hot sweaty kitchen as a baker.

Lindlahr also included rational dress in his return-to-nature lifestyle. He crusaded against the corset, recommended suspenders instead of belts, and made a neighborhood cobbler "moderately well-to-do" by referring patients with chronic musculoskeletal problems to him for properly built and fitted shoes. He was an early opponent of tobacco use and blamed the "deplorable health of the English army" on cigarette smoking. In fact he saw the pre-World War I ascendancy of Germany as a direct result of that nation's "return to nature" (H. Lindlahr 1924, 425).

Finally, nothing in this category of therapy was more important for Lindlahr than rest and relaxation. He felt that convalescence allowed nature to make "the real cure," and often sent his patients on vacations up into the Michigan woods. Outpatients of the sanitarium had to spend their weekends in bed. This was to economize the vital force. He informed new sanitarium patients that their cases would be handled by Dr. Diet and Dr. Quiet. (V. Lindlahr 1973, 189-191).

Lindlahr's second category of natural therapy was elementary remedies such as water, air, light, electricity. The basement of the sanitarium was given over to water therapy. Both the men's and the women's sections were made up of small cubicles lined with tin, equipped with a short length of garden hose with a three- or four-way nozzle and a tin sitz bath. As the sanitarium prospered he replaced these with tiled rooms and elaborate water-projecting installations. The same excellent results were obtained in toning the patient's circulation regardless of the sophistication of the equipment.

All the sanitarium's ambulatory patients had to appear for their water treatments each morning. It was initially difficult to talk them into the cold water therapies, but once they experienced their benefits, they would "indignantly refuse to take other treatment if there was to be no cold water" (H. Lindlahr 1922, 242).

Lindlahr also used hot hydrotherapies. He employed fever baths to treat syphilis and gonorrhea. Later he experimented with the blood-washing-shower, or marathon bath, of Christos Parasco, which Lust introduced to him on his visit to Chicago in 1923. He studied its effects on blood pressure, blood counts and urinalyses, and finding beneficial results, instituted a modified, more intense version of the extended hot showers (H. Lindlahr 1924, 425). He plausibly explained this peculiar hydrotherapy's mechanism of action as follows:

> The continual dropping of hot water on the body draws the blood to the surface and discharges its impurities through the relaxed and open pores. The morbid excretions are then washed away by the constant flow of hot water (H. Lindlahr 1923, 528).

Lindlahr believed that the human being was an "air animal." He himself was a "fresh air fiend" who always quizzed his patients on the ventilation in their sleeping and working rooms and who occasionally came to blows with fellow streetcar riders over the issue of whether or not to open the windows. He foresaw that "If we get a few more million automobiles in this country, the air in cities is going to be so poisoned with their fumes that we're going to have a whole new crop of diseases to deal with" (V. Lindlahr 1973, 86).

Lindlahr felt fresh air was important not only for the lungs but also for the skin. He routinely prescribed air baths, exposing the naked body to moving currents of air, because he believed a properly functioning skin would excrete waste products. He felt the skin must be free several times each day to breath, detoxify, make vitamin D and regulate water and salt balance. He found air baths effective for hot flashes, low blood pressure, weight reduction and chronic fatigue. After his conversion to nature cure Lindlahr took three air baths every day of his life. He felt an air bath was "as important as a bowel movement" (ibid., 74). He claimed that the open-air sleeping porches and sun parlors, which we can still see today on houses built during his era, were the result of his air bath propaganda.

During his travels in Europe, Lindlahr studied with Niels Finsen, a pioneer of ultraviolet therapy. One of the first improvements he made on the sanitarium was to construct sunbathing areas on its roof. With separate sections for men and women, patients could exercise and rest with full exposure to the sun. While sun baths would be commonplace in decades to come, Lindlahr's rooftop solarium caused a scandal in his respectable Chicago neighborhood. Lindlahr treated many skin and joint conditions with sunlight and even used water and olive oil pre-exposed to the sun as medicine. He used ultraviolet lamps when they became available, as well as phototherapy and chromotherapy. Another elementary remedy used at the sanitarium was electricity. Lindlahr employed high-frequency and Morse wave among other electrical modalities.

Lindlahr's third category of natural therapy was chemical remedies. By these he meant herbs and homeopathic remedies. While he used these skillfully in his practice, he did not emphasize them in his writings, probably because he felt the necessity for their use could be avoided by following his other natural precepts.

The fourth category of natural therapy was mechanical remedies. Lindlahr was familiar with osteopathy, chiropractic, naprapathy, neuropathy, Swedish movement and massage. He "reconciled the divergences of the various spinal methods by incorporating the best of them in his system of Neurotherapy" (Davidson 1923, 452).

Lindlahr was not a big fan of the physical culture craze which other naturopaths had embraced because he found that the average patient would not stay with it. "A hobby will stick," he would say, "gymnastics won't" (V. Lindlahr 1973, 93). He employed F. H. Behncke for eighteen years as "physical director" of the sanitarium. Behncke's job was to interest the patients in croquet, gardening, bicycle riding, horseshoes, bowling or some other activity that they would continue once they left the sanitarium. Behncke's talent for this added greatly to the success of the sanitarium.

Lindlahr understood and utilized the psychoanalytical techniques of Jung and Adler. Due to an apparent misunderstanding on the part of the public, who may have equated the term "sanitarium" with the term "asylum," Lindlahr had ample opportunity to practice these techniques. Most of the patients brought to his institution during its early years were insanity cases. He appreciated their effects on the health of the mentally ill, but he realized that many mental conditions came from abnormal physiology and chemistry. He claimed a fifty percent success rate for "all so-called incurable nervous disorders" (Lindlahr 1910, 458).

Lindlahr was also a student of New Thought, a philosophy which emphasized the power of the mind in achieving health and happiness. In his writings he liberally quoted Emanuel Swedenborg, the Swedish philosopher and patron saint of the New Thought movement. Although Lindlahr was a strong critic of Christian Science because of its neglect of the physical aspects of health, he respected its insight into the mental and spiritual influences on health, and made use of them in his methods.

Lindlahr recognized fear as the great emotional enemy of health. "Fear is faith in evil," he wrote, showing a gift for the apt epigram. He considered the fear habit to be committing slow suicide through psychical refrigeration. To him cheerfulness was "the best of all tonics and love the greatest physician. " He likened anger to "psychological phthisis" (tuberculosis). He tried to demonstrate to his patients that "the best way to help yourself is to help others," and employed "positive affirmations" to establish healthy conditions in the mind so that they could be "conveyed to and impressed upon the cells" (H. Lindlahr 1922, 403). These techniques remain popular to this day.

New Thought was often associated with spiritualism. Lindlahr had a mild interest in spiritualistic phenomena and was not afraid of the ramifications this might have on his reputation. "As a 'Nature Cure Doctor,'" he wrote, "we are already so hopelessly 'irregular and unscientific' that a few more sins added to our already long list of medical and scientific heresies matter but very little" (H. Lindlahr 1910, 459).

No aspect of mental and emotional health was more important to Lindlahr than self-control. He observed that many of his patients were sick because their minds were disorderly and they lacked the will power to do the things necessary for health. He believed that disease was "brought on by violations of Nature's laws" and that "it can only be overcome by compliance with the law." "Obedience to the law" was the only means of cure (H. Lindlahr 1922, 29-30). To comply with these laws required self-control, self-mastery and unselfish personal effort. "The demoralizing effect of health law-breaking . . ." he wrote, "does not depend so much upon the enormity of the deed as upon the loss of self-control" (V. Lindlahr 1973, 231). He did not limit the necessity for self-control to physical practices but rather emphasized its importance for controlling mental and emotional habits as well. "The brain is a musical instrument," he wrote, "under the absolute control of the will of the ego" (H. Lindlahr 1981, 189).

Lindlahr geared his sanitarium therapies to instill these qualities in his patients. A rigid, unvarying daily schedule was followed. Former pleasures were given up and beneficial hardships endured. The orderliness of the sanitarium was to demonstrate and teach discipline. The laborious efforts required by the therapies necessarily involved the patients in their own cures. While the hydrotherapies, dietetics and other natural therapies were strong forces for health, Lindlahr admitted that the greatest benefit of his program was the "strengthening of will power and self-control, the learning of obedience" (H. Lindlahr 1973, 231).

> We cannot cheat Nature by any means whatsoever—not by Christian Science, electricity, blood washing or any other therapeutic measure. We still have to comply with Nature's laws or take our spanking (H. Lindlahr 1923, 529).

He believed that "life is a school for personal effort. If it were not so, life would be meaningless" (V. Lindlahr 1973, 208). He inspired in all his patients a strong faith in the "wonder-workings" of nature. He "seared deeply into their minds the thrilling and comforting knowledge that there is a physician within all of us; that Nature's healing powers are automatic and need only to be encouraged and fostered" (ibid., 199). He added: "Once we have learned the laws of living and have mastered self-control, all that Nature holds in store for us in health matters is at our command" (ibid., 231).

Lindlahr was apparently successful in utilizing these mental and spiritual remedies. Visitors frequently commented on the cheery, happy atmosphere in the sanitarium. At times, as many as twenty percent of the patients were "permanent guests," men and women who chose to live there "because it gave them hope and courage, because it was a peaceful haven for them." One doctor who made repeated inspections of the sanitarium was intrigued by the natural therapies and amazed by the attitudes of the patients. "I've never seen such patients," he said. "I think they're all hypnotized by Dr. L." (ibid., 199-200).

Still, Lindlahr realized that the heart of his health message was also his biggest public relations problem. "The greatest drawback to the spreading of the Nature Cure idea," he wrote, "is the necessity of self-control which it imposes" (H. Lindlahr 1922, 419).

Lindlahr was the first naturopathic doctor to distinguish himself as a scientific diagnostician. His own health experiences caused him to be repelled by what he perceived as the allopathic idea that disease resulted from unpredictable accidents. He believed that every disease had a cause and, if it had not already done irreparable harm, that it could be cured by removing its cause. He was obsessed with finding the causes of his patients' conditions. He often told them: "We are going to pull your disease out by the roots" (V. Lindlahr 1973, 33). He hated the concept of "idiopathic" conditions which was in as common use then as now. "Don't send me diagnosis reports with idiopathic on them," he once flared. "If you don't know why a patient is sick, it's not a diagnosis" (ibid. 1973, 85).

As a consequence of this concern, the Lindlahr Sanitarium's diagnostic department was, by one estimate, "the most complete in any medical institution of this country," and its personnel "of highest caliber." The department was run by three medical doctors who had no other duties but diagnosis. They gave every patient a thorough examination from head to foot, which lasted from two to four days. They used "up-to-date allopathic methods" as well as osteopathic and chiropractic methods for spinal analysis. The x-ray department contained "the latest and best equipment for Roentgen ray and fluoroscopic examinations," and an "expert dentist" examined the mouth and teeth of every patient (Davidson 1923, 455). "There is no backwardness at Lindlahr's," an impressed Benedict Lust wrote, "everything is progressive and up to date" (Lust 1922, 500).

Lindlahr also employed iris diagnosis at his sanitarium and wrote a book on the topic. He had studied iris diagnosis under Henry Edward Lahn, M.D. (1864-1921), also known as H. E. Lane, who had come to America from

Bohemia in 1899. About 1905, Lahn founded the Cosmos Institute and Sanitarium in Chicago, a European-style nature cure. He introduced iris diagnosis to America with his book *Diagnosis from the Eye* (1904). Lust praised him as "a real true Naturopath who stuck to principles and was the only genius in Iridiagnosis we have yet had in America" (Lust 1921, 558).

While detractors claimed that "the methods of diagnosis used in the Lindlahr institution were preposterous" (Fishbein 1932, 119), there is no reason to believe that the sanitarium did not enjoy first-rate diagnostic services. Lindlahr established a strict division of labor between the diagnostic and therapeutic departments of the sanitarium to avoid even the appearance of a conflict of interest. As many as one third of the patients visiting the sanitarium came exclusively for diagnostic purposes.

What kind of results did Lindlahr achieve with his sanitarium patients? For acute conditions the answer appears to be very good. One writer noted:

> Thus in the Lindlahr Sanitarium during the flu epidemic of 1918-1919, three hundred cases were successfully treated without a single death; while at the Cook County Hospital just across the street, fifty-four deaths occurred of three hundred cases treated by medical methods (Hale 1926, 218).

Lindlahr claimed never to have lost a case of typhoid, diphtheria, smallpox, or scarlet fever, and to have lost only a single case each of cerebrospinal meningitis and lobar pneumonia (H. Lindlahr 1922, 188). He also held "a continuous record of more than 20 years successful treatment of appendicitis without surgery and without a death, although some of the cases received came with the usual alarming prognosis of 'abscess and threatened infection of the peritoneal cavity'" (Hale 1926, 218).

Lindlahr's confidence in natural treatment of acute conditions was built early in his career when he was studying nature cure in Germany and he visited some friends in a neighboring village. He found the housewife in great anxiety about her husband who had just been diagnosed with a serious case of pneumonia, accompanied by a high fever. "Carried away by my enthusiasm for Nature Cure," Lindlahr wrote, "I explained to the friends the difference between natural and medical treatment. They both insisted that I should give him the water treatment." Lindlahr may have gotten in a little over his head, but he went ahead and gave a wet sheet pack followed by a cold ablution, then put the man to bed. After the man generated a good sweat, Lindlahr gave him another cold ablution, a brisk towel rub and then let him sleep. The next morning Lindlahr "found him working in the meadow. The family doctor, who called early in the morning, was greatly surprised to find the bird had flown . . . . It was my first experience of treating a serious case of acute disease" (H. Lindlahr 1981, 41-42).

Lindlahr's record with chronic conditions was necessarily less spectacular, yet good. "Certainly we fail," he wrote, "but our failures are usually due to the fact that sick people, as a rule, do not consider Nature Cure methods except as a last resort" (H. Lindlahr 1922, 223). He realized that he had gotten himself into the unenviable situation of trying to prove the value of natural healing methods on chronic, terminal cases. Certainly he had opened the sanitarium in hopes of proving the viability of natural methods against chronic disease, but he obviously got more than he had bargained for. Patients sometimes arrived at the sanitarium in a dying condition, and seventy-five of the patients were of the "so-called hopelessly-incurable kind" (V. Lindlahr 1973, 27). He was especially rankled by patients with chronic disease who wanted to be cured right away. "To cure you quickly," he liked to quote Priessnitz, "I should have started with your grandmother" (H. Lindlahr 1918, 123).

Lindlahr soon realized that prevention was the answer to his predicament. If disease had causes, so did health. Natural therapeutics have "something better to give than the treatment of disease," he wrote, "and that is prevention of disease" (H. Lindlahr 1981, 191). He lucidly articulated the principles of prevention.

> The preventive method does not wait until diseases have fully developed and gained ascendancy in the body, but concentrates its best endeavors on preventing, by hygienic living and by natural methods of treatment, the development of diseases. By these, it endeavors to put the human body in such a normal, healthy condition that it is practically fool-proof against infection and the inroad of germs, bacteria and parasites (V. Lindlahr 1973, 28).

He was encouraged that others were acknowledging his message that it was "cheaper and more advantageous to prevent disease than to cure it." "The successful doctor of the future," he wrote," will have to fall in line with this plan and do more teaching than prescribing" (ibid., 29).

It is hard to assess the impact of Lindlahr's emphasis on prevention, but the success of the sanitarium bespeaks a certain level of success of his treatment methods; even in the face of so many difficult chronic cases. Over a twenty-year period he treated 50,000 patients. During that time he wrote fewer than one hundred prescriptions and never used aspirin. The sanitarium was generally full to its 200-bed capacity. As one writer said, the Lindlahr

Sanitarium was "the most eloquent testimony possible to the potentialities of Nature Cure" (Davidson 1923, 454). The same writer felt that Lindlahr himself was the best proof of his methods: "There is no better testimonial to the efficiency of Nature Cure than the inexhaustible vitality and unfaltering endurance with which Dr. Lindlahr bears up under this tremendous burden of responsibility and labor" (ibid., 456). Lindlahr arose at 5:30 each morning and performed a full day's work by noon. He lectured daily for over twenty-five years and personally supervised all departments of the sanitarium.

He had absolute faith in nature cure methods. This was illustrated in 1914 when his son Otto was struck by a car while playing ball in the street. Lindlahr discovered the accident minutes after it had happened, walking home from the sanitarium. He found the boy unconscious and barely alive. He examined his son's skull and found a large mid-line swelling at the back of his head which he diagnosed as a blood clot. He consulted with several allopaths who recommended trephining, i.e. cutting a piece out of the skull to relieve the pressure on the brain caused by the clot and administering stimulant drugs, such as strychnine, to rouse the boy from his unconsciousness. Lindlahr rejected their advice and gave his son cold salt water rubs and osteopathic manipulation. After eighteen hours, his son partially revived only to fall into a raving delirium which lasted for several days. The consulting physicians urged sedative drugs such as morphine to quiet the boy's hysteria, but Lindlahr chose to give him wet packs, cold ablutions, "inhibitive manipulation," and soothing suggestive and magnetic therapy.

After a week, the delirium went into spinal meningitis, complete with high fever and opisthotonos, i. e. spastic backward bending of the body. The other doctors recommended antipyretics, such as belladonna and potassium bromide and a lumbar puncture so that spinal fluid could be let out and meningococcal serum injected. Instead, Lindlahr fasted the boy and continued with wet packs, cold ablutions, manipulation and magnetic therapy. In another week the boy's temperature fell below normal, and he was found to be completely paralyzed and totally blind. At this time the allopathic physicians suggested powerful stimulants and a nourishing diet of meat, eggs, etc., which Lindlahr did not follow. He continued with a light diet and natural treatments. For six weeks there was no change in the boy's condition. Then one morning when Lindlahr examined his eyes, the boy said that he could see something moving in front of him. From that time on his vision and paralysis improved. After another year he was able to go back to school. He grew up to be "the proverbial 'picture of health.'" Lindlahr admitted it was his most challenging case. "The greatest difficulty," he said, "was to maintain an attitude of 'masterful inactivity'—to be able to look on patiently and allow nature to have her way in and throughout the most serious reactions" (H. Lindlahr 1981, 37-38).

In 1914, Lindlahr acquired the Lathrop family homestead, an eight-acre, park-like country place in Elmhurst, Illinois, which would become "one of the most beautiful 'back to nature places' in this country." He remodeled the manor into the "Lindlahr Health Resort" and made additions in the way of cottages, bungalows, tent houses, treatment rooms, water works, and electrical equipment. To enhance the property, Lindlahr successfully transplanted full-grown elm trees at the expense of $400 each. Like the earlier facility, this one was a success. During one mid-winter season there were over 500 outpatients taking two to six treatments per week.

By this time, Lindlahr had started his own college to train doctors in natural health methods. During 1922 a fireproof three-story building was erected for the growing school and the Lindlahr Health Institutes, consisting of the Lindlahr Sanitarium and college, occupied two hundred and fifty feet and nine separate buildings on 509-529 S. Ashland Boulevard in Chicago. There were some 200 employees at the sanitarium and school, including twenty-five clerical workers such as typists and stenographers. Lindlahr was a responsible, "exceedingly democratic" employer and always saw to it that his employees were treated with dignity and fairness. Lindlahr continued his literary pursuits. He had inaugurated *The Nature Cure Magazine* early in his career and authored a number of noted nature cure texts. During 1922, over 10,000 books and 63,000 magazines were produced and distributed at a cost of $30,000 (Davidson 1923, 452-455).

The school was originally called Lindlahr College of Nature Cure & Osteopathy, and later became the Lindlahr College of Natural Therapeutics. Finally it was changed to the Progressive College of Chiropractic, "chartered and operating under state regulations." Lindlahr assembled a solid faculty. He himself taught iridology, natural therapeutics, dietetics and Nature Cure philosophy. The dean of the school was a Harvard graduate and medical doctor. The college boasted graduates practicing throughout the United States as well as Canada, Argentina, Chile, Australia, India, Japan, China, Portugal, England and the Philippines (ibid., 456-458). Lindlahr frequently advertised his school and sanitarium in Benedict Lust's magazine, *The Naturopath*. In 1926, the Lindlahr College was purchased by the National School of Chiropractic, the liberal rival of the Palmer School of Chiropractic. In 1930, it changed its name to the National School of Drugless Therapy. Later renamed the National College of Chiropractic, it granted its last N.D. and D.D.T. (Doctor of Drugless Therapy) degrees in 1952.

In 1923, at the very pinnacle of his career as a naturopathic practitioner, Lindlahr decided that he was "at the wrong end" of his work. He had just hosted one of the greatest naturopathic conventions of that era. His sanitarium, with $50,000 of newly installed equipment, was an "unqualified success." It frequently had a waiting list of one hundred patients. The outpatient department consumed the efforts of five doctors and regularly handled 200 patients every day. But Lindlahr was dissatisfied, because people, in their ignorance, "live a lifetime of mistakes. They violate every law of Nature and then come to us expecting to be freed of so-called incurable disease in a few weeks or a few months." To act on his conviction that prevention was the best form of natural medicine, he decided to liquidate his practice and devote all his efforts to teaching preventive health methods to the public through lectures, books, and other publications. However, within a year of this fateful decision Lindlahr would be dead, the victim of "a fatal bit of carelessness" (V. Lindlahr 1973, 217-218).

Lindlahr planned to kick-off his new crusade with an extensive lecture tour. En route to his first stop in Mobile, Alabama, he slipped on the steps of a train and stubbed his toe. Lindlahr did not realize that he had sustained a flesh wound in his foot until he removed his shoe at the end of his busy day. Then he merely wrapped it in a clean handkerchief. He proceeded with his lecture the next afternoon but was soon forced to cancel the rest of his engagements and to head back to Chicago. By the time he arrived home, the toe showed signs of blood poisoning. The next day the leg was so swollen that amputation seemed imperative. Lindlahr died March 27, 1924, two hours after the operation.

As Lust wrote in his obituary, Lindlahr "died in the saddle" (1924, 359). The immediate cause of his death was "post-operative pneumonia and shock." These circumstances may have come to pass because of Lindlahr's semi-exhausted state "due to his unceasing labor and total disregard of his own comfort" (V. Lindlahr 1924, 1009). Death from such a neglected wound is ironic, to say the least, for someone who wrote: "The natural and most efficient treatment for wounds and open sores consists of exposure to air and light, and . . . the best of all antiseptics is lemon juice diluted with water" (H. Lindlahr 1918, 124).

Lindlahr's unexpected death was a shock to the naturopathic profession. His son, Victor, an osteopathic and medical doctor, carried on the work for a number of years. Although he was a successful practitioner, curing over 350 "rheumatic" cases in 1928, and would become well-known for his popular radio health shows, Victor never achieved the profound influence and authority of his father.

Henry Lindlahr was a family man and despite his busy schedule always had time for a rich family life. The indulgence and assistance of his family also played a big part in his success as a doctor and teacher. His wife, Anna, was "able and energetic," and her "sacrifices and loving labors made possible many things not otherwise to have been considered." She was modest and unassuming yet "most gracious and charming." She "adapted herself with the sweetest possible grace to the unusual demands upon her time and talents as dietician, hostess and adviser." She frequently had to put up with having her home converted to a hospital and office for weeks at a time.

> Without the patient and loyal co-operation of Mrs. Lindlahr and the entire family, Dr. Lindlahr's most important work would have been impossible (Davidson 1923, 457).

But Anna Lindlahr was not just another sweet disposition. Her knowledge of nature cure was "peculiarly extensive" (Davidson 1924, 1014). Interestingly, Mrs. Lindlahr had not always been so "able and energetic." In fact, she had been an invalid for years before she married Henry. And after they were wed, she was rejected by the New York Life Insurance Company, because she had Bright's disease. As Lindlahr described it: "The examining physician for the company assured me it was no use to try again and pronounced her case incurable."

Of course, having already embarked on the nature cure, Lindlahr could not accept this verdict, and he challenged the insurance doctor saying, "you will take her within two years." "Never," the doctor insisted. "Once albumin, always albumin." Of course, the doctor had to retract his prognosis.

> After another year of natural living, not a trace of albumin was to be found and the New York Life Insurance accepted the risk without hesitation. I may add that she has ever since enjoyed perfect health (ibid., 440).

Lindlahr had an interesting relationship with his son, Victor, whom he groomed to carry on and expand his work by sending him to osteopathic school and medical college. Victor was an apt student but he was more inclined toward the modern orthodox medicine than the old-fashioned nature cure he saw practiced at home. With typical filial skepticism, often marked by "the scoffing of youth" and the "contempt of familiarity," he would challenge his father's quainter beliefs, but he was up against the most formidable nature doctor of his day. As Victor later confessed:

> I saw him prove in countless cases the wisdom of his teachings, and I saw the awe and respect I held for orthodox medicine

> crumble before the simple truths he espoused (V. Lindlahr 1924, 1010).

There are those who suggest that Lindlahr was deeply disappointed in Victor, but if this is true, he apparently never vented any dissatisfaction to his son. As Victor related:

> When I made mistakes he would say, "that's all right, I had to learn." When I came to him in trouble—no rebuke, just, "I went through the same things," and when I failed to comprehend his ideas in the higher philosophies there was not impatience, only this, "Well, I didn't see these things until my thirties. I guess you won't either." Such a father was he! (ibid.).

Although his temper was evident when patients did not follow his instructions, Lindlahr generally showed the same kindly indulgence to others that he did to his son. He wrote: "Serenity, patience and cheerfulness are the primary requisites of the Nature Cure physician" (H. Lindlahr 1981, 236).

If any jealousy existed between Lindlahr and Lust, it didn't keep Lindlahr from publishing and advertising in Lust's publications, or keep Lust from always giving Lindlahr good press. Lust referred to Lindlahr variously as "our true friend and hearty co-worker" (Davidson 1924, 1013), "a Naturopathic Physician of the first order" (Lust 1908, 94), and, at Lindlahr's death, "a personal friend for the last 25 years . . . a very able man who cannot be replaced" (1915, 54). Lust called the Lindlahr Sanitarium "the greatest center for the Nature Cure movement in America" (1924, 359), and referred to Lindlahr's school as "great," noting that it was "phenomenally successful" (1922, 500). After visiting Lindlahr during a 1912 lecture tour, Lust wrote:

> Dr. Lindlahr is a man who has the necessary enthusiasm and vigor and works without getting tired. His personal qualities fit him especially for this great work. His institution is a model institution where all the different agencies of the nature cure are used and the best proof of his success is the large business that is going on at his two establishments. Patients and students are so numerous and prosperity is all over the place. It is wonderful what Dr. Lindlahr has accomplished in the eight or nine years since he has been in this work (1909, 2).

Lust's assertion that Lindlahr was introduced to nature cure through his magazine does not square with Lindlahr's autobiographical account which credits the book by Kuhne, but this is the only suggestion of a possibly self-serving intent in any of Lust's associations with Lindlahr. A curious fact is that Lindlahr never used the term "naturopathy" in his writings but preferred the older German terms "nature cure" or "natural therapeutics." A less flattering view of Lindlahr and his work came from Morris Fishbein, editor of the *Journal of the American Medical Association,* in his book, *Fads and Quackery in Healing.*

> The evidence available indicates that Henry Lindlahr fell early in life for the strange notions of health and disease exploited by Bernarr Macfadden in the moron's bible, *Physical Culture,* and also for the schemes of Benedict Lust (Fishbein 1932, 118-119).

The fact that Lindlahr came to nature cure in his thirties, rejected Macfadden's physical culture as ineffective, and had no business interests in common with Lust suggests Fishbein had very little "evidence available." Fishbein went on to call the treatments at the Lindlahr Sanitarium "ridiculous," and, to prove his point, he offered the following list which he apparently considered self-evident:

> The methods of treatment used include strange diets, air baths, water cures, light treatments, chiropractic, osteopathy, homeopathy, herbals, psychoanalysis, and other monkey business that any strange healer might bring temporarily into the limelight (ibid., 119)

As noted earlier, Eugene V. Debs was once a patient at the Lindlahr Sanitarium. After one of his stints in federal prison, Debs fell sick and entered the sanitarium for treatment and eventually died there. Fishbein felt that Debs' susceptibility to weird ideas made him an easy mark for Lindlahr's weird health ideas. Fishbein said he visited Debs at the sanitarium on two occasions and claimed to have witnessed improper treatment which contributed to his demise (ibid., 119). Victor Lindlahr gave a different version:

> The famous leader [Debs], suffering from a variety of chronic degenerative ailments, made a satisfactory recovery but left the Sanitarium under strict orders to take things easy. The injunction was disobeyed, and in spite of his subsequent return after a breakdown, Debs' health had been so severely impaired that he passed away at the Sanitarium after a long period of coma, on October 19, 1926 (V. Lindlahr 1973, 83).

It should be noted that these incidents occurred after Henry Lindlahr was dead.

In evaluating Lindlahr's career, one must acknowledge Lindlahr's apparent self-doubt about his own effectiveness. He seemed never to have doubted nature cure or his abilities to employ it effectively, but he made a number of significant shifts in his career strategy because he felt he was failing to have a big enough impact on the general quality of health care in this country. His goal was to demonstrate that chronic ailments were indeed curable so that all doctors would learn how to prevent and treat them. At first he hoped to influence the orthodox medical community directly because he was a legitimate medical doctor, one of them. But he was soon dissuaded from that notion by the ridicule and enmity with which he was welcomed into the medical community. Then he decided that a better tactic was to train young doctors in natural methods before they were indoctrinated in the usual fashion. He put about forty through medical school, but once they completed their studies, many went their own way. That is when he started his own school, but eventually found that this was not effective on any meaningful scale because his graduates had no real standing in the ranks of regular medicine. In 1918, he wrote of these educational efforts, "It has been a very slow, arduous, and from the worldly standpoint, a thankless work" (1918, 123). Finally, he set upon the idea of teaching the public directly. How satisfied he would have been with the results of those efforts we do not know because his death intervened. Drugless practice, which included naturopathy, chiropractic and other natural methods, did gain considerable popularity during Lindlahr's lifetime. One writer claimed that at least fifty percent of the United States population of that era went to drugless practitioners (Davidson 1923, 450).

If Lindlahr's work did not achieve the hoped-for changes in American health care, it did have a tremendous impact on naturopathic medicine. His accomplishments in the scientific practice of naturopathy on a large scale were unprecedented. His writings, including *Nature Cure,* which went through at least twenty editions by 1922, were clear, concise and comprehensive expressions of naturopathic philosophy. In 1914, *Nature Cure* was advertised as "the best work ever published in Nature Cure literature," and this statement may still be true. Lindlahr's emphasis on the mental and emotional aspects of health made naturopathy one of the most complete approaches to health, decades before the concept of "holism" evolved. His insistence on prevention as the ideal form of health care was a timely innovation that continues to be validated. The distinction he made between organic diseases, full blown pathologies such as diabetes and cancer, and functional illnesses, disturbances in metabolism which presage the organic changes, is still usefully employed by naturopathic physicians and other holistic practitioners to guide them in preventing diseases during their incipient phases. His 1919 statement, "I would also warn strongly against amalgam fillings," may have been one of the earliest expressions of concern about the nature of dental material, which has recently emerged as an important health care issue (1981, 273). Lindlahr was an early enemy of circumcision, another health issue of current concern; to him "the mutilation of the sexual organ seems inexcusable" (ibid., 147). Lindlahr was also a champion of bowel regularity and cleanliness, and he suffered ridicule for the notion that toxins can be absorbed into the body from the bowel, a concept which has long since been verified and currently represents one of the most intense areas of research in gastrointestinal medicine. Modern atomic theory was being formulated during Lindlahr's era, and he appears to have been influenced by it. He regarded life and matter as vibratory, defining disease as "disturbed polarity" and health as "satisfied polarity" (1922, 38, 44). The validity of these concepts remains undisputed, and they continue to guide some of the most forward-looking medical research today, especially in the field of cancer.

The Inventor of Constitutional Hydrotherapy

Otis G. Carroll

(1879 - 1962)

Otis George Carroll had a close personal link with Father Kneipp as had other great American nature doctors of the twentieth century. He was born in Illinois, February 17, 1879. As a boy he suffered from rheumatic fever and juvenile arthritis so severe that the nails on his crippled fingers lacerated his palms. Although he never met Kneipp, the boy finally found help in New Orleans from Alex LeDoux, a medical doctor who had studied with Kneipp and who founded the LeDoux Institute of Natural Therapy in 1895. After his cure, the young Carroll returned home to Illinois, studied botanical medicine with a Thomsonian doctor and was said to have learned 750 herbs by heart. Later he returned to New Orleans to study with LeDoux. From 1904 to 1908 he formally trained in Chicago at the Cleveland College of Chiropractic and with Dr. Henry Lindlahr. At the request of LeDoux, who considered it of strategic importance for nature cure to establish a beachhead in the Pacific Northwest, Carroll moved to Spokane, Washington in 1908 and set up a practice which he maintained until his death in 1962.

Dr. Carroll's approach to health, summarized in the following excerpt from his writings, echo the teachings of his mentor, Henry Lindlahr:

> Health must at all times come from and be maintained by digested foods. Naturopathic physicians understand this principle and use it to repair the damage done to organs, tissues and cells which have become depleted of the necessary constructive elements. These necessary elements can come only from digested foods. After a food is digested, it goes through a process of assimilation which converts it into nutrition which is carried by the circulation to every organ, tissue and cell. Remember, this process begins first with the digestion of food, and no drug yet offered can rectify damage done by failure of digestion (Scott 7/15/1992).

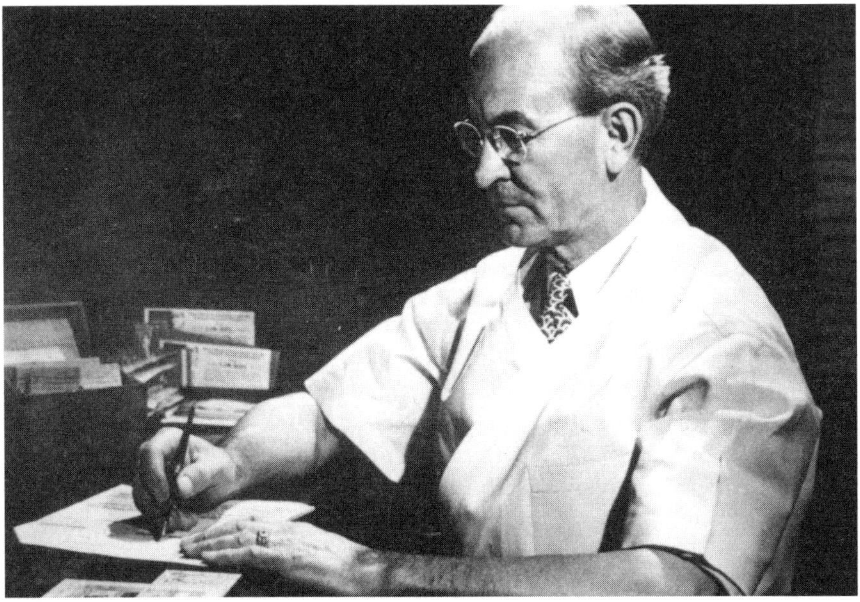

Otis G. Carroll
(Courtesy of William J. Carroll, N.D., D.C.)

Dr. Carroll is remembered for originating constitutional hydrotherapy and developing one of the first means for discerning food sensitivities. Both these methods were aimed at building health through enhanced digestion. He is also remembered as a fearless practitioner who didn't shrink from even the most hopeless cases. This resulted in many legal actions against him with consequences for the profession, which are still debated today.

Constitutional hydrotherapy, Carroll's greatest innovation, is a series of hot and cold compresses to the chest, abdomen and back during which the patient is wrapped snugly in wool blankets. In certain phases of the treatment gentle electrical stimulation is applied to the abdomen and back. It is a modernization and intensification of Priessnitz' wet sheet pack which is suited to a busy office practice. By manipulating the circulation via the body's reactions to heat and cold, this treatment gently stimulates the function of the digestive tract, immune system, spinal column, respiratory system and other vital centers underlying the treated areas. With various timings, sequences and temperature combinations, this therapy is almost infinitely variable to suit individual clinical situations. Carroll felt that the treatment improved digestion and helped the body to break down and eliminate toxins which were obstructing healthy function. He found it especially adapted to

Meditation in Hydrotherapy

Six hours a day I lay me down
Within this tub but cannot drown.

The ice cap at my rigid neck
Has served to keep me with the quick.

Within this primal element
The flesh is willing to repent.

I do not laugh; I do not cry;
I'm sweating out the will to die.

My past is sliding down the drain;
I soon will be myself again.

Theodore Roethke (1908-1963)
(Roethke 1975, 248)

respiratory conditions such as asthma and colds, GI tract problems such as dyspepsia and constipation, circulatory problems such as hypertension and varicose veins, and other ailments such as diabetes, arthritis and infertility (Boyle 1988, 135-145).

By 1923, Carroll had perfected constitutional hydrotherapy, and it remained unchanged for the next 40 years. Patients often needed a series of 50 or more treatments before the desired results were obtained, but Carroll's success with this therapy was considerable, and his confidence in it was infinite. John Harvey Kellogg, the great American authority on hydrotherapy, brought in his asthmatic wife, and Carroll promptly cured her. Carroll promised his proteges that this hydrotherapy would work for them in every case. "If the water treatment fails you," he told one of them, "you are doing something wrong"(Saine 12/8/1982).

Constitutional hydrotherapy was kept alive in Spokane after Carroll's death by Dr. Leo Scott and Dr. Harold Dick, who had trained and worked with him. But it was only in the 1980s that it was brought back into the mainstream of naturopathic medicine through the efforts of Dr. Andre Saine.

In the 1930s, Carroll had a number of difficult patients he could not cure even with constitutional hydrotherapy. His physical exam, which included subtle differentiations of the heart beat as heard through a special stethoscope, usually indicated that the stomach was involved in these cases.

Exposed during his training to Lindlahr's idea that some patients had bad reactions to certain foods, Carroll experimented with different foods to find which were causing the problems. Through trial and error he succeeded in solving these difficult cases and concluded that every person had a "food enemy," as he first called it, or an intolerance to certain foods which had to be avoided in order to maintain good health (Scott 1989).

Dissatisfied with the cumbersome and lengthy trial-and-error method of determining a patient's food intolerance, he experimented with Albert Abrams' apparatus. Abrams, despite the brilliance of his early medical career, was considered "the most notorious quack of the twentieth century" (Gevitz 1988, 7). Carroll adapted Abrams' controversial device, originally designed to diagnose and treat various pathologies, to detect what he considered constitutional or inborn food intolerances. While Abrams' machine was attacked and generally discredited by medical authorities, and Carroll's method of using the machine has never been scientifically validated, his clinical success with it was indisputable. Some doctors could not "get the same answer twice," using the machine, but Carroll was "very gifted" in its use (Bastyr/AANP 11/3/1989). Former patients of Dr. Carroll bear witness to his success.

> An 82-year-old farmer of Umatilla, Oregon, was recently seen at Dr. Leo Scott's clinic in Spokane. He said that forty years previously he could not walk from his house to his tractor without getting out of breath. At that time he had diabetes, hypertension and heart failure. His doctor had told him to sell his farm and stay in bed, as he had less than six months to live. He then went to see Dr. Carroll in Spokane where he received constitutional hydrotherapy and was taken off his food intolerance which turned out to be dairy products. He recovered rapidly and went back to farming. Afterward, he had his wife and children evaluated for their food intolerances, and, through the years, his grandchildren also. He said that in forty years neither himself, his wife, his children nor his grandchildren had ever been sick. Moreover, he feels better at 80 than he did at 40 (Boyle 1988, 169).

Like the European nature doctors, Carroll believed that disease was caused by an overload of toxins in the body. These toxins were frequently the result of faulty digestion. In constitutional hydrotherapy, he had a treatment that hastened the elimination of toxins as well as reduced their formation, and in the constitutional food intolerance test he had a method to prevent the creation of the toxins.

> Naturopaths practicing hydrotherapy have a treatment which changes the chemistry of digestion. A better quality of gastric juices is produced which results in a better digestion of foods. With the constitutional food intolerance removed from the menu there are no interferences with this digestive process. It is little wonder that the patients become enthused with the treatment even though they themselves may not understand it. Their family and friends notice the dramatic differences in their mental and physical attitude as well (Saine 1983).

In his original work in the 1930s, Carroll found seven major food intolerances: dairy, fruit, meat, eggs, sugar, potatoes and grain. In the 1940s, he determined that most people also had a combination intolerance between cereal products and dairy, fruit, eggs, potatoes and sugar. Later he added mine salt to both categories. He believed that these intolerances were unchanging. His own food intolerance was fruit. Dr. Carroll's son, William, a naturopathic physician who worked with his father for years, continues to refine his father's technique for food intolerance detection, hoping to make it scientifically acceptable.

Carroll was an accomplished herbalist who made extensive use of botanical medicine in his practice in addition to hydrotherapy and nutrition. He believed each herb was a complex medicine compounded by nature, and therefore kept his formulas, which were strongly influenced by Father Kneipp, quite simple. One of his most famous and frequently used formulas was the "42," which was four parts wormwood and two parts cape aloes. As one might expect, these and most of the other herbs he employed acted strongly on the GI tract to improve digestion and elimination.

Carroll also used iris diagnosis on every patient. He had studied iridology with Lahn and Lindlahr during his training in Chicago. He used it as much for prognostic purposes as for diagnostic purposes. By noting changes in the iris during therapy, he could predict when and in what organ systems healing crises would occur and prepare his patients accordingly. He became so accomplished at this that many of his patients considered him to be psychic. In one instance he told a patient she would develop shingles as part of her healing process, and she did. In another case he told a patient that she would vomit worms, and she did. As one of his colleagues related to a meeting of younger naturopaths: "I'd like to see some of you fellows do that." (Bastyr/AANP 11/3/89).

Carroll was a master of healing crisis management, fasting his "crisis" patients for seven, fourteen or twenty-one days or more according the "law of sevens." This was based on Lindlahr's teachings of Pythagorean numerology and the Hippocratic "law of crisis" (Lindlahr 1922, 226-240). "It took a lot of confidence on the patient's part, too. He would preach of the reaction to them, so they'd know, they'd expect it."(Bastyr 1989, 72). Carroll would never discharge a patient until they had had a reaction. Carroll made his preceptors take the water treatments and go through their own healing crisis as part of their training. It was "no fun." But the results with patients were good. It was not uncommon for patients to come to Carroll with uterine tumors, take the treatments, go through a crisis and be rid of their tumors. Men with serious prostate problems would pass copious shreds of mucus and pus while going through their crises. However, before allowing patients to enter healing crises, Carroll carefully checked to make sure their urinary specific gravities rose after their hydrotherapy treatments, which meant that their bodies could handle the toxins released during a crisis (Bastyr/AANP 11/3/89). Before World War II, Carroll usually needed 20 treatments to bring his patients into a curative crisis. After the war it often took as many as 100 treatments. He and his followers attributed the difference to decreased patient vitality due to farm chemicals, pollution, suppressive drugs and other postwar changes.

Carroll knew Benedict Lust and worked with him within the American Naturopathic Association. Whenever Lust traveled to the Northwest he always visited Carroll. Carroll's wife, the former Angela Lorang whom he married in Idaho in 1906, was of German heritage. She would converse with Lust in the language of the Fatherland and always cooked him big German meals. As Lust himself recounted after one of his trips:

> We enjoyed the hospitality of Dr. Carroll at his home, had dinner there and Mrs. Carroll surprised us with our favorite dish prepared in the old German style: good old sauerkraut (Lust 1925, 368).

The relationship between Carroll and Lust, however, went beyond the social and culinary. Lust had great respect for Carroll as a practitioner and admired the success of his clinic.

> If naturopaths would visit Dr. Carroll's institution, where men and women are treated all day and all evening, they would see fine equipment, efficient management, cleanliness and propriety, and many would be inspired and urged to do better. Diet, hydrotherapy, electric therapy, phototherapy and massage are the special features of his institution (ibid., 368).

Carroll was equally impressed with Lust, and wrote to him in 1925:

> You certainly made a hit with our boys. They agreed that you were the fairest minded man who had ever lectured to them. I

> haven't had time to sign them up, as I have been extra busy. My work seems to grow larger every day, and my obligations with it. I haven't really time to devote to organization work, but I have grown so tired of the situation in my state that I am determined to do something to make it better. I am going to go among them before your influence wears off and sign them up (1925, 170).

Here, Carroll makes reference to the political and legal climate in Washington state regarding drugless healing: generally one of persecution and prosecution. One of the earliest and most notorious cases centered around Linda Burfield Hazzard (1850-1939), an osteopath who specialized in fasting and other natural methods. In 1912, she was charged with willfully causing the death of one of her fasting patients through starvation. She was eventually tried and convicted of manslaughter and sentenced to a minimum term of two years in the state penitentiary. After some time in prison she was granted a full pardon by a sympathetic governor, only to continue to have run-ins with the medical authorities, including a serious one in 1925 when Carroll wrote the above to Lust.

Hazzard was an osteopath, but in her letters to Lust appealing for help in her legal travails she signed herself as "N.D."(1925, 472). For his part Lust always gave strong support to Hazzard and referred to her as a "wonder woman" and "one of the pioneers of Naturopathy," and made a point of visiting her at her fasting retreat on his trip to the Northwest (Lust 1926, 401). Hazzard claimed to have gotten into trouble due to sensational attacks from the newspapers which were common at the time. In one instance, O. G. Carroll played a role in quieting such assaults. While the newspapers were competing with each other in their vehement denouncements of drugless practitioners, O. G. Carroll secretly treated and cured the ailing wife of the head of a prominent newspaper. Anonymous articles favorable to the drugless doctors began to appear in the paper. No one could figure out who was writing them, but it turned out to be the head of the paper. This defused the uproar against the natural practitioners and allowed them to practice in peace, at least temporarily (Saine 8/29/ 1983).

Naturopathy also had an identity problem in the state of Washington. The term "Sanipractic" was coined and advanced by Dr. John Lyden, a graduate from Lust's school, to distinguish the drugless practice in Washington, at least in name, from naturopathy, possibly for purposes of public relations or personal gain. Not all of the problems faced by the drugless doctors came from without. Conflict among the sanipractors reached such unseemly proportions that even *The Naturopath,* usually reticent in its criticism of the various drugless groups, was forced to condemn the in-fighting as "creating a very unfavorable impression," and "certain to leave the name of Sani-Practor under a cloud" (Kipnis 1926, 409). Carroll's intent in his letter to Lust, may have been to establish some order and coherence in the Washington situation by bringing everyone under the same umbrella of Lust and the American Naturopathic Association.

Carroll was the most prominent and influential drugless practitioner in Washington during this time. His was the only listing in the "Drugless Directory of the American Naturopathic Association" in 1922. In 1926, Lust nominated Carroll to the Board of Directors of the American Naturopathic Association as representative of the state of Washington. When Lust died in 1945, Carroll wrote concerning the proposed permanent memorial to Lust:

> No greater honor could be bestowed upon our beloved leader, Dr. Lust. Everything we do now, will be a shining beacon to those who follow us. We must not think of ourselves as of today, but we must build for those who will follow in our footsteps (Gehmann 1947,19).

O. G. was not the only Carroll important to the naturopathic profession. His brother, Robert V. Carroll, who died in 1951, was a prominent naturopath in Seattle who did yeoman service in making the Washington Naturopathic Association a viable organization. He also played a controversial role as the first president of the Western American Naturopathic Association and leader of the group responsible for the split of Lust's organization. He was the main target for the acrimonious attacks of the leaders in the old Lust organization who accused him of "pseudo-medicalism" and to have betrayed the old nature cure principles and teachings of the pioneers by imitating allopathic medicine.

Robert V. Carroll's son, Bobbie, O. G.'s nephew, also became a naturopath and was instrumental in founding the National College of Naturopathic Medicine in Seattle which later moved to its present home in Portland, Oregon.

O. G. had a tormented relationship with this brother since they held opposite views and stood in opposite camps. He implored his brother not to destroy the unity of the organization Lust had built. In 1947, he attended the separate conventions of both groups in Detroit and in New York. In New York, where the parent organization held the Golden Jubilee Congress, he spoke the following words:

> I was born a naturopath. It is in my blood. I belong to this association, but I was dragged into the pseudo group by an act of the state of Washington; not because I wanted to be in that group, but because I pay money into it, I am a member of that group, so

> I cannot help myself that I am a member of both. I want to warn you of something, and that is what I have come here to tell you.
>
> You are either all going to get together or you are lost: I want to warn you that when I attended the convention in Detroit, I found the best group of high pressure salesmen that any group has. They have all withdrawn from us. They don't argue with me, but I am a brother of the president of that association, and there is no better high pressure salesman than he is. He has a sales group of men around him who are just as good as he is and they are going to overcome you.
>
> Now what are you going to do about it? Committees and arguments will get you nowhere. You are going to have to stay with naturopathy. Remember, that group of people are pseudo medical men and just as soon as they get power they are going to be no better. I mean that the naturopaths will be known as "no group" as the osteopaths are today I . . . . Hydrochloric acid application and oxygen under the skin, etc. That belongs to the medical profession. That doesn't belong to our group at all. I don't practice this kind of thing. I have never had to and I am not ashamed of my practice . . . . (cited in Freibott 1990, exhibit D, 49).

Despite his misgivings about his brother's "pseudo-group," he never stopped urging both groups to amalgamate. O. G. offered his own amalgamation plan in 1948, "to bring the American Naturopathic Association, Incorporated, of which Dr. Jesse Mercer Gehman is now President, and the American Naturopathic Association, Incorporated, of which Dr. Robt. V. Carroll is now President, to a clear and firm understanding of our needs for furthering the cause of one and only one Great Naturopathic Organization" (cited in Freibott 1990, display D, 39). Even in 1951, when he was the 2nd Vice President of the Western ANA, he didn't give up hope.

> I led off with an attempt to draw the two groups together more than two years ago, and my attempt met with disaster. But that attempt did not break down my hopes. It enkindled the flames within me, for I could easily see that the troubles lie in personal feelings, which I know could be overcome. This was consummated and I personally went to the convention at St. Louis with the intention of aiding in unifying these two groups . . . .
>
> To those of you who hold back because you think a small group, who will be known as "die-hards" tell you that they are the one and only organization, please forget it. Let's all get together and have a strong unified group. You should know by this

> time that we haven't made the progress which would permit you to feel proud. Fifty-five years have been wasted. We haven't, in most instances, convinced our lawmakers that we are any better than masseurs. Your judges, generally speaking, don't know our qualifications and capabilities (Carroll 1951, 5).

Carroll wouldn't have been pleased with the curriculum of the modern naturopathic college and its emphasis on a thorough medical training. Instead he preferred an intensive training of students in nature cure methods and in nothing else.

> Your schools are the backbone of our profession. Comb your hair up out of your eyes. Can't you see? Can't you hear? You are all being charged with knowing little or nothing. And your legislators believe that you know nothing. This makes me think some, too; but in a different vein. If we all can take the business away from the medics, with as little knowledge as they say we have, compared to their super master knowledge, then why spend so much time on super education when one can get by on so little. There is a vast difference between curing and treating. There is a vast difference between doing something *for* the patient and just merely doing something *to* the patient. We need schools to prepare our doctors to use our methods. You don't need their methods at all, and if you did know all about it you couldn't use it to any better advantage than they are using it. So why don't we tell the legislators to put us upon an equal basis with allopaths and let "survival of the fittest" reign? (1949, 10)

Carroll played an important role in helping train naturopathic doctors by accepting many of them as interns at his clinic. Already mentioned was Dr. Harold Dick, a former Boise, Idaho auto mechanic whose hopelessly sick brother was saved by a single visit to Carroll's clinic in Spokane. Impressed with Carroll's skill, Dick undertook naturopathic studies in Oregon. While he was a student, his young daughter had a fulminant reaction to poison oak and went into a coma. Unsuccessful in obtaining help from the top professors at his school, Dick contacted Carroll, who guided her dramatic recovery long distance over the phone. "Guess you know who I thought was the doctor," Dick said in describing the situation (Dick 4/9/1983). After his graduation, Dick would spend three years, from 1955 to 1958, working with Dr. Carroll.

Dr. Leo Scott was Carroll's other main protege. As a very sick twenty-year-old, and after fruitless visits to ten other doctors in the previous eleven months, Scott visited Carroll. Carroll's food intolerance diet and constitutional hydrotherapy cured him, and Scott was inspired to pursue his own naturopathic training. He went to work with Dr. Carroll from 1958 to 1962. Dr. John Bastyr also spent six months with Carroll in 1933.

Carroll's clinic was housed in the downstairs of a large, beautiful mansion that provided a comfortable, homey atmosphere for his patients. He and his family lived upstairs. Besides various examination and treatment rooms there was space for ten tables for constitutional hydrotherapy. An "unbelievable number" of patients would receive the complete one-hour treatment in the course of a day (W. Carroll 1/4/1991).

There were no appointments at Carroll's clinic which was run on a first-come, first-served basis. His patients referred so many of their friends and family to him that the clinic was often flooded to the point of paralysis. On one occasion, the clinic was overrun; patients sitting on every inch of the floor and stairways. In desperation the staff had to lock the doors to cope with the situation. Because the clinic could not handle the large number of patients, Dr. Carroll gave many of them instructions for home treatments. He endeared himself to his patients by being available every workday morning for 1½ hours of telephone consultations.

Carroll was an indefatigable practitioner, always equal to the challenges of a busy practice. His daughter Margaret, who worked as a nurse at the clinic for fifteen years, said that as a young man Carroll was badly crippled in one leg by typhoid. He promised God that if his leg was healed, he would devote the rest of his life to helping others. His leg did get better, so that later in life he was able to run up and down the sanitarium stairs, ice skate, and rough-house with his children. And Carroll clearly dedicated his life to healing. He loved his practice and worked day and night with no apparent breaks, not even to go to the bathroom. He was always pleasant and upbeat, constantly singing or humming a tune. He exuded hope and confidence, and he never gave up on a patient.

Carroll feared no disease or medical authority. As one of his students noted, Carroll "treated germs like they didn't exist"(Dick 4/9/1983). Carroll once had a case of diphtheria. He took a culture, sent it to the state health department and treated the patient. By the time the culture came back positive and the authorities "came out to quarantine the patient, the patient was well. And they couldn't understand that" (Bastyr 1989, 72-73).

Carroll had a reputation for helping hopeless cases, and he often attracted patients away from allopathic doctors who wanted to operate. This prompted many legal actions against Dr. Carroll which, according to his son, were brought by patients at the instigation of the medical profession. Carroll seemed to thrive on these conflicts. He declared with great self-confidence:

> Long ago we could have had naturopathic laws in every State had we been able to show that we have a philosophy

> different from allopathy. Too many of our men are trying to mimic the medicos. Anyone leaving my workroom knew that they received nothing that even resembled the treatment they would have gotten in an M.D.'s office. And I have built a practice, in spite of 'knocking,' unequaled in the Pacific Northwest. The M.D.s used to haul me into court but they found that I had a clever way of telling the jury who had my patients before they found me. Naturopathic methods are sufficient in themselves, to put the allopaths out of business in a single generation (Freibott 1990, exhibit D, 41)

"One of his hobbies, it seems, was fighting the M.D.s" (Saine 1983). He would never give up the battle, and was still fighting when he died. The bitter enmity between the medical doctors and Dr. Carroll persists even today more than thirty years after his death. When his daughter Margaret meets some of Carroll's old allopathic rivals in public today, a distinct chill falls over the situation. "They still dislike me greatly," she explains (McReynolds 12/8/91).

Carroll's wife's death in 1952 was a devastating blow but he still carried on. He had diabetes all his life and suffered from a rheumatic heart, and in 1959, at 80, he was forced to curtail his practice. He and his wife had three children, a son and two daughters. His son and one of his daughters worked with Carroll in his clinic. The other daughter, Virginia, was not connected with the practice, although she lived in a separate wing of the home. In the big, rambling mansion, they did not have contact every day. In 1961, unknown to Carroll and his son, Virginia became ill, and instead of seeking help, she secluded herself in her wing of the mansion. After three days they became suspicious, and Bill, the son, broke down her door, but it was too late. It was just a matter of minutes before she died. Her death at age 50 came as a sudden shock which devastated Carroll. The loss of his "favorite creation" sapped his will to live. According to his son, Carroll decided to see things through to his birthday and then died a week later on February 24, 1962, of complications of dropsy.

His obituary in the Spokane paper noted that he had practiced naturopathy in Spokane for 49 years, was an officer of the International Society of Naturopathic Physicians and a Fourth Degree Knights of Columbus (Spokane Spokesman-Review 2/26/1962).

Before Carroll died, he had a phone conversation with Dr. Harold Dick and asked him how he would treat the kind of edema Carroll was experiencing. Dr. Dick thought hard and mentioned various diuretic herbs and nutrients which might help. "I thought I taught you better than that," Dr. Carroll roared. "Don't you know there's no cure in those vitamins and herbs? The cure is in those (water) treatments." With that Carroll hung up the phone. He died the next day (Dick 4/9/1983 & Saine 5/5/85).

Of course, Carroll had no intention of taking any treatments. This conversation was his oblique way of telling his friend goodbye, that the water treatment could save him, but he did not want to be saved, and not to forget the treatment but to carry it on.

Like many naturopathic practitioners, Carroll was a poor teacher but a good demonstrator. He loved to talk about natural healing and would do so day and night, but his interns learned his methods from following him around and observing him closely rather than from instruction. He was known for talking at length around a topic without ever quite coming to the heart of the matter. He would stay up till three or four in the morning discussing naturopathic medicine, even on his wedding anniversary, but imparted few hard facts. Even his soft-spoken friend, student and admirer, John Bastyr, was led to call Carroll "the most evasive, round-the-mulberry-bush person I ever knew" (Bastyr 1984).

O. G. Carroll remains a controversial figure in the history of naturopathic medicine, especially in the state of Washington. To many, he was a hero who fearlessly pioneered the field of naturopathic medicine in the Pacific Northwest. To other naturopaths, who felt the sting of oppressive crack-downs which they believed were brought on in response to Carroll's bold methods, he was a villain who played recklessly with the privileges of his profession. Perhaps the most telling criticism of Carroll comes from Dr. John Bastyr, who had great respect for his mentor. "He would never follow up and corroborate his findings with standard tests." Bastyr pushed Carroll to use standard tests to protect his patients medically and himself legally, but Carroll's supreme confidence in his methods and his stubborn individualism led him to reject this advice. It was also too great a concession to conventional medicine which he fought tooth-and-nail throughout his career. In most cases, Carroll's exceptional abilities carried the day, but he was not infallible. He once missed a case of acute appendicitis by not taking the routine blood tests, and the patient died. It was the husband of his own nurse (Bastyr 1989, 70-72).

Of course, thousands of Carroll's patients idolized him. Dr. Leo Scott related:

> I recently talked with several of Dr. Carroll's patients from years gone-by. Most of them are up in years now, anywhere from 60 to 90 years of age. Some of their comments included: "Great," "Brilliant," "Independent," "Knowledgeable," "Deep insight," "Outgoing," "Proud, but humble," "Very brilliant, yet basic and down to earth" (Scott 8/27/1989).

Dr. Scott's own comments are telling.

> It is hard to describe someone whose insight and talents go beyond the ordinary. Unquestionably, his dedication and work came first. He unhesitatingly would have lived his life over again doing the same work. He was never too busy to care for those in need or for that matter to simply sit and visit. Even in the most serious situation he always inspired hope. During the 22 years I knew him I never saw him openly put anyone down. In my humble opinion he exemplified greatness few ever attain (ibid.)

O. G. Carroll is indisputably one of the premiere figures in the history of twentieth-century American naturopathic medicine. He achieved greatness not as a teacher, writer or organizer but rather as a "pure" practitioner. His origination of constitutional hydrotherapy preserved a permanent place for the tradition of Priessnitz in modern naturopathy. His pioneering work with food intolerance gave naturopathic medicine valuable insight into helping patients with food sensitivities. He helped transplant naturopathy from the East Coast to the Northwest where it flourished despite its near demise in the East. Despite a lack of teaching skills, his willingness to serve as preceptor to numerous doctors led to the best of his methods being adopted by several influential naturopathic physicians of today who are passing them on to a new generation of doctors.

Perhaps the last word on Carroll should go to his son, William Carroll, who got naturopathy in his blood from being dragged all over the country by his father to naturopathic conventions. As a young man he spent every day for over twelve years beside his father at the clinic. "Dad was a great man but from the old school, never pretentious. He is my unforgettable hero, and best friend in this life" (W. Carroll 4/8/1989).

The Scottish Nature Cure Pioneer

James C. Thomson

(1887-1960)

As a young man in his native Scotland, James C. Thomson enjoyed browsing the Edinburgh bookshops for popular health books, written by "crazy advocates of water treatment, physical culture and dietetic reform." He read the most "odd and freakish" sections to his friends in medical school and listened with glee to their "authoritative debunkings." He couldn't have known that in a few short years he would be rereading these books "in a different frame of mind: instead of looking for laughs he was desperate for any glimmer of hope" (C.L.Thomson 1987, 3).

Thomson was born July 18, 1887, at his family's farm, Eastertown of Gagie in the county of Angus. He claimed such distinguished relations as David Livingstone, the explorer, and William Thomson, the inventor of the pneumatic tire. Thomson was eleven when his father died, and shortly thereafter his mother took him and his two sisters to Edinburgh where he attended Daniel Stewart's College. His mother was "a striking character, of formidable presence and with an unwavering faith in her own rights and judgment," characteristics she shared with her son and which would serve him well in his future career as a naturopath (ibid., 2-3).

At sixteen, Thomson joined the Royal Navy, but eighteen months later he "went down with an acute lung condition," tuberculosis. In the Naval Hospital he deteriorated so drastically that he was discharged as incurable. His doctor sent him home with no more than three months to live. The sick young man interpreted the hearty slap on the back which accompanied this news as a challenge, and he decided at that instant to fight for his life, "just to spite you, you . . . . (nautical expression)." He stated many years later: "The most active therapeutic agent of which I know consists in a determination to get well at all costs" (1954, 192).

With nowhere else to turn, Thomson dug out the popular health works he had read before only for sport. "In a crude and groping way, he formulated a regimen for himself and stuck to it with determination." He retired to a cousin's farm where he could devote himself full-time to the job of fighting

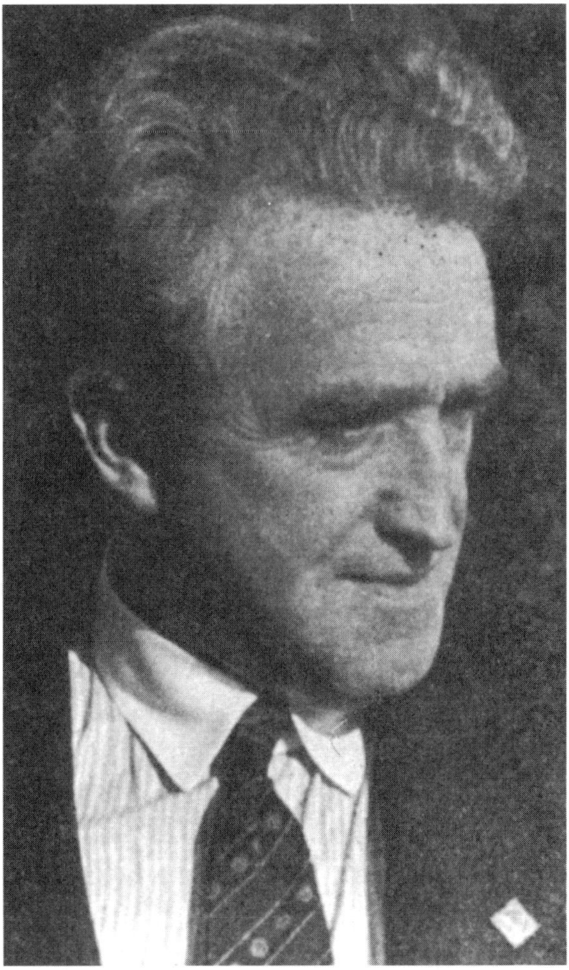

James C. Thomson
(C. Leslie Thomson 1987)

for his life. He prayed daily that the bleeding from his lungs would stop. One day he realized that he had been so engrossed in prayer that he failed to notice that he hadn't bled for a week. He continued to build up his health and to educate himself as much as possible in the ways of natural healing. To study further, he decided to set off for America.

His first destination was Battle Creek, Michigan, where he worked at Bernarr Macfadden's natural health sanatorium. He treated the famous American writer Sinclair Lewis and met C. W. Post, who became rich marketing the coffee substitute Postum and the breakfast cereal Post Toasties. Initially, Thomson was quite impressed by the results he witnessed from Macfadden's regime, primarily fasting and daily enemas. He saw "disease of almost every type fade away under treatment as morning mist does before the summer sun." However, he noticed over time that the patients "did not stay cured." As his enthusiasm "began to wilt a little," he came across an article by Henry Lindlahr, pointing out the dangers of injudicious fasting and bowel cleansing (ibid., 6-7). Thomson promptly left Battle Creek for Chicago to join Lindlahr, "who seemed to be producing more stable results." Thomson realized that he had found what he had come to America seeking, "a comprehensive system of natural methods of treatment, bound together by a philosophy and resting firmly on a scientific basis" (C. L. Thomson 1987, 4).

If he needed further convincing that he had come to the right place, an unusual incident on his trip provided it. During a dangerous mid-Atlantic storm, Thomson stood on deck of the steamship and watched "the enormous waves build up, far above deck height." Then, suddenly:

> . . . as he was gazing at a great green wall of water, he saw in the midst of it, a clear picture of a brightly lit room, through an archway, in which sat a middle-aged man surrounded by a circle of people . . . . The scene was nothing like any place he had previously seen, and the people were unfamiliar (ibid.).

Thomson gave this no further thought until his first visit to Lindlahr's sanitarium in Chicago, which was on a Sunday evening.

> As he entered the main hallway, he looked through an archway and there was the scene exactly as it appeared to him in the Atlantic storm many months before. It was Dr. Lindlahr seated amidst his patients at a Sunday Evening health talk (ibid).

Thomson and Lindlahr found that they had many interests in common, and a strong mutual respect developed. Thomson was such an "eager pupil" and "tireless worker," and Lindlahr eventually made him manager of the sanitarium. Thomson carried out his duties with distinction, especially in his work with psychiatric cases. However, not all of Thomson's activities at Lindlahr's were serious and health-oriented. Thomson often accepted friendly challenges from co-workers to see who could eat the most ice cream in a sitting, the loser having to cover the cost of the confections. According to his son, Thomson "never had to pay." Although Thomson left Lindlahr to strike out on his own after "frictions within the Lindlahr menage developed to an uncomfortable degree," Thomson always adhered to the principles and practices he learned from his mentor and constantly quoted his teachings (ibid., 8).

From Chicago Thomson traveled to Missouri where he set up a successful practice long enough to become known locally as the "Sunshine Doctor." From there he went to Florida, but he found its climate too warm for his health. In 1912 he decided to return to Scotland for a rest.

Back in Edinburgh he established a small practice and accepted as one of his first patients a Miss Jessie Hood, secretary to a famous eye specialist at the Royal Infirmary. Miss Hood, skeptical at first, soon had to admit "there was something lovable about the young quack." When he healed her of a condition her boss had assured her was incurable, she was even more impressed. For his part, Thomson began to find that Edinburgh had more than its agreeable climate to recommend itself. In June, 1913, he and Miss Hood were married.

Shortly after their son, Leslie, was born in 1914, World War I broke out. As a staunch pacifist, Thomson refused induction into the armed forces and had to appear before a panel of judges. Thomson presented his case with uncompromising militancy. Instead of imprisoning him, as he expected, the tribunal unanimously agreed to exempt him. He went home "utterly deflated and with a feeling of having been cheated" (ibid., 9-10).

Against the earnest advice of Lindlahr who had warned him against the "difficulties and heartbreaks" of a residential practice, Thomson decided to establish a sanatorium in Edinburgh. However, he could not afford the estate he desired and moved into a large house in the West End of Edinburgh, 11 Drumsheugh Gardens, "right in the middle of the medical world." For the next sixteen years "Drumsheugh" would be "a hive of industry." It housed his family, school, growing practice and publications office. He established a free clinic for needy children, founded the magazine *Rude Health*, and imported the first mercury vapor lamp for ultraviolet therapy. He experimented extensively with x-rays and received so much radiation exposure that he developed nodules on his arms. By 1938, when the estate he had originally hoped to purchase came back on the market, Thomson could now afford its considerable price. The magnificent old mansion of Gothic proportions, made of a rare pinkish orange sandstone, cemented with putty instead of mortar, was in dire need of rehabilitation.

In April of 1939, after massive renovation, Thomson opened the doors of "Kingston," his beautiful new in-patient facility; but shortly thereafter, World War II broke out. The resultant rationing, call-up of staff, blitzes and invasion scares were a challenge to the development of the new clinic, but Thomson and his wife, with the help of their son and daughter, both naturopaths, managed to overcome these difficulties. Additionally, various legal and medical authorities did their best to close Kingston down under numerous pretexts. But Kingston stayed "open and active." Thomson represented himself during these prosecutions "with more than credit," having previously suffered from incompetent legal counsel in an alleged traffic violation, for which he went to prison and staged a thirteen-day hunger strike rather than pay a fine for an unjust conviction. During this time Thomson was diagnosed with radiation sickness from his exposure to x-rays and given only two years to live, but he managed to overcome this too (ibid., 14-15).

Thomson became one of the greatest nature cure philosophers of the mid-twentieth century, and his practice, the "Kingston system," was directly descended from Lindlahr.

> In our philosophy and practice we keep the word 'cure' firmly attached to its original meaning . . . cure in its original form, implied a combination of care and curiosity. Care for the ailing person and curiosity about why he became ill (1960, 50-51).

"Anyone who offers a short cut to health, ignoring cause," he noted elsewhere, "is a quack" (1954, 89). Like Lindlahr, he was a staunch believer in the *vis medicatrix naturae*.

> I cannot understand why we should be so distrustful of the forces which built our bodies out of an almost invisible speck of protoplasm. . . . If they can build a body, they should be able to repair it (1938, 46).

He was a purist in his nature cure philosophy, insisting that healing came from within, not from without. "Genuine Nature Cure," he wrote, "has no use for medicaments or 'remedies' in any form" (1960, 59). He believed healing occurred only within living tissues. It was as much a function of the living body as breathing. He considered the idea that one person heals another person "a pitiful superstition" (ibid., 28) "It is no more possible for one human being to cure another human being," he wrote, "than it is for one person to breathe for another" (1950, 5). As he told a very sick patient who overcame "terminal" tuberculosis, "I cannot cure you, but you can probably cure yourself if you do as I tell you" (1960, 58).

This strict attitude, of course, led to many conflicts with "mixers" who employed herbal, nutritional and homeopathic remedies in their naturopathic practices, and who, Thomson felt, had an "inadequate understanding" of natural treatment. Their patients had little faith "in their inborn self-healing powers, and feel the need to lean upon some variety of bottled remedy" (1954, 19). Because the *vis medicatrix naturae* was intolerant of toxic tissues, Thomson taught that real health was rarely placid. To emphasize this point he entitled his magazine *Rude Health*. The body underwent periodic detoxifications, or as Thomson liked to call them, "house cleanings," which unburdened it from the poisons that made it sick. These detoxifications were easily misinterpreted. Most people became upset when they got sick, but Thomson preached an alternative point of view:

> When your body decides upon a spring cleaning, instead of becoming emotional and afraid, you should be thankful to your body for making such an excellent effort on your behalf (1950, 3).

Like Lindlahr and his predecessors, Thomson believed that chronic disease resulted from suppression of acute disease. He was fond of quoting the famous Summerhill educator, A. S. Neill, who agreed with nature cure practices:

> I believe that Nature Cure people are right when they apply to physical disease the same method that we apply to psychical disease. Just as a buried wish should be lived out, so should a buried poison be allowed to find its way out (1939, 65).

Thomson often invoked John H. Tilden's "intelligent leaving alone," as the best course for working with the *vis medicatrix naturae* during a healing crisis (1938, 50). If the body's efforts to expel toxins were suppressed, he believed, one could eventually expect "the long suffering and lingering death from cancer" (ibid., 17). Thomson even went so far as to suggest that the drawn-out agony so often seen in modern death was less attributable to life-saving devices than to debilitating medicines given throughout life, which left the body without the vitality to accomplish its own natural, peaceful demise. Because all disease resulted from accumulated toxins and was in fact the result of the body's attempts to get rid of them, Thomson did not believe in "conferring titles upon conditions of ill health" (1947, 11). Conventional diagnostic names promote the mistaken idea that the "disease" has to be suppressed and that only one part or system of the body is affected. "Disease is never only local," he wrote. "Your body is either all healthy or all unhealthy" (1950, 11). Conventional diagnosis also imparted a sense of hopelessness to patients with "terminal" diseases. Thomson believed that "incurable diseases do not advance without supplies. Withdraw the cause and the body is self-healing" (1954, 18).

The prevention of intoxication through natural living and the allowance for detoxification by not suppressing acute disease were the keys to vibrant health which Thomson believed were available to every person. "Healing is essentially a 'do-it-yourself' phenomenon," he wrote late in his career (1960, 51). Like Lindlahr, he believed that maintaining healthful habits by strong self-control was of utmost importance. "There is but one cure," he wrote, "break the habit" (1954,71). The secret to a long, healthy life was "to live within one's physiological limits at all times." This simple goal is rarely attained due to the worst human habit of all, "the daily adventure to see how near to disaster we can go without being caught."(1960, 28).

> What is wrong with most people is that they want to eat things that are not good for them, they want to drink things that are not good for them, and they want to do things that are not good for them (1954, 18).

In short, they wanted to enjoy life, not only health. Most of them didn't want to be the health puritans prescribed for by nature cure.

The therapeutic mainstays of the "Kingston system" were diet, hydrotherapy and spinal manipulation. Thomson's dietary philosophy was summed up in a Lindlahr statement he liked to quote: "One-third of what we eat enables us to live; the other two-thirds enables the doctors to live" (1954, 24).

Thomson prescribed a mostly raw food vegetarian diet and railed against denatured foods, especially those with artificial preservatives:

> We now have food that "keeps" indefinitely . . . which means that germs cannot live on it and that, in turn, means that we would be well advised not to try to do so either. If the additives are so poisonous that they will kill bugs, it is only a matter of time before it does the same to the human consumer (1960, 29).

Thomson also practiced judicious, short-term fasting on his patients and promoted the drinking of Koumiss, a cultured raw milk product, as a source of healthful bowel flora.

He regarded hydrotherapy as "one among several equally important parts of Nature Cure practice." His hydrotherapy practices fell squarely within the tradition of Priessnitz, Kneipp and Kuhne. One of his favorite therapeutic baths was the "squat splash," a modification of Kuhne's friction sitz bath suitable for home use, where the patient squats in a tub with three to four inches of cold water and splashes the lower abdominal and perineal areas (C. L. Thomson 1970, 11).

Unlike some predecessors and contemporaries, Thomson did not advocate internal hydrotherapy. His experience at Macfadden's sanatorium convinced him of the disadvantages of enemas and colonic irrigations, and he used them only in special circumstances. He was also against copious water drinking.

> For the majority of the chronically ill persons with whom we have had to deal, the most common physical peculiarity has been a long-established tendency toward flabby, water-logged tissues—very often derived from following medical advice to drink so many pints of water daily (1960, 4).

While he was a strong advocate of detoxification, he believed the popular idea of flushing the system out with water was misguided. "Elimination is of a chemical and not a mechanical nature," he wrote (1970, 14). Thomson was convinced that excessive water intake diluted the intestinal juices, caused the intestinal tissues to "lose their tensile strength," and promoted constipation by causing a rebound dryness (1950, 21). One of Thomson's books was entitled *Two Health Problems: Constipation and Our Civilization,* which indicted laxatives, enemas and excessive water drinking as causes rather than cures of chronic constipation. While water drinking to overcome intestinal dryness could achieve immediate relief of constipation, it was at the expense of the body's future well-being and regularity. Instead of secreting its own mucous fluids to lubricate its membranes, the bowel learned to rely on massive water intake to artificially wash its contents through. In the tradition of Kneipp, who believed the body should be hardened by judicious challenges, Thomson advocated keeping the bowel as dry as possible. "Dryness of faecal matter is stimulus for the secretion of mucous fluids," he quoted from Lindlahr. "When the stimulus is lacking the intestines become less active" (1954, 13-14).

Additionally, Thomson believed that excess water increased the absorption of toxins from the intestines into the bloodstream, because "the bowels are distended, and their walls accordingly stretched and thinned, therefore becoming more easily permeable to the bowel contents" (1970, 15). This is an intriguing theory in light of the intense research which is currently being conducted on the relationship between gastrointestinal mucosal permeability and disease (Crissinger 1990, 145-154).

Thomson believed manipulating the spine was essential for achieving and maintaining healthy organs and tissues. He used it skillfully to correct nerve and circulatory imbalances which hampered normal function.

Although often accused of extremism because of his radical devotion to nature cure, Thomson saw himself as striving for the "sweet reasonable" in all things (1960, 4). This tendency was manifest in his approach to iris diagnosis, which others had taken to extremes. He favored common sense iridology "shorn of glamour" and not "obscured with romanticism" (1970, 17). Common sense described much of his approach. He made a dramatic cure of gangrene of the foot in a patient by, among other things, having her quit smoking. Concerning her previous doctors she told him:

> I used to lie in bed talking and smoking all the time they were examining me. You are the first person who ever said that tobacco could have anything to do with my condition (1960, 32).

He also used common sense to invent natural treatments of stunning simplicity such as the "T. K. Wriggle."

> Sitting or standing, have the subject place both feet flat on the floor. Then the toes of one foot are raised as high as the footwear will allow—keeping the sole of the foot firmly pressed down. Then lower the raised toes and raise the lowered ones alternately, at about the speed of walking. Keep that up during all your waking hours and, providing the wriggler's nutritional and other habits are reasonable. . . practically all ulcers, skin eruptions, intermittent claudication, etc., should quietly fade away.

In the tradition of the earliest nature doctors, Thomson learned this "trick" by watching horses, cows, elephants and other large animals. "The healthy ones all keep wriggling," he wrote, "the unhealthy ones keep still."

> It adds that little push to defective circulation which can decide the issue . . . . These results have been obtained over and over again in cases pronounced 'impossible' by all kinds of leading authorities (1960, 34-35).

Of course, Thomson was a strong advocate of prevention. Even though he had good success treating advanced disease, he repeatedly emphasized, "We cannot hope for results by treating the end-effects of wrong living" (1938, 8). He roundly condemned vaccination and food pasteurization as misguided public health measures which caused far more sickness than they prevented, and he was a strong critic of conventional pharmaceutical medicine. He felt drugs were poisonous substances which could only intoxicate the body, and that placing official medicine's "Rx" before their names did nothing to change the nature of these harmful remedies. He pointed out the irony of the stern media warnings to burglars which always followed thefts of drugs from a doctor's car or pharmacy: "I would say that any material which is likely to damage a healthy thief is even more likely to harm an unhealthy invalid" (1960, 46). When a heckler interrupted his "Belfast Lecture" with the question, "What would you put in the place of drugs?" Thomson answered, "Surely if we get rid of a bad thing, it is unnecessary to put anything in its place" (1950, 9). He felt pharmaceutical medicine had turned health care on its head.

> The drug-doper studies human habits and tries to alter natural laws to suit them; the Naturopath studies natural law and corrects the individual habits till they harmonize (C. L. Thomson 1983,10).

Thomson felt there was an unseemly profit motive operating in the promotion of drugs by physicians. He liked to quote Lord Horder on pharmaceutical corruption: "Formerly the chemist was the servant of the doctor; today he tends to become the doctor's master" (1960, 20).

Thomson advanced the provocative theory that chemical pesticides such as DDT and chlordane played a role in the etiology of infectious diseases such as polio and hepatitis by intoxicating tissues and making them susceptible to viruses. He went so far as to suggest that the large chemical companies made out nicely by selling the cause of disease and then marketing its supposed cure. He repeatedly made radical links between health and politics, condemning the war machine and the drug machine as co-conspirators in keeping the world sick. "The healthy man," he wrote, "has no desire to damage or destroy anything; not even his fellow man!" (1960, 39). In addition, Thomson despised all specialization in medicine. He considered a specialist someone "who knows nothing else" (1947, 14).

Of course, the medical establishment returned Thomson's harsh criticism in kind, and Thomson spent a lot of his time and energy testily answering his allopathic critics. He was especially irked by established medicine's unwillingness to acknowledge nature cure's successes. He claimed a conspiracy between the news media and the "medical junta" kept naturopathic successes out of the press, and that medicos were primed with pat answers such as "amusing explanation" or "misdiagnosis" when confronted with naturopathic successes (1960, 5). Thomson found this latter device maddening. "Could it be," he wrote, "that in some peculiar way only people who have been wrongly diagnosed and advised gravitate toward Kingston?" He related the case of a female surgeon with breast cancer who was certified as incurable by the top eight British specialists in the field. In desperation she came to Thomson and was cured on his program. Upon return to the specialists, she was certified by all eight of them to be cancer-free and wrongly diagnosed. Enraged by such hypocrisy, she embarked on a bitter campaign against orthodox cancer therapy and "held it up to ridicule in a most uncompromising way." She died mysteriously of a gunshot to the back of the head (1960, 42-44).

Thomson was also rankled by established medicine's eagerness to exploit the death of any nature cure patient as proof of the ineffectiveness of its methods—even if it occurred many years after allopathy had given up on the patient. He wrote:

> The only way we could overcome that recurring criticism would be to arrange for our patients to live forever. Ultimately they all die and just as surely as this happens we learn that still another Nature Cure failure has been registered' (1960, 41).

Thomson became keenly aware of the hidden hand of organized medicine working behind the scenes. He was once enthusiastically received by a Glasgow University medical society and eagerly invited back to speak again, only to have the invitation rescinded when the medical society was reprimanded by a higher body for allowing him to speak the first time. He also cited instances where tuberculosis patients, cured by naturopathic treatments, were not given a clean bill of health required in order to return to work after they disclosed the method by which they were cured.

Besides his practice and his promotion of health reform through his many books, Thomson was the principal of the Edinburgh School of Natural Therapeutics, which he founded in 1913. For over two generations this school was "the only place in Britain at which a truly professional and adequate understanding of training in Nature Cure could be obtained" (C. L. Thomson 1967, 9). Thomson continually upgraded the instruction available at his school. His eventual insistence upon four full years of training led to "an unhappy difference of opinion with Stanley Lief." This resulted in Thomson's leaving the Nature Cure Association in 1927, an organization which both he and Lief had helped start in 1922. He then established the Society of Registered Naturopaths. Just because students graduated from the Edinburgh School did not mean that Thomson was finished with them; he was famous for traveling all over the country to check on them and help them build good practices.

Indeed it was the furious pace that Thomson, who "refused to relax," kept up which lead to his demise. He worked "at full pressure right up to the onset of his last illness" (C. L. Thomson 1983, 15). One day in his workshop he was "struck violently in the diaphragm by a heavy piece of metal." Possibly due to his over-exposure to x-rays decades before, and to the scar tissue on his lungs from his tuberculosis, the injury did not heal as expected, and complications set in. He died March 27, 1960. Alluding to his father's saying that, "the only way we could prove the success of Nature Cure would be to keep all our patients alive forever," his son, Leslie, wrote:

> He gallantly approached that ideal in his own life, by extending an expected three months of wasting existence into fifty-six years of vigorous activity, during which he taught thousands of people how to extend their own lives and usefulness (ibid., 15).

Thomson was eulogized by the son of his first Edinburgh patient:

> He is finished with his earthly body, which for so long was held together by his courage, his determination and his will, but our remembrances of him and the blessings of countless numbers, who owe so much to his help and guidance and who took strength from his dominant personality, will never die (ibid., 16).

Along with Stanley Lief, Thomson helped transplant Lindlahr's scientific version of nature cure to the British Isles, and his dynamic personality ensured that it took root and thrived. His successful clinical practice, books, and respected school were the fruits of a Herculean labor. Thomson's son called him "the first physician to base his methods on proven facts, and not at all on mystery and superstition" (1970, 4). Perhaps the highest tribute paid him came from a long time colleague:

> Without his strength, ability, power and inspiration, the Society (of Registered Naturopaths) might never have existed, nor would we as practitioners have been here (Harrison 1969, 5).

James C. Thomson was fortunate to have a son of equal stature. Charles Leslie Thomson (1914-1992) followed his father as the Director of the Kingston Clinic, which he ran for 30 years until its demise. He was an outstanding practitioner, teacher and author. One of his admirers summed up his accomplishments as follows:

> He was a literary descendant of Dr. Lindlahr, whom he once described as a "great collector of information." His father honed this down to a pragmatic or workable format, and Leslie improved its literary and scientific credibility through extensive research, his ongoing clinical experience and homely parallels (Fenton 1992, 2).

England's Foremost Naturopath

Stanley Lief

(1892-1963)

Stanley Lief and James C. Thomson set the standards for naturopathy in the British Isles the way Lust and Lindlahr defined naturopathy in America. Lief was born in Lutzen in the Baltic state of Latvia on October 9, 1892. He was one of five children of Isaac and Riva Lief, whose Jewish surname was shortened from a much longer version. His father was a soldier in the pay of the Russian czar. When Lief was quite young, his family emigrated to South Africa to escape poverty and persecution in their homeland. They settled in Pretoria, where Lief spent a boyhood "ridden with illness." As one writer stated bluntly: "He was too fat and had a weak heart" (Day 1979, 84). Receiving little help from the doctors who treated him, he grew shy and introspective. He obtained a basic primary school education, helped his father with the family grocery store and later studied engineering.

He often sat watching the African natives at work. When they got sick, "they just lay in the sun and refused to eat till well again." He eventually copied this "instinctive fasting" and vastly improved his own poor health. He was also influenced by friends, who were physical culturists, to work out and develop his body. When he chanced upon a copy of Bernarr Macfadden's magazine, *Physical Culture*, he decided then and there to travel to America and study with Macfadden. His family roundly ridiculed his intention to devote his life to natural healing, but at age eighteen he worked his way to America as a ship's steward.

In America, he enrolled at Macfadden's International College of Drugless Physicians in Chicago, became Macfadden's star pupil, and graduated with honors. In addition to academics, the course of study at Macfadden's required Lief to become a "first-rate physical specimen" (Wood 1963, 600). He built up his physique to the extent that he became a wrestling champion of Illinois.

After his studies, Lief traveled throughout the states broadening his knowledge at various health establishments. According to his son, Peter, one of these establishments was Lindlahr's sanatorium in Chicago where Lief

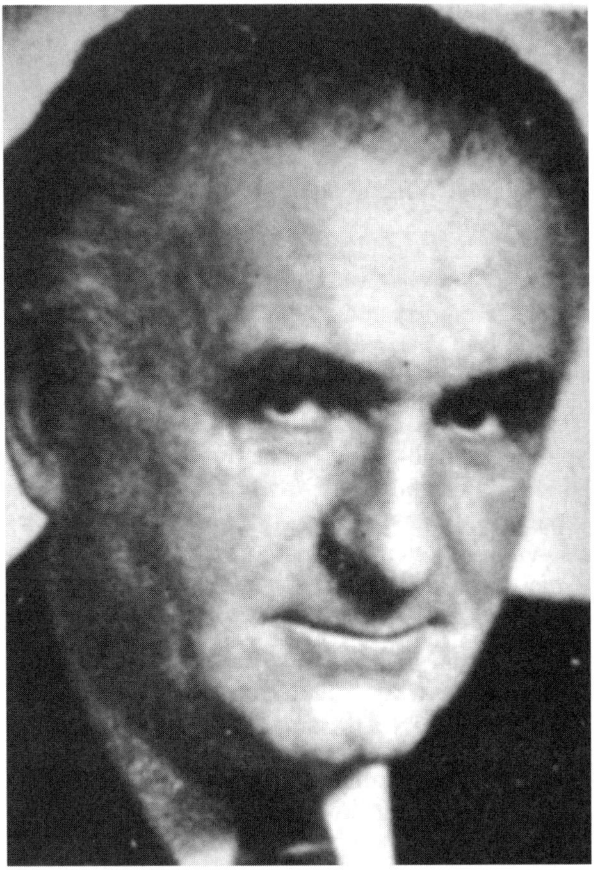

Stanley Lief

was exposed to Lindlahr's teachings (Edwards 1992, letter). Lief then returned to England qualified both as a chiropractor and naturopath, and became manager of Macfadden's "Healthatorium" at Brighton, the name of which prompted one British writer to exclaim, "Oh, these American appellations" (Wood 1963, 601).

Unlike J. C. Thomson who refused service as a conscientious objector, Lief volunteered for World War I. The British Army appreciated his prior experience and made him a physical training instructor, there being a liberal spirit within the British forces at that time. There was even an "Almeric Paget Massage Corps," a troop of young women certified in massage and employed by the War Office in treating the injuries of wounded soldiers. Lief eventually saw action in France and was wounded by shrapnel in the arm. He was released from service in 1918, and told by surgeons he must have his arm amputated. In the tradition of other nature doctors, Lief refused to accept their verdict and, after six months of a vegetarian diet, occasional fasting, and diligent exercise, he regained the full use and mobility of his arm.

After the war Lief resumed practice. To reach a wider public, he moved nearer to London and established a small health home at Chesham in Buckinghamshire. He attracted a great number of "incurables," and was able to heal most of them. One such patient was Mr. C. M. Trelawney Irving, a government official forced to retire at age forty due to a chronic "incurable" illness. Using natural methods, Lief restored his health, and to show his gratitude, Trelawney Irving helped him purchase Champneys, a large, elegant estate which Lief converted to the first natural health retreat in England. Trelawney Irving maintained his support of Champneys for over fifty years, helping it to become one of the largest nature cure establishments in the world. He never tired of boasting that, thanks to Stanley Lief, he was "the State's longest surviving pensioner!" (White 1992, 1).

Champneys had a distinguished history going all the way back to its founding in 1307. During the sixteenth century it was owned by the Archbishop of Canterbury, and later by the famous Rothschild banking family. The Champneys mansion which Lief took over was built in 1874.

At Champneys, Lief established his reputation as "a daring and pioneering healer" (Chaitow 1987,12). He achieved "spectacular results" and developed a huge following, including many in fashionable society who regarded him as a "new Messiah" of an alternative medicine. Champneys soon became known as the "Mecca of those who distrusted the medical profession" (History of Champneys, 1989 Leaflet).

Lief constantly sought to position himself advantageously for the promotion of nature cure. In 1927, to achieve a wider acceptance of his health beliefs among the general public, he recruited a journalist and fellow physical

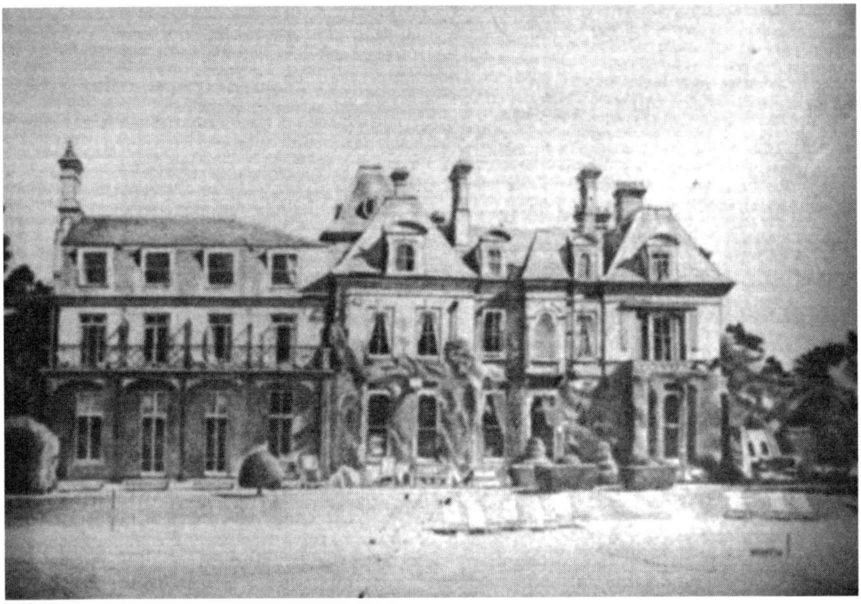

Champneys Mansion

culture enthusiast, John Wood, to help him launch a popular magazine. So important did he consider this publication, *Health For All*, that he mortgaged Champneys to finance it. Lief himself was a frequent and talented contributor. He advertised *Health for All* as "a practical magazine edited by a practical man for practical people." As one writer put it, "His delightfully lucid writing was truly superb journalism" (Franklin 1963, 671). Within three years *Health For All* was being published monthly in 13,000 copy runs. Within ten years, it claimed a readership of 50,000 and enjoyed a worldwide distribution, with advertisers receiving orders from Zanzibar, Burma, China and Sweden. It was "by far the best health magazine in the country" (Day 1979, 85).

The philosophy Lief espoused in his magazine and put into practice at Champneys was pure classical nature cure. He subscribed to the time-honored intoxication theory of pathology as articulated by his naturopathic forebears. "Disease," he wrote, "is nothing else but a state of toxaemia brought about by eating habits—food in excess and food of wrong quality" (Lief 1932, 67). Elsewhere, he repeated Lindlahr's four primary causes of disease: lowered vitality due to overwork and stress; abnormal composition of blood and lymph due to improper diet; accumulation of waste material; and "mechanical interference" with circulation due to strain or injury (Lief 1931, 17).

Because disease represented the body's attempt to expel excess toxins, Lief considered it "a friend in disguise" (Lief 1963, 407). Like Thomson, he frequently compared sickness to "a physical house-cleaning." He embraced the nature cure tenet that suppression of the detoxification efforts of acute disease leads to debilitating chronic ailments. He called the germ theory of disease a "prize bogy," and regarded germs "not as a primary cause, but as a secondary manifestation of disease" (Lief 1931, 18). He claimed that naturopaths treated basic causes, while medical doctors trifled with effects. He also advocated a holistic approach. Believing that disease was a systemic disturbance, he felt "the only form of treatment which will succeed and be lasting is that which will affect the body as a whole" (Lief 1962, 271) Like Thomson, he put little stock in conventional diagnosis, especially as practiced by what he called "learned M.D.s," who appeared to feel that by naming the patient's illness "they have done their full duty by him, and are justified in washing their hands of him" (Lief 1931, 18).

Lief's attitude toward the common cold illustrates his basic outlook on disease. He wrote, "No ailment is produced in the body by chance nor is it caused by an outside influence. Ill-health always arises from a condition within the body." (Lief 1931, 342) To avoid colds, he warned, "keep the body free of toxins." He believed, that "A cold purifies the system if properly treated" (ibid., 343).

Lief had a five point plan for treating colds: stop eating; flush the bowels; take warm baths; get plenty of fresh air; and rest in bed. This strategy represented his therapeutic approach to most problems. He successfully adopted the fasting and enema approach of Macfadden which Thomson found wanting. He believed that fasting overcame disease by enabling the body to rid itself of toxins, allowing vital organs to rest and recuperate and by allowing the individual to develop normal hunger. Although Lief employed hydrotherapy, massage, spinal manipulation, electrotherapy, milk diet and heliotherapy at Champneys, fasting was his favorite therapeutic tool. When asked by a patient what good the various treatments did her, he replied, "If you want to know, very little. It is the fasting that gets you well" (Gorst 1963, 670). He found enemas "really indispensable during the fast" and recommended they be taken every other day (Lief 1932, 70).

Ignoring the admonitions of Lindlahr and Thomson, Lief took therapeutic fasting to new lengths. As his editorial partner John Wood wrote, "No other healers have ever conducted such long therapeutic fasts, simply because none had such a profound experience of the method" (1963, 600). Wood described orange juice fasts of seventy-two and ninety-three days as among the longest conducted by Lief, and described the results as "spectacular" in such varied conditions as elephantiasis, rheumatoid arthritis and pernicious anemia. Regarding the last condition Lief wrote: "In cases of pernicious anemia, where the blood count is a third of its normal number, double the number of red corpuscles have been produced in so short a period as seven days' abstinence from food " (Lief 1930, 125). In cases of rheumatoid arthritis, which he considered to be caused by an accumulation of toxins, Lief usually prescribed a fifteen to twenty-five day fast, Epsom salts baths and a fruit and vegetable diet which excluded eggs, fat, meat and starch. The diets of all his patients consisted "largely, if not wholly, of raw foods" (ibid., 85).

A look at Lief's own personal health habits gives further insight into the nature cure approach he followed with his patients. He slept on an open veranda year round. Upon waking, he shaved naked in front of an open window, drank two glasses of cold lemon water, performed fifteen minutes of exercise, then gave himself a friction rub and cold sitz bath, which he topped off with a general cold water body splash. Such regimen put him in "extremely good fettle" for his day's work. He believed that "few human beings need more than two meals per day," and that these meals should not be regular. As for meat products, he partook of these maybe three times "in a fortnight." He was very strict with this program. As he wrote: "When I say daily regime, I mean daily, 365 days in a year. That is the only way to keep fit. Regularity, except in eating, tells the whole story" (ibid., 165).

Besides championing the time-honored methods of classical nature cure, Lief also added novel treatments of his own. As a chiropractor and osteopath he was a gifted manipulator of hard and soft tissue. He invented what became known as Lief's neuromuscular technique which was a "methodical, sequential, systematic, controlled combing" of muscles for trigger points, areas of abnormally high contraction and sensitivity (Chaitow 1991, 67). Because it reduced the abnormal contractions, this technique was at once diagnostic and therapeutic. Working with other practitioners, Lief developed it into what is known today as NMT (neuromuscular technique). Lief was influenced to work in this area in the 1930s by Dr. Dervanchand Varma, an Ayurvedic practitioner in Paris, who employed a rudimentary neuromuscular technique he called "pranotherapy" (ibid. 113/114).

Lief developed a special variation of neuromuscular technique, which came to be known as "bloodless surgery," for breaking up post-surgical abdominal adhesions. He performed these soft tissue manipulations under subdued red light to induce deep relaxation in the patient (Turner 1984, 101). These techniques were reminiscent of the work of Adolf Lorenz (1854-1946), an Austrian orthopedic surgeon who used manipulative methods.

Lief was extremely successful in his practice. His followers attributed this to his strict adherence to nature cure and his instinctive ability to heal. Lief never deviated from the early teachings he was exposed to in America.

He had no use for any "fringe therapies" or "so-called remedies" (White 1992, 3). While he would travel the world to investigate any new natural treatment, his basic message remained the same: "There are no substitutes for obedience to the never-changing laws of life" (Lief 1963, 670). Despite the luxurious appointments of Champneys, he offered a simple, straightforward nature cure program without "frills, complementaries or supplementaries" (Moule 1963, 599).

Lief also possessed a remarkable instinctive understanding of the human body. As one admirer noted, "His powers of diagnosis were extraordinary and his skilled manipulation uncanny in its accuracy. That he possessed healing powers and could transmit healing energy by touch I have no doubt." (Gorst 1963, 670).

Lief's success was more noteworthy because of the difficult nature of many of the cases he took on. As a longtime housekeeper at Champneys recently pointed out, he often took patients who had been told to "learn to live with their condition." She remembered the dramatic case of a woman "in a terrible condition" being treated for Parkinson's disease. Lief examined her and found a problem in the spine which, after he corrected it, resulted in "no P.D. at all." The same former employee recounted the history of a young boy of eight who was scheduled to have his spleen removed. Lief prescribed a special diet for the child who "grew up well and strong" and joined the Royal Navy "spleen intact" (Dixon 1992). A man employed at Champneys for fifty years as head porter recalled many patients brought in on stretchers who, after treatment, were able to walk out under their own power (Spencer 1992).

Lief constantly warned his patients against expecting quick cures for their chronic illnesses. "No one should expect to be cured of a disease that has been in process of development for many years, in a few weeks or a few months" (Lief 1930, 249). Still, he was very slow to give up on even the most apparently hopeless cases. "Health is natural and sickness is not," he wrote. "Nature fights for a man's life long after he gives up the struggle." He felt there was hope even in the most serious conditions, because "it takes more energy and power to run the human machine in sickness than in health" (Lief 1930, 205).

Lief's best work went largely unnoticed by the general public, but it came into the limelight whenever a celebrity would be found "taking the cure" at Champneys. Two of his most famous patients were Paul Robeson, the great American singer, and Amy Johnson, the noted British aviatrix.

In 1930, the medical establishment began to pay him closer attention. Lief was set up with a planted patient who complained to the authorities of being misled to believe he was being treated by a "registered" medical practitioner. Although Lief was often referred to as "Dr." in the press, he never used the term himself. Nonetheless, at the conclusion of the highly publicized trial the charge was upheld on technical grounds, but: "to register its disapproval of the manner in which the case had been brought the court awarded a derisory 'one farthing' damage—i.e., the smallest coin of the realm at that time" (White 1992, 2). Lief's reputation and the principles of natural healing were enormously enhanced by the testimony of many famous people on his behalf. In the 1940s, Britain's National Health Service tried to thwart the practice of naturopathy by refusing medical care to any patient who followed non-medical approaches. Lief successfully led the fight to block this restriction.

Lief was a complex character. Like many predecessors, he was a charismatic personality with little tolerance for those who would not follow his health prescriptions. A long-time employee described him as a "dominant personality" who turned his patients out of the nearby Orchard Cafe if he found them disobeying him and having tea there. Lief was also "a bit of a showman." On Sunday evenings he would gather all his patients together and "perform" for them, "showing off his body and his great muscles!" (Spencer 1992). He was a strict disciplinarian who kept both staff and patients in order, but showed his appreciation for work well done. While some described him as "buoyant" and never shrinking from controversy (Gorst 1963, 670), others considered him quiet, kindly and "generous to a fault" (White 1992, 3). He often treated the local people free or at reduced charge. When a grateful patient once told him, "I will see your secretary about the fee," all Lief said was, "She does not want to see you" (Gorst 1963, 670). Despite his many run-ins with the medical authorities, he "never bore any malice" (Parnell 1963, 670).

His resilient vitality and apparently easy success prompted many to call him "Lucky Lief," but as his associate, John Wood, noted, Lief's success came from "his absolute faith in himself and his cause and his unremitting self-sacrificing work" (Wood 1963, 600). Despite his many achievements, Lief was "singularly modest." (Powell 1963, 602).

An interesting assessment of him comes from Mary Williamson Macfadden, the wife of his former teacher and boss, Bernarr Macfadden. She described him as "extremely capable," adding that he "despised fanaticism in anything." "There was no textbook dogma in his ideas of working with nature to cure the sick," she wrote. She commended him for his "common sense" and eclecticism, saying, "If he thought doctors had good ideas he used them." She went on to describe, among other things, his baby-sitting abilities with her daughter:

> I would miss the brilliant Stanley Lief. He was the only one I trusted with Baby Byrnece when I had to take my walking exercises on the Sea Terrace. I finally came to the conclusion that he changed her diapers better than I did. No tender mother can pay a greater tribute! I agreed with his intelligent ideas on curative fasting. He would never have reduced a patient to starvation. He had taken what was good in the Macfadden method, and improved on it. (Macfadden 170-171).

Besides his busy practice, Lief contributed to the growth of naturopathy in Great Britain through his educational and organizational efforts. In 1936, he launched an appeal for funds to establish a naturopathic college and was able in 1938 to open the Nature Cure Association and Clinic. This school, which became the present-day British College of Naturopathy and Osteopathy, was destroyed by bombs in World War II and in 1954 moved to its present site in Hempstead on property donated by Hector Frazer and his wife who were grateful patients treated by Lief. In 1945, Lief was instrumental in forming the British Naturopathic and Osteopathic Association (BNOA), a merger of the National Osteopathic Association of Great Britain (founded 1915) and the British Association of Naturopaths (founded 1925). He served three terms as president of the BNOA and functioned as dean of the college from its foundation until his death.

Throughout most of his career, Lief saw an average of 5,000 patients a year. In 1958 he cut back his practice. A year later, while he was giving "an eighteen-stone patient a heavy osteopathic manipulation, 'something went,'" which turned out to be his heart. He died four years later in 1963 (Wood 1963, 601). As his colleague, Arthur White, eloquently wrote:

> His inability to refuse the constant professional and social demands of his time meant that in later years he was able to devote little or no time to the physical and recreational activities which had so dramatically transformed a puny and sickly youth into a robust and dynamic adult. It is ironic, therefore, that through ignoring his own oft-repeated dictum that 'What you do not use you lose' the heart weakness of his youth should have reasserted itself and caused his untimely death in the 72nd year of his remarkable life (White 1992, 3).

After his death Lief was hailed variously as "the best-known and greatest personality in British Nature Cure" (Powell 1963, 602), a "veritable genius in healing" (Barker 1963, 671) and "one of the most dynamic and gifted personalities who ever worked in the field of unorthodox healing" (Wood 1963, 601). He was credited with bringing nature cure into the limelight and making it respectable via *Health For All* and with making more converts to nature cure than any other naturopath. As early as 1936, Harry Benjamin dedicated his book, *Everybody's Guide to Nature Cure*, to Stanley Lief "who has done more to forward the work of Nature Cure in this country than any other man." Oddly enough, a review of "The Growth and Development of the Naturopathic Movement in Great Britain," published in America in 1938 managed to sum up all naturopathic activities in the British Isles to that date without mentioning Lief or Thomson (Lucas 1938, 4).

Champneys limped along after Lief's death, but by 1972 it was "no longer viable." It was eventually refurbished and turned into "a medically based health resort" which "operated according to the principles of preventative medicine" (History of Champneys, 1989 Leaflet). While Champneys remains a luxurious health center in a class of its own, it is now a business venture owned by Guiness PLC rather than a healing venture run by a naturopath. It is renowned as a country retreat where the urban health set, including the Prince of Wales, can relax and recharge their batteries. Lief's lengthy fasts and other stern nature cure practices have been replaced by "Tummy Trimming/Body Firming" and "Hydro Fitness." The new Champneys acknowledges Lief's popularity, but not wanting to be identified with health "cranks" or risk "caricature," it repudiates the "pseudomedical" and "mystical" naturopathy of its founder (History of Champneys, 1989 Leaflet).

Lief was a true pioneer of naturopathic medicine. He founded the first and largest natural health retreat in England, developed musculoskeletal treatments which are highly valued today, and published a successful natural health magazine which effectively presented naturopathy to the British public. Although his work is no longer carried on at his beloved Champneys, it lives on through the school and organizations he helped to establish, the doctors he trained, the patients he cured and the public he educated in the principles of nature cure.

Canada's International Ambassador for Naturopathy

Arno R. Koegler

(1898-1991)

Arno Rudolph Koegler was a prominent and colorful Canadian nature doctor. Like so many of the early nature doctors, he was of German origin. Like Lindlahr and Lust, he was converted to nature cure by one of the great German nature doctors, not Father Sebastian Kneipp but the younger Pastor Emanuel Felke. Koegler's sphere of influence was not confined to Canada. As President of the International Society of Naturopathic Physicians, he was a leading international spokesman for naturopathy and he established contacts with colleagues and naturopathic organizations all over the world.

Koegler, the oldest of five children, was born in Planitz, a town in the German province of Saxony, on May 1, 1898—as he used to put it, "the first day of a sun month, in a sun year, on a Sunday" (Bender 1991, 1). This gave him the feeling that he was chosen to be a special person.

His childhood memories were of hiking in the mountains and especially of food, the beautiful fruit trees in Saxony and the wonderful chocolate that his favorite grandmother gave him. He said that she was responsible for his being "addicted" to chocolate. He became such a connoisseur of foods that he would not hesitate to tell the cook of a restaurant if the food was not done just right and give helpful hints on how it should be done. He was a passionate cook himself. Later on in his life, as a widower, when an interested widow who was a good cook herself said, "you know cooking is the most important thing," he retorted, "I know, that's why I do my own!" This was characteristic of him, that he was completely his own man and self-sufficient (ibid., 2).

He entered World War I as an x-ray and laboratory technician. Staying in Macedonia, he got to know the local people and helped them with their various ills. He felt compassion for them because they were poor and couldn't afford medical care. When a Gypsy woman offered to read Koegler's palm for payment, he conceded because he thought it would be interesting. She told him he would be in a terrible accident and would come close to death,

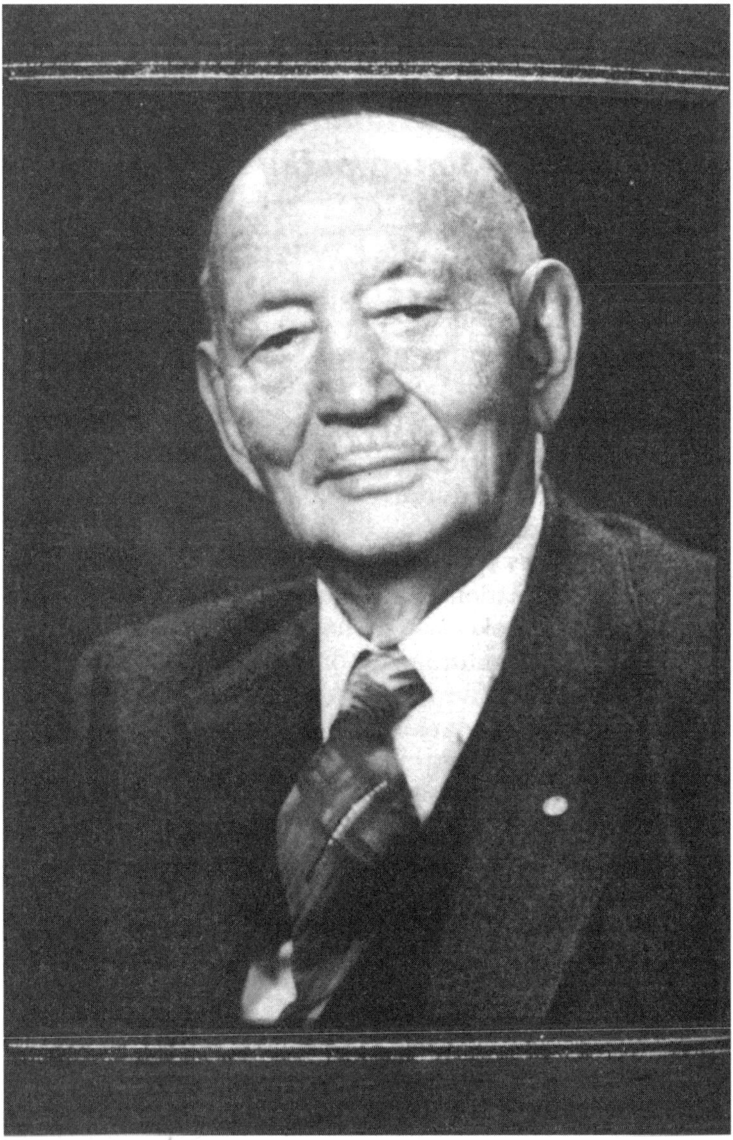

Arno R. Koegler
(Courtesy of John Bender, N.D.)

but would eventually recover and go to America and become a famous doctor. This seemed like an utter impossibility to the young German soldier but it came to pass when he was severely injured in a train accident. Facing death directly changed his life forever, because he lived each day as if it were his last. And the pain and suffering he went through enabled him to have more empathy for the people who later came to see him as a doctor.

Eventually the famous nature doctor, Emanuel Felke, restored Koegler to full health, and this experience led him to become the healer that he was. Felke was the most eclectic of the German nature doctors, developing his own brand of homeopathy and becoming a master in iris diagnosis. Koegler's own special interest in homeopathy and iridology had their roots with Felke.

In 1923, Koegler left for Canada with "his wife, two children and five dollars" (ibid., 2). He immigrated to the Kitchener area where he set up practice in 1926 after taking courses in several American naturopathic schools. During 53 years of practice in Waterloo, Ontario, he participated in the naturopathic profession at practically every level possible. He worked tirelessly on the licensing board, served as board member and president of international and Canadian naturopathic associations and was literally responsible for the naturopathic law in Ontario. He trained the founding members of the Board of the Ontario College of Naturopathic Medicine, established in 1978, when he was a teacher at the Canadian Memorial Chiropractic College which offered a naturopathic program. He was 81 when the Board appointed him as president of the first college of naturopathic medicine in Canada. After being located in Kitchener for a few years, the college moved to Toronto and changed to Canadian College of Naturopathic Medicine in 1992.

Koegler became well-known in naturopathic circles as President of the International Society of Naturopathic Physicians (ISNP), a position he held from 1956 to 1972. The ISNP was founded in 1938 by a group of Californian naturopathic physicians, foremost among them Dr. Arthur Schramm, who had a special interest in botanical medicine. Schramm had been associated with Dr. Carl Schultz, the "Father of Naturopathy in California." Schultz was the founder of California University of Liberal Physicians in Los Angeles which became Emerson University shortly after his death. Schramm was Dean of the Naturopathic Department at CULP which offered a four-year-training program until 1944. Dr. Mario T. Campanella, who had a rich European background and received his first medical training at the Royal University of Turin, was the next President of the ISNP. After his term, Campanella edited the *Journal of Naturopathic Medicine*, its official publication. His office in Graham, Florida, served as the administrative headquarters of the ISNP, which Koegler visited each year during his term as president.

The International Society failed in its attempt to unite the different competing organizations that claimed to be the true representatives of the naturopathic profession after Lust's death, but it stood above the feuding factions enough to attract members from the different camps; and the membership fee was low, $10.00. Thus Dr. Paul Wendel of Brooklyn, N.Y., President of the Eastern American Naturopathic Association, was member of the Board of Trustees of the ISNP. So was Dr. A. R. Hedges of Medford, Oregon, President of the former rival Western ANA, the American Naturopathic Physicians and Surgeons Association. In its heydays it had over 3,000 members, and its 1955-56 Directory lists 40 affiliated national and international associations. The annual conventions were attractive events with an array of speakers representing the best in naturopathy at this time. For example, at the 1953 convention in Salt Lake City, Otis G. Carroll spoke about "Hydrotherapy and My Success in its Use," Dr. Charles Gesser about "Naturopathy and its Modalities," Harry M. Hoxsey about "The Solution to the Cancer Problem," Bernard Jensen about "The Science of Iridology in General Practice," Herbert M. Shelton about "Essential Hypertension," Norman W. Walker about "Juice Therapy and Raw Foods," Paul Wendel about "Asthma and its Cure" and Koegler about "Homeopathy" (Convention issue of the *Journal of Naturopathic Medicine*, June 1953).

The ISNP wanted to be more than a national organization and proved it by its naming of international vice-presidents, among them Dr. Vincente L. Ferrandiz, "the Benedict Lust of Spain" and President of the Naturopathic Association of Spain. Ferrandiz (born 1894) received his Doctor of Naturopathy from Lust's American School of Naturopathy, then continued his studies under the direction of Dr. Carl Schultz at the Naturopathic Institute of California in Los Angeles. After returning to Spain, he set up practice in Barcelona, published the nature cure magazine, *Salud y Vida* (1923), and founded schools of botanic medicine, massage and physiotherapy. The naturopathic profession today has lost this international dimension.

Within the ISNP, specialty councils existed on naturopathic medicine, botanic medicine, obstetrics, bloodless and manipulative surgery, hospitals and sanitaria, naturopathic education and research. President of the International Council on Iridology was Dr. Bernard Jensen, who made it his life-long mission to establish iris diagnosis as a serious science in this country. Jensen studied iridology with Henry Lindlahr, Dr. F. W. Collins and Dr. J. Haskel Kritzer before he became a popular lecturer and author on the subject. Thousands of patients flocked to his health ranch in Escondido, California, where he treated them with a detoxifying and rejuvenation diet. Even today, at 86, an example of vibrant health, he is a prolific writer of books on natural health and longevity and travels all over the world lecturing to enthusiastic listeners.

Also still alive is Dr. William A. Turska who was the chairman of the International Council on Naturopathic Philosophy. Now at the age of 84, Turska, the grand old maverick among the naturopathic physicians, is still practicing in Mist, Oregon. Like Koegler, a true eclectic who does not shy away from methods, even those controversial among his peers, such as ozone therapy, hernia injection therapy and the Wet Blood Drop Test, he became a prototype of the modern naturopathic physician.

Koegler was also President of the International Council on Homeopathy, and considered it his main task to encourage his fellow naturopathic physicians in the use of homeopathic remedies. He wrote a series of articles, "Homeopathy for the Naturopathic Physicians," in the *Journal of Naturopathic Medicine* which explained the action of the more important remedies such as *Pulsatilla, Carbo Vegetabilis* and *Apis Mellifica*, what potencies to use and how to prepare them. Koegler made many of his remedies himself in his own laboratory. Since he knew that many naturopathic colleagues were deterred from using homeopathy because it was a complex and complicated system, he wrote an article titled "Simplified Homeopathy."

> As I studied homeopathy, I was discouraged, as I never realized that homeopathy was so complicated. The more I studied—the more I found out how little I knew. As I progressed, I aimed to the development of the system so that any physician—of any school—could simplify the application of homeopathy without going into the complicated symptomatology . . . .
>
> I first simplified the system by cutting down the number of remedies to about 60—which was one great help. It is easier to concentrate upon 60 remedies than one hundred, or six hundred. Then, after studying the system of Dr. Felke, I realized we could simplify the complex system by using a certain combination of remedies (by this I do not mean a complex mixture of remedies, but using two, or in some exceptional cases, three remedies alternately. Remedies which will work in harmony with each other). The results were amazing. After trying this out for 25 years and treating successfully more than 100,000 patients from coast to coast, and since I found so many naturopathic physicians interested in homeopathy . . . I decided to put my observations and simplification of homeopathic remedies in writing. I do not want any of you to think for a single moment that I want to change a great system which was able to withstand the test for over a

> century. I want to make it plain that my attempt to simplify homeopathic prescribing was done so that any doctor, of any school, could apply the worthy remedies of the homeopathic school without spending a lifetime to learn the whole system (1951, 20).

Koegler also challenged the profession to come forward with its own research. In an article titled "Can Naturopathic Medicine Take the Place of Antibiotics?" he wrote:

> While many individuals have carried on research in many fields of naturopathic medicine, very little of this information has been made available to the profession at large. So, let us all pull together; we have a Journal and let us publish all our findings in any field of the natural healing art . . . . Let us not depend on what the medical men find out for us; let us do our own research and see if we can develop better ways and means to help suffering humanity. We Naturopaths are wonderfully equipped to help the sick but let us not rest on our laurels. There is a lot more to be found out.
>
> In the search for natural antibiotics we have found some in our vegetable kingdom . . . . The most practical and best antibiotic in the vegetable kingdom has been found in cress, either water cress or garden cress . . . . This is usually the first thing I plant in my garden in the spring. It is easy to grow and does well in almost any soil and it is a wonderful table green and tasty even if eaten with bread and butter alone (Koegler 1959, 13).

Koegler was a superb gardener. He grew and held the record for the largest cabbage in Kitchener-Waterloo. People would come from miles around just to see his showcase garden.

After Campanella's death, the ISNP faltered due to lack of support from its members. In a 1972 letter Koegler summarized the reasons for its demise:

> We had to discontinue all our activities because we can't find anyone who would spend the time and money we spend on this Association. It has cost me thousands of dollars and a lot of my time, and Campanella had to spend even more to keep this Association going. We had over 3000 members and only a small percentage were able to pay dues, as some countries will not allow money out of the country. In some countries the value of their

> money is so low, that even if we would charge only a small fee, it still would be a fortune for these people. We had 40 countries represented in our Association. So it is impossible for me to carry the load all by myself; first of all I can't afford to spend the money any more and secondly I am getting too old to carry on and have to think about myself for a change as I don't know how long I will be able to carry on my work and have an earning from my practice (June 14 to Dr. Kyaw Zan, Burma).

Koegler's accomplishments as a naturopathic physician were legendary. Patients came to him from virtually every state in the United States and every province in Canada. He built up a record of a quarter million patients. His favorite saying was, "I'd rather be a 'quack' and do something than a specialist and do nothing." He was extremely hard-working. In the beginning of his practice he worked for seven years before taking a vacation, working seven days a week, often making house calls at night and never turning anyone down, even though in the early years he was not allowed to charge a fee. He saw an incredible 50-200 patients a day! In a 1979 letter to a fellow homeopath he explained why he had never found the time to write books:

> For 40 years they asked me to write some textbooks, but when you work 16 hours a day there is not much time left. In fact when I started I was on a twenty-four hour call all year around. In the days when the M.D.s lost 29% of all their pneumonia cases I never lost one, so I was called on most of these cases. Now they are quite proud of themselves because they have antibiotics; they don't die right away but instead they get ill more often while in my day you either lived or died; if you did live, you never had it again, you were immune to it (Oct. 21 to Rayana Ryane. C.H., Vancouver, B.C.).

When a medical doctor approached him on the street, chided him for curing so many patients, and asked if he wasn't afraid of going out of business, his quick-witted reply was: "As long as there are medical doctors around, there'll be lots of work" (Bender 1991, 3-4).

As a physician he was a keen observer. He once visited a dying young girl and noticed plenty of peaches in the house. When he asked the mother if the girl liked the fruit, she replied that the girl was very fond of them; the peelings being her favorite part. Koegler immediately recognized that the girl was suffering from acute Arsenic poisoning and quickly antidoted the Arsenic. He literally brought her back from her death when other doctors had given up.

Koegler had a practical, no nonsense approach and was always looking for better ways to solve problems. In fact, when told something was impossible, he made it a special point to make sure it could be done. He was an inventor ahead of his time and held many patents, among them a homeopathic mixing machine still used by his successor and a calcium fluoride toothpaste. Later he would get a great kick out of the government officials telling him that fluoride had nothing to do with healthy teeth. "Of course," he would say, " not the junk sodium fluoride that they put in now." He would often remark: "I was born 40 years too soon" (ibid. 1991, 4).

Koegler's great passion was travelling and, as the President of the ISNP, he had ample opportunity to indulge. In 1957 he went on a trip through Europe, speaking before the affiliated naturopathic associations in Germany, France, Spain, Portugal and other countries. He was presented with the Prix Hippocrate in Paris for research work in Natural Medicine and was appointed Honorary Professor of Botanical Medicine at the University in Barcelona. Two years later he toured South America. Finally, he went on an extensive speaking tour to New Zealand and Australia and even met the Queen. The National Australian Naturopathic Association reported about the successful trip in the *Journal of Naturopathic Medicine.*

> Many points of progress have arisen from Dr. Koegler's visit to Australia .... A tremendous number of Australians are now convinced that Naturopathy is an organized force growing very fast on an educational basis and are prepared to help in every way .... The theme of Dr. Koegler's visit, "Legislation by Education" proved a popular one and sums up the aims and the efforts of our Australian Naturopaths affiliated with the International Society of Naturopathic Physicians (May 1961, 22).

Koegler's favorite get-away was Hawaii. How many Canadians can claim to have gone to Hawaii 41 times?

> When he went to Hawaii the last time, I think all of us tried to discourage him because we felt he wasn't physically fit to go. When I said to him, "what would happen if you got up in the middle of the night and fell and broke your hip, you could be there for days before anybody would ever notice!" He looked right at me and said, "so what, it's paid for." In other words, he was more interested in not being a burden than he was in his own welfare.

> So, he did get his wish to go to Hawaii one last time but of course he fractured his hip and this was to be the beginning of the end (Bender 1991, 4-5).

His last six months were difficult for him. He suffered a stroke during a prostate operation that he didn't want and didn't know that he was getting. He was not able to speak and was not interested in communicating. Still his death on February 23, 1991 came earlier than expected. Perhaps one reason for this was that he was unhappy and didn't like the rehabilitation hospital he was in. He was a proud man, in charge all his life. All of the sudden, he was helpless.

Koegler had five children. He was probably disappointed that none of them followed his calling although his oldest son became a well-known pediatrician. But it must have given him some consolation that he found a worthy associate and successor in Dr. John Bender, a 1979 graduate of the National College of Naturopathic Medicine.

Dr. Koegler was one of the naturopathic physicians who kept the flame of naturopathy alive during dark years when the naturopathic profession in America suffered its deepest decline. Later he became a role model and inspiration for the new generation of students who would rediscover and revive naturopathy in the late 1970s.

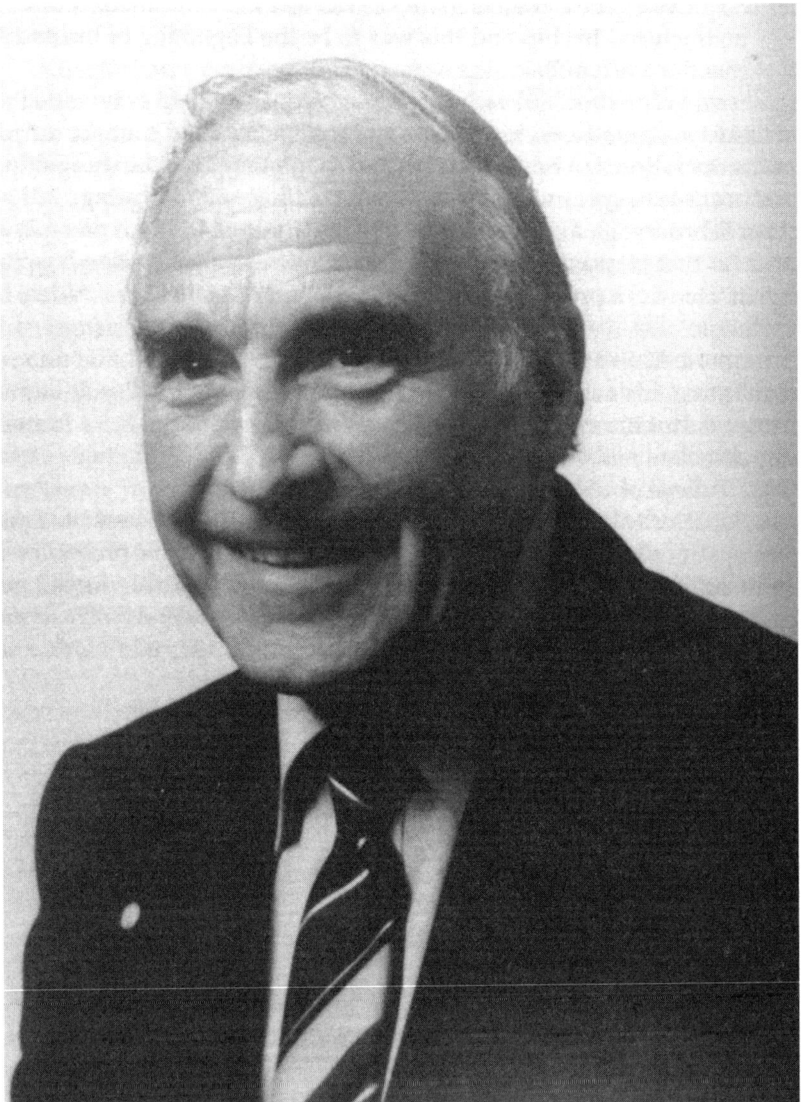

Joseph A. Boucher
(Courtesy of Robert Fleming, N.D.)

An Inspiring Teacher of Naturopathy from Canada

Joseph A. Boucher

(1916-1987)

Joseph A. Boucher, a highly respected naturopathic physician of the last half of the twentieth century, like many earlier nature doctors had first embarked on a career far from the health field. A serious illness cured by natural treatment converted him to naturopathic principles and led him to become a practitioner. He is one of the premier figures in Canadian naturopathy and also has had considerable influence in the United States.

Born on October 27, 1916 in Edmonton, Alberta, Boucher was the eldest of eight children. He received his primary education at parochial schools and attended Vancouver College in Vancouver, British Columbia and St. Anthony's College in Edmonton. True child of the depression, he once jumped a freight train for a ride home from Vancouver for summer vacation. He worked variously as a golf caddie, cook, and construction worker and drove a dairy truck while attending business college at night. Eventually he went to sea as a deckhand on a small freighter which supplied the coastal fish canneries. Later, working as first mate on a fishing boat, his knee was seriously injured during a heavy storm and required surgery. A further misadventure occurred when he returned to duty and his boat was boarded by U.S. officials for allegedly drifting into territorial waters. Boucher was put in jail overnight while his boat, left unattended, dragged anchor and sank. This resulted in the loss of all his personal belongings.

He took a break from sea life long enough to work his way up to sales representative for a large wholesale grocer. There he met his future wife, Pat Curry, the beautiful daughter of one of his customers. They were married in 1941 and had five children, including two foster children.

In 1939, as World War II approached, Boucher joined the Royal Canadian Artillery Militia, which required his participation on weekends and at summer camps. In 1941, after hostilities broke out involving Canada, he was transferred to active duty in the Royal Canadian Navy and stationed at Victoria with the rank of Petty Officer. He spent the next two-and-a-half years patrolling the west coast of Canada, sometimes in the same merchant ships, now "bristling with armaments," he had sailed previously during his civilian maritime days. His ship was the first to investigate the shelling of the Hesquiet by an enemy submarine.

Boucher was eventually discharged from the Navy due to a severe ulcerative colitis. Despite a successful return to the business world, his colitis worsened. Medical care failed to help him, and he was told that surgery was the only option left. Twenty-nine years old at the time, he decided to investigate another therapeutic approach before consenting to a colostomy. He sought out a naturopathic physician who helped him obtain a total remission within a year's time.

Impressed with these results, Boucher began to attend lectures, and read everything he could find on natural healing. In 1949, he moved with his family to Portland, Oregon to attend Western States College of Chiropractic where he would earn doctorates both in naturopathy and chiropractic. Boucher worked forty hours each week at a grocery store while attending school full-time, in addition to being class president and student-body president. During the summers he attended Lewis and Clark College where he received a degree in psychology. He graduated from all three programs with honors.

Boucher opened his practice in Vancouver in 1954. During the first eighteen months, while building up his practice, he worked nights and weekends as a first-aid attendant at a sawmill. He was also elected to the Board of Governors of the Association of Naturopathic Physicians of British Columbia during this time. For the next 32 years, he held various offices, from Chairman of the Examining Board to President. In 1955, the Canadian Naturopathic Association was chartered and Boucher immediately became its Executive Secretary. In 1976 he served as its President.

Boucher was a naturopathic idealist and purist. To him, the patient's regaining of true health through adherence to natural principles was paramount, overshadowing social, political or legal considerations. "After all," he wrote, "it's the results that count in the long run; not popular acceptance or official recognition" (Boucher 1982, 24). He was a ready critic of suppressive allopathic treatments:

> Man is now taken from a conscious point of suffering or malaise into oblivion where the ashes of disease smolder only to burst forth again with greater velocity and chronicity later on (Boucher "Detoxification").

He believed that true cure resulted only when the cause of disease was removed. In the time-honored tradition of Priessnitz and Kneipp he believed there was only one cause of disease.

> The essence of all disease is the accumulation in the system of waste matter and impurities due to wrong habits of living. The elimination of this toxic matter from the body is what nature is striving for all the time. . . . It is through detoxification . . . that the healing latent within all of us can be given a free hand to function (Boucher 1982, 23)

Boucher emphasized the *vis medicatrix naturae* in every aspect of his teaching and practice. He felt it was what made naturopathy work and what distinguished it from all other healing disciplines. He decried attempts by the profession to blend in with orthodox medicine at the expense of its firm allegiance to the *vis*. "We can only justify our existence by the fact that we are DIFFERENT," he wrote. He strove for a profession united by a deep loyalty to the *vis*, rather than "a group of mavericks split into factions, quarreling and bickering . . . a hodge podge quilt on the bed of the healing arts" (Boucher 1981, 40-41).

Boucher was a devotee of Stanford Kingsley Claunch, a California naturopath and student of John H. Tilden, and republished two outlines of Claunch's provocative teachings "The Polarity System" and "Exploding the Germ Theory," as well as applying them in his practice. He was one of the few North American naturopathic practitioners who utilized the Schroth system, especially the unfashionable thirst method, in which "incredibly as it seemed, the more the patient thirsted the more rapidly the acids and toxins accumulated in the diseased body were loosened and expelled from the system, with a consequent more rapid return to health and vigor" (Boucher "Schroth System").

Although a Canadian, Boucher played an important role in the development of naturopathy in the United States. In 1956, he joined John Bastyr and others in founding the National College of Naturopathic Medicine in Seattle. After the school moved to Portland, Boucher traveled from Vancouver, Canada to Portland every Friday for years to teach classes at the college. He was involved as a teacher, board member and board chairman of the school for twenty-seven years. His strong leadership helped guide National College through many financial crises. Boucher was instrumental in forming the Northwest Association of Naturopathic Physicians, a joint American-Canadian association that has sponsored the largest and longest-running annual convention in North America for over 35 years. (Farnsworth 1990, 49).

For many years Boucher had a regular column called the "The Nature Doctor" in *The Naturopath* where he expounded his philosophy of health and prevention of disease. There he wrote about the role of the naturopathic physician:

> The Naturopathic Physician considers disease as the inevitable result of or the body's reaction to an unnatural condition . . . . After we have determined the cause, and in most instances it is autointoxication in one form or another . . . it behooves us as Naturopathic Physicians then to set about correcting it.
>
> When viewed in this light, the function of the Naturopathic Physician becomes one of "DOCTOR" in the fullest sense of the word. The word itself is derived from the Latin "*Docere*" meaning not to treat, but to TEACH. In effect, to teach people how they. . . acquired the condition of which they are complaining, and what now must be done to overcome it, then "going their way and sinning no more." In other words, the Naturopathic Physician discerns the laws of physiology and takes the physiological approach (Boucher 1964, 8)

This "official publication" of the National Association of Naturopathic Physicians (NANP) and the Oregon State Association of Naturopathic Physicians was edited by John W. Noble, N. D. (1906-1976), a driving force in the establishment of the National College of Naturopathic Medicine in Portland and in naturopathic politics of Oregon from 1956. His friend Boucher called him the "'Horatio at the Bridgehead,' not only in college administration but for the Oregon Association of Naturopathic physicians as well" (1976, 2). *The Naturopath,* a small tabloid started in 1963, was, until 1980, the only outlet left where naturopathic physicians could express their views and advertise their practices.

Boucher, a man of many interests and talents, was a sought-after speaker who taught public speaking at the University of British Columbia and Vancouver Community College for a number of years. He was a natural athlete, being especially accomplished at badminton, squash, racquetball, tennis and cross-country skiing. He was a robust outdoorsman, whose interests ranged from vegetable gardening to mountain climbing. He became the unofficial hiking guide to hosts of people in Garibaldi Park, frequently climbing its challenging Black Tusk, and always priding himself on being first to the top. At age sixty-seven, he hiked nonstop to the floor of the Grand Canyon, then hiked nonstop back to the top. He was also an amateur cinema producer, making two feature-length films, "The Four Faces of Garibaldi" and "Graveyard of the Pacific," both shown throughout British Columbia.

When Boucher died on March 22, 1987, it was a palpable loss to the international naturopathic community. He inspired the naturopathic profession through his successful practice, his staunch support of naturopathic education and the thorough application of naturopathic principles in his own life. When National College had dual campuses, one in Portland for clinical instruction and the other in Wichita, Kansas for basic science instruction, Dr. Boucher would fly to Wichita with Dr. Bastyr to give encouragement to the beleaguered, isolated students there, and to show them what "real," established naturopaths looked like. Indeed, to prove to them that such beings still existed. He was an idol and guiding light to thirty years of graduating students. Some of the busiest naturopathic practices in British Columbia are now conducted by doctors brought into the profession by Dr. Boucher and who have modeled themselves on his example.

Boucher was an altruist in the tradition of Lindlahr. To him helping people was "what life is all about, what naturopathic medicine is all about" (Boucher 1986 video). His selfless spirit made him one of the most revered figures in modern naturopathic history.

> A friend to all, he never refused help. When older colleagues fell on hard times, he shared his office space with them, sometimes for years—at times to his financial detriment, and later when young doctors needed a place to begin practice he reduced and rearranged his office hours so they could use his facility. He gave everything he had to whatever he attempted, and would have been financially more comfortable if he had collected the multitude of 'loans' he made to those less fortunate. He couldn't say no to his friends and had no enemies ("Joseph A. Boucher" 1987, 4).

Joseph Boucher is not remembered for new diagnostic and therapeutic techniques or revolutionizing naturopathic practice. He is remembered because his "strong shoulders and gentle heart helped carry Naturopathy through some of its hardest years" (Matsen 1987, iii).

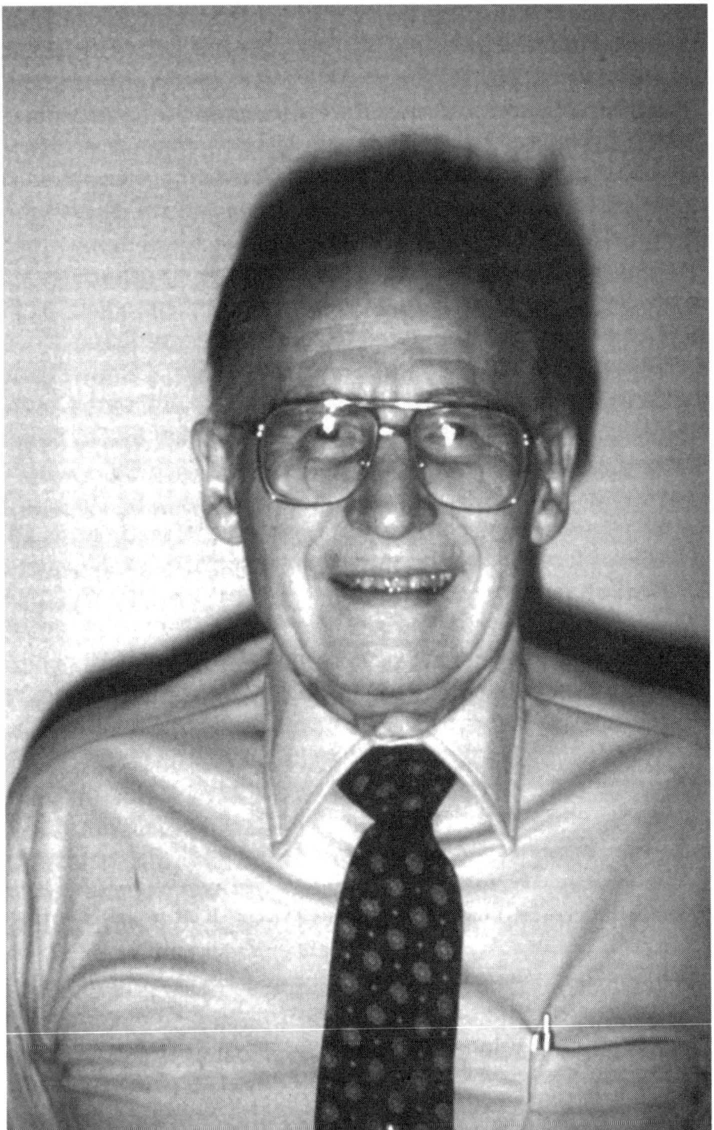

John Bastyr
(Courtesy of Karen Boyle)

Father of Modern Naturopathic Medicine

John Bastyr

(1912-1995)

Dr. John B. Bastyr is the most important link between the old-fashioned nature doctor, diagnosing by close observation and collecting his own plant medicines, and the modern naturopathic physician, who uses the latest laboratory techniques and employs standardized extracts of "phyto-medicines."

Bastyr was born at home May 16, 1912 in New Prague, Minnesota, a Bohemian (Czech) immigrant community. At an early age he moved with his family to North Dakota where his father pursued work as a pharmacist. His mother was an able gardener and a knowledgeable herbalist who had learned these skills from her mother. Like most of her contemporaries in that locale, she was a follower of Father Kneipp. She had one of his books that she read constantly and applied its recommendations when occasions arose. When at age nine Bastyr had an appendectomy, and his incision opened up and started to drain while he was outside climbing trees, his mother "went out and got some plantain and put it on the wound and it healed up inside of a week. She knew what to do" (Bastyr 1989, 6).

Bastyr was educated at parochial schools and worked as a farm hand and telegraph boy. In 1928, as the Great Depression hit, his family sold their house, bought a Pike's Peak Chandler car and headed west to seek better times in Seattle. There he worked in his father's drugstore where, in addition to tending the soda fountain, he learned the basics of botanical and homeopathic pharmacy. In 1932, after obtaining his high school diploma from Seattle Prep, he considered entering a seminary. However, his mother had been consulting Dr. Harry F. Bonnelle, a chiropractor and sanipractor, who had an office nearby. He influenced Mrs. Bastyr to interest her son in enrolling at the Seattle College of Chiropractic where he taught.

Upon graduating from chiropractic college, Bastyr interned at Grace Hospital, a rare, thirty-bed "open door" hospital. Grace allowed medical doctors, osteopaths, chiropractors and naturopaths to admit patients there and to treat them within the legal scope of their practices. Also in 1936, Bastyr enrolled at Seattle's Drugless Institute. In all, Bastyr went to school for six years.

Head Surgeon at Grace Hospital was C. P. Bryant, a medical doctor and homeopath. Bryant had studied homeopathy with Walter James, a student of Adolph Lippe. Lippe had been a student of Constantine Hering, who had been a Hahnemann student. Bastyr studied homeopathy intensively with Bryant for three years putting him fifth in line from Samuel Hahnemann, the founder of homeopathy.

Bastyr's experiences sold him on homeopathy.

> I remember one lady, she was having bladder trouble; she was in pain; and she was looking at all the medicines . . . and I said, "I'll tell you what I'll do." I was studying homeopathy. "I'll give you a remedy if you will take it." I gave her Sepia 200, that was in crystal form, #10 pellets. So she came in the next day; she had no trouble, nothing. She couldn't believe it. She said, "Whatever you gave me was like a miracle." And I was really encouraged to continue studying homeopathy . . . we were studying different homeopathic remedies. So that's how I really began to get serious about homeopathy. That was one of the cases. (Bastyr 1989,18-19).

Bastyr's conversion to homeopathy was an important move for the modern naturopathic profession. Homeopathy had been part of naturopathic medicine for decades, but its role had been more or less peripheral. The majority of practitioners had not received such intensive, classical instruction as Bastyr. In the 1950s, when Bastyr became involved in establishing and teaching a naturopathic curriculum, his balanced emphasis of homeopathy as a therapeutic modality coequal with nutrition, hydrotherapy and botanical medicine assured its place in the ongoing development of naturopathic science. That's one of the reasons that naturopathic physicians are in the forefront of the current homeopathic revival in this country.

As a chiropractor and a naturopath, Bastyr relied heavily on manipulation in his practice. After fifty years of practice he considered it his most important therapy, because he could "bring about immediate improvement and establish physical contact."

> You convey your confidence in what you're doing. You get an insight into what they need. You somehow transfer your energy to theirs, and the patient senses it. You have an interchange of energy (Bastyr 1986, 3).

During his training, still working in his dad's pharmacy, Bastyr had an early experience with manipulation similar to his one with homeopathy:

> An old man with corns came into the store and said, "My feet sure do hurt." And I showed him all the [Dr.] Scholl's stuff. He said, "'We tried all that and none of them do any good." I said, "Tell you what I'll do. You let me work on your feet and see if it'll help." So I worked on his feet . . . on one foot . . . and I said, "You come back and tell me if this foot is any better than the other one." He came back the next day and said, "That one foot sure do feel good. Would you mind doing the other one?" That was my introduction to manipulation (Bastyr 1989, 19).

When Bastyr first opened his practice in Seattle, it was at the depth of the Great Depression. He only charged fifty cents to one dollar for office calls, but was always able to cover his sixteen dollar per month rent. After referring a number of patients with uterine fibroids to Dr. Otis G. Carroll in Spokane and having them come back cured, he closed his practice for six months and went to study with Carroll. When he returned, he adapted some of Carroll's methods to the practice of obstetrics, a field to which he had been introduced in what can only be called a baptism by fire.

Early in his days as an intern at Grace Hospital, Bastyr was scheduled to meet Dr. Bryant there to assist in the delivery of a baby. Bastyr arrived first, and the prospective mother immediately began to deliver. As Bastyr relates, the attending nurse, whom he called "Surgical Suzie," was:

> . . . someplace else, and I was yelling for her to come. I'd never seen a birth in my life. I didn't know what was going to happen. And she (the mother) kept saying, "That's alright, Sonny, that's all right," and sure enough, out pops one. She said, "There's another one coming," and sure enough, another one did come. "Just take it easy, Sonny," she says, and I kept hollering, "Susie, Susie!" And pretty soon there was the third one. By the time he (Bryant) got there, I had three babies and by that time Susie had arrived. They were all okay (Bastyr 1989, 35).

Despite the fact that the mother was calmer than the young doctor, an unassisted triplet delivery was no mean feat. From these auspicious beginnings, Bastyr went on to become the premier naturopathic obstetrician in America.

Bastyr managed thousands of successful home births. "In one family," he said, "I delivered three generations." At one point he had four obstetrical nurses who attended women at home in various stages of labor. "Some days," Bastyr said, "we'd have two deliveries at the same time" (Bastyr 1989, 32). Somehow he always managed to guess which birth would happen first and be there when he was needed. One of his most memorable deliveries was of a frank breech (bottom first) baby, another doctor's patient he had never seen before, who lived on a remote Washington mountain top. He drove up the mountain in the dead of winter as far as the bad roads allowed, hiked the rest of the way, and accomplished the difficult delivery with no problems. "It's kind of delicate," he explained. "You have to be careful with a frank breech baby, not to break an arm or leg" (34). In another case, he delivered an eclamptic woman prematurely of a two-pound, four-ounce baby, who survived nicely under the care of his assistant, Mrs. Baxter, an old English nurse. Bastyr delivered so many babies that the Seattle Selective Service Board declined to draft him into the army for World War II despite his 1-A classification.

Bastyr's success in obstetrics can be attributed to the meticulous preparation of his patients. To minimize fear, he educated the women thoroughly about the birth process. To deal with pain he taught them relaxation exercises. To prepare the uterus he made various cold hydrotherapeutic applications. To ensure a flexible birth canal he manipulated the woman's pelvis. To insure a healthy baby he put the mother on a nutritious diet. To prevent erythroblastosis, long before its genetic basis was understood, he employed light therapy from a cobalt blue lamp. To make sure the baby was in a favorable position prior to labor, he would turn a breech baby from bottom-first to head-first by external version. To minimize maternal discomfort he often conducted the later stages of labor in a warm water bath, either delivering the child under water or, more often, removing the mother to the kitchen table as the baby's head crowned to complete the delivery. To ensure that the babies got a healthy start, he insisted the mothers nurse their children until their teeth came in, which signaled the appearance of ptyalin, the amylase enzyme necessary for complicated digestion. Bastyr had mastered these techniques, standard practice in the current "natural childbirth" movement, over fifty years ago. As he modestly stated, "We had very little complications" (Bastyr 1989, 31)

As any who saw him at work could tell, Bastyr "loved birthing" (Overton 1989,15). But its demands took a toll. "I remember going maybe a week, seven days, without getting horizontal to sleep," he said. "I'd just stand up in a corner and sleep a bit" (Bastyr 1989, 32). Finally in the 1960s, Bastyr's wife put her foot down. "Either them or me," she said (Wardrip 1989, 15). With that, Bastyr's illustrious obstetrical career came to an end.

In the early years Bastyr's days were "very, very long," and his fees "ridiculously low" (Wardrip 1989, 7). He would start at 8 a.m. and frequently go to 10 or 11 p.m. He would attend to "everything from a broken bone to delivering a baby. That would break up the day. When you'd have to go to deliver the baby" (Bastyr 1989, 46).

Given his busy, unpredictable schedule, his utter lack of a sense of time, and his desire to give everyone the best possible care, Bastyr's many patients became used to lengthy office waits. With five calls an hour from doctors all over the country seeking Bastyr's advice, chaos often reigned. "It was crazy," one observer noted. "They maintained only one phone line, and they took it off the hook a lot" (Pizzorno 1989, 3).

Bastyr was famous for his house calls. As one of his patients and associate who was nursed back to health by a long series of his evening house calls related:

> After he'd worked hard all day, then he would get in the car and he'd make house calls. Time never meant anything to Dr. Bastyr. He always needed somebody to keep time for him. But people, where he would make house calls, would save food. They knew he hadn't stopped to eat anywhere, so many times they would save something for him to eat (Overton 1989, 8).

For his part Bastyr was in his element. "I used to enjoy the house calls," he said. "Never even charged the patient. I loved to go to their houses"(Bastyr 1989, 46). The relationships which developed between Bastyr and his house call patients were exceptional as the following description of one of his elderly patients shows.

> He would come and see her no matter what time he got off work . . . . She worshipped him. She just loved him. Everybody does. He has such a healing energy about him . . . . Just talking to her—just touching her—you know, she'd feel better. And that's what I hear all the time . . . . Even if he doesn't do anything—just talks to them—they feel better (Wardrip 1989, 2).

Somehow in his busy schedule Bastyr still found time to gather and prepare many of his own herbal remedies. One of his mentors, Dr. Elizabeth Peters, who had studied with Father Kneipp and who Bastyr regarded as a "matriarch of natural therapy," told Bastyr how the priest would go out in the field in the morning wearing an apron, pick the different herbs and put them in the apron, and come in with the herbs for the day. Perhaps inspired by this example, Bastyr made many forays into the mountains surrounding Seattle to gather herbs which would not otherwise have been available for his patients. Even today Bastyr still makes up a number of "his own little formulas."

The key to Bastyr's legendary clinical success lay in his basic philosophy of naturopathy. In a 1985 interview, asked to distinguish between naturopathy and conventional medicine, he said, "The basic difference is that in naturopathy it's not the doctor that does the curing. It's the patient" (Katz 1985, K 3). While skillfully applying natural remedies to assist the patient's recovery, Bastyr subtly shifted the responsibility for getting well to the patient. He did not preach to them about their duty to take responsibility for their own health, but rather gave them the confidence that they could actually do it. Besides the "transfer of energy" mentioned in his discussion of manipulation, this crucial shift was brought about through Bastyr's listening skills. As his long-time office manager noted, "He listens with his heart" (Wardrip 1989, 4). Besides the sympathetic confidence his listening engendered in his patients, it also often clued him to the correct diagnosis. As Joseph E. Pizzorno, one of Bastyr's students and a founder of the Bastyr Naturopathic College in Seattle, noted, the patient usually knows what's wrong but may not have the insight or terminology, or be given an opportunity to tell someone who does.

> So many times we'd be seeing a patient in clinic who would be quite seriously ill, and all the clinicians feeling some fear about the whole thing . . . and he'd come in and examine the patient, he'd talk to him gently, start communication, and it seemed half the symptoms would clear up by the time the interview was over (Pizzorno 1989, 6).

While Pizzorno and his colleagues were contemplating grave and complicated diagnoses, Bastyr would show them that it was "something much more simple and much more easily taken care of. I think much of medicine comes down to what we're all aware of now as the placebo effect, the ability of the physician to stimulate the recognition in the patient of their health, rather than concentration on illness. He did this very, very well" (Pizzorno 1989, 6). Pizzorno concluded: "I think he's developed some pretty fundamental insights into why people are sick and how they can be helped"(9).

Despite his busy practice and educational commitments, Bastyr found time for a rich home life. He was married in 1937 to Aletha Persis Laroude, an English instructor at the University of Washington, whom he met when he was a student in her phonetics class. So as not to jeopardize her teaching position, they kept their marriage secret for some months. Bastyr explained: "We had special jewelry made—a locket—and her wedding ring was in the locket. Gunderson, the jeweler, made it for her" (Bastyr 1989, 24).

The Bastyrs did not have children. Their two great passions were music and gardening. Bastyr "always sang" and belonged to the Ralston Male Choir. Although he claimed not to have had "a particularly great voice," he was occasionally invited to sing at weddings. "I always had my wife in the audience," he acknowledged, "and I would sing to her" (ibid., 26). The Bastyrs loved opera and attended the Seattle Opera faithfully. Bastyr had many opera singers as patients and enjoyed being invited backstage. He helped a number of opera stars who lost their voices. At home, his wife played the piano, and Bastyr accompanied her on the fiddle. They also loved to dance. Their "very close" and romantically alive marriage lasted over 52 years, until Mrs. Bastyr's death in 1989, at the age of 95. Even in the last year of her life she and her husband would "put on the stereo and dance around the house"(ibid.).

Both Bastyrs loved to garden, and between them managed a veritable mini-farm at their home in Kent, Washington, with fruit trees, goats, ducks, geese and even a calf. Bastyr stayed fit by working hard in the garden and yard and doing his own carpentry work on their house.

Bastyr is famous as a naturopathic practitioner, but his role in the development, even the survival, of naturopathic medical education is inestimable. The state of naturopathic schools was rather dismal in the 1950s. The University of Utah, at the request of the Utah State Medical Association, conducted a thorough investigation of naturopathic schools throughout the United States in 1958.

> Of the twenty six schools investigated during this study, only nine were still in existence in the fall 1958. Of these nine, only three schools are now granting naturopathic degrees and two others are teaching naturopathy (University of Utah. The Bureau of Economic and Business Research 1958, 4).
>
> A comparison of naturopathic schools now in existence with certain other types of professional schools, shows that naturopathic schools do not appear to have the faculties, equipment or physical facilities which would adequately train their students to engage in a complete practice of healing arts . . . .

> Most of the schools reviewed were located in remodeled stores, clubs or residences. At one school, only one classroom exists with the rest of the space being used for an out-patient clinic.
>
> One school [Harry Riley Spitler's Central States College of Physiatrics in Eaton, Ohio, accredited by the National Association of Naturopathic Physicians] reported that since no cadavers were available, the school sent its anatomy students to an embalming school for the dissection part of the course. However, when the embalming school was contacted, it stated that no students from the naturopathic school had ever been registered for the embalming school's anatomy class (ibid., 6).

Naturopathic education in the Northwest had been under the protective guardianship of Dr. William A. Budden (1884-1954), President of Western States Chiropractic College (WSCC) in Portland, Oregon, from 1929 until his death. Graduates in chiropractic could go an additional two years to receive a diploma in naturopathy. Budden's sympathies for naturopathy stemmed from his time as a student and faculty member of the National College of Chiropractic which had absorbed the Lindlahr College of Natural Therapeutics. While Dean of the National College, he raised the standards of education and extended the course of study to a four-year program. The modern naturopathic colleges followed his example when they upgraded the quality of their education to a four-year program.

After years of "fellow traveling," when chiropractic schools all over the country taught naturopathy, chiropractic, in its drive for greater respectability, wanted to disassociate itself from naturopathic medicine. Many chiropractic schools stopped granting naturopathic degrees in 1955 when the National Chiropractic Association stated that it would only give accreditation to schools that only granted chiropractic degrees. After Budden's successor, Ralph W. Failor, resigned as the president in 1956, the naturopathic program at WSCC was dropped.

Without a school to educate a new generation of naturopathic physicians and to insure the survival of the profession, a handful of naturopathic doctors took matters in their own hands and founded the National College of Naturopathic Medicine, incorporated by Frank G. Spaulding, W. Martin Bleything and Charles R. Stone in Portland, May 23rd, 1956. In 1959, the college moved to Seattle where better facilities were available. Bastyr served as the "Executive Director" and taught obstetrics and gynecology. After the college moved back to Portland to benefit from the more liberal Oregon naturopathic law, Bastyr and other Washington and British Columbia naturopaths traveled to Portland every weekend for lengthy teaching sessions.

Bastyr served as the president of the college for many years in a more nominal than administrative position. When he retired in 1979, his comrade Dr. John A. Boucher, praised him as the "bellwether of Naturopathy . . . . Dr. Bastyr has, in all these 23 years, gently, firmly, efficiently, lovingly, professionally, guided the flock. And like the bellwether of the karakul world, has always brought the flock through safely to its destination" (Boucher 1979, 1).

Bastyr's medical knowledge made him valuable in the classroom, and his instruction in the clinic was unparalleled. He taught specific techniques of diagnosis and treatment and instilled in his students the more general wisdom to "always touch the patient," and to read at least one article about medicine each night before going to bed (Pizzorno 1989, 4). Always current on the latest research in nutrition, he taught an unusual clinical relativism in diet, claiming that what one eats is not so important as one's attitude about what one eats. "I don't believe there's an ideal diet," he said in a 1986 interview. "The nutrition we believe in is what's important." (Bastyr 1986, 3).

In 1978 the John Bastyr College of Naturopathic Medicine, now Bastyr University, was founded in Seattle by Bastyr's former students, Joseph E. Pizzorno and William Mitchell, to carry on the educational heritage of their mentor. Bastyr himself remains an avid attender and occasional presenter at continuing naturopathic education courses. He is President Emeritus of National College of Naturopathic Medicine in Portland.

Bastyr has curtailed his practice in recent years and takes no new patients, but continues the active practice of naturopathic medicine. Some of his patients have been with him for over fifty-five years and have been treated by him in seven different decades. He has observed many changes through the years and now finds his patients more prone to sickness than before due to poorer food quality and increased exposure to environmental toxins, electromagnetic radiation, and suppressive medications. He finds his allopathic colleagues more tolerant and appreciative of naturopathic methods. "I remember," he said, "when we would give a diet to a patient, and the medical men would just laugh" (Bastyr 1989, 45). He also saw a tremendous expansion in both allopathic and naturopathic medical knowledge, and he played a major role in making sure the best of both were integrated into naturopathic medical education. Bastyr greatly admired O. G. Carroll, a successful practitioner of old-fashioned empirical naturopathy, but he felt strongly that naturopathy's empirical successes should be documented and proven by scientific methods. Bastyr became the prototype of the modern naturopathic doctor, who culls the latest findings from the scientific literature, applies them in ways consistent with naturopathic principles, and verifies the results with appropriate lab studies. Bastyr met Benedict Lust on two occasions, and was closely tied to the nature cure tradition of Kneipp through his mother and Dr. Elizabeth Peters. He effortlessly reconciled the empirical tradition of naturopathy with the latest scientific studies and helped create a truly new and original form of clinical care, naturopathic medicine. He has spent the twentieth century preparing the nature cure of the nineteenth century for entry into the twenty-first century.

Bibliography

One of our primary sources was Benedict Lust's journal *Naturopath* which went through several title changes. It started as *Amerikanische Kneipp-Blätter* (1896-1901), in English as *The Kneipp Water Cure Monthly* (1900) and *The Kneipp Water Cure Monthly and Herald of Health* (1901). It continued as *The Naturopath and Herald of Health* (1902-1915) with a German parallel edition, *Der Naturopath und Gesundheits-Rathgeber,* until 1912. The next titles were *Herald of Health and Naturopath* (1916-1922), *Naturopath* (1923-1927) and, after an interruption of six years, *Naturopath and Herald of Health* (1934-1944). The gap between 1927-1934 was filled by *Nature's Path* which Lust had started as a lay magazine in 1925 and which was published until 1953. Thereafter, no other periodical of the American naturopathic profession in America equalled Lust's publication with respect to breadth, depth and duration. In 1990 the American naturopathic profession launched *The Journal of Naturopathic Medicine,* the first naturopathic journal devoted to scientific research. Several national and state associations and naturopathic schools issued their own publications which seem to be more or less lost. People tend to hold on to books longer than to journals and newsletters that are often more valuable as historical documents because they report about the activities of the profession such as conventions and new legislation and contain biographical articles and obituaries. Therefore we appeal to anyone who finds such historical treasures hidden away in some attic or basement of an old-time naturopathic doctor to send them for their preservation to the library of the National College of Naturopathic Medicine, 049 SW Porter, Portland, OR 97201

Abbreviations

AKB	*Amerikanische Kneipp-Blätter*
HHN	*Herald of Health and Naturopath*
KWCM	*Kneipp Water Cure Monthly*
N	*Naturopath*
NCNM	*National College of Naturopathic Medicine*
NHH	*Naturopath and Herald of Health*
NP	*Nature's Path*

Anonymous. 1897. "Father Kneipp's Successors." *AKB* 3:281.

———. 1901. "Wedding Bells." *KWCM* 2:163.

———. 1905. "A Percursor to Father Kneipp." *N* 6:357.

———. 1924. "Training of Followers, Life Work of Doctor." *N* 29:766-767.

———. 1924. "Nature School Sued by Senator Straus." *New York Times. January 30, p. 8.*

———. 1925. "Benedict Lust—The Man and His Work: By One to Whom He Gave a Lift in Life" *N* 30:943-945.

———. 1927. "The Johann Schroth Cure: Its Use at Home, by an Anonymous Nature-Curist Who Was Saved By It."*NP* 338-339, 348-349.

———. 1931. "Anecdotes from the Life of Pastor Kneipp." *NP* 36:109.

———. 1943. "Fire Destroys Yungborn Main Building at Tangerine, Florida." *NHH* 48:46.

Asbeck, Friedrich. 1977. *Naturmedizin in Lebensbildern (Natural Medicine in Biograpies).* Leer: Verlag Grundlagen und Praxis.

Baer, Hans A. 1992. "The Potential Rejuvenation of American Naturopathy as a Consequence of the Holistic Health Movement." *Medical Anthropology.* 13:369-383.

Barker, Florence. 1963. "Stanley Lief: More Personal Tributes. *Health for All* 37:671-672.

Baruch, Simon. 1892. *The Uses of Water in Modern Medicine.* Detroit: Davis.

———. 1895. "Kneipp's Water Cure in the Light of Medical History." *New York Medical Journal* 1:522-525.

Bastyr, John. 1984. NCNM lecture. Audiotape.

———. 1986. "Update Interview." *Update* Fall: 3.

———. 1989. Personal interview by Alma Howard. JBCNM. 14 & 25 April. Audiotape.

———. 1989. *Treatment of Chronic Disease.* Personal Interview by André Saine. AANP Annual Convention 3 Nov. Audiotape.

———. 1990. Personal communication. 28 April.

———. 1992. Personal communication. 1 March.

———. 1993. *Evolution of a Naturopathic Practice.* Audiotape. 36th Annual Northwest Naturopathic Physicians' Conference, Seattle, May 14-16. Redmond, Wash.: Tree Farm Communication.

Baumgarten, Alfred. 1898. *Sebastian Kneipp: Biographie.* Berlin: Becker.

———. 1909. *Die Kneipp'sche Hydrotherapie.* Wörishofen: Buchdruckerei und Verlags-Anstalt Wörishofen.

Behnke, F. H. ca. 1921. *Pioneer Teachers.* Elmhurst, Ill: Published by the author.

Beller, Adele Beth. 1979. *A New Lease on Life: A Tribute to the Late Dr. Otis G. Carroll and Dr. Leo Scott, Doctors of Naturopathy.* Kalispell, Mont.: Published by the author.

Bibliography

Bender, John. 1991. *In Memoriam, Arno Koegler, N.D., May 1, 1898 to February 25, 1995.* Eulogy delivered by John Bender, N. D., March 1, 1991. Mimeographed. Waterloo, Ontario.

Benjamin, Harry. 1961. *Everybody's Guide to Nature Cure.* 14th ed. Croydon, U.K. Health for All Publishing Co.

Benzecry, Frances. 1913. "What I Have Found Out as a Medical Detective?" *Ladies Home Journal* 32 (4):14.

Bergner, Paul. 1993. "Wade Francis Boyle, N.D.: In Memoriam." *Medical Herbalism* 5(3):11.

Bilz, F. E. 1898. *The Natural Method of Healing: A New and Complete Guide to Health.* 2 vol. Leipzig, London: Bilz.

Boden, Dr. med. 1901. "Louis Kuhne und das Reibesitzbad vor Gericht (Louis Kuhne and the Friction Sitz-Bath in Court)." *Der Natur-und Volksarzt* 39:51-52.

Boderwein, J. A. Henry. 1959. "Kneipp—The Man and His Work." *Naturopathic Practitioner* 4:7-10.

Bohn, Wolfgang. 1922. "Kneipp and the Kneipp Method." *HHN* 14:215-222.

Boucher, Joseph A. *Detoxification.* Patient handout. Vancouver, B.C.

———. *Health for Those Want it . . . Enough.* Pamphlet. Vancouver, B.C.

———. *Schroth System of Detoxification.* Patient handout. Vancouver, B.C.

———. 1964. "The Nature Doctor" *The Naturopath* 2 (10):8.

———. 1976. "John Wesley Noble (1906-1976)." *Reflections*

———. 1979. "Faith Can Build Colleges." *Natural Health World and the Naturopath* 18:1.

———. 1980. *The Future of Naturopathy.* Audiotape. Highland, Ind.: Creative Audio.

———. 1980. *Naturopathy: The Science and Art of Natural Healing.* Mimeographed. Vancouver, B.C.

———. 1981. "The Future of Naturopathy." *Journal of the John Bastyr College of Naturopathic Medicine* 2:40-44.

———. 1982. "Patient, Heal Thyself." *Alive: Canadian Journal of Health & Nutrition.* No. 43:23-24.

———. 1982. "How to Be a Naturopath." *Alive: Canadian Journal of Health & Nutrition* No. 44:24-25.

———. 1986. *Naturopathy according to Hippocrates.* Videotape. Tape 2 of the NCNM Symposium held at the National College of Naturopathic Medicine, Portland, Or., at June 6-7.

———. and Richard Liebmann. *History of the National College of Naturopathic Medicine to 1973.* Audiotape.

Boyle, Wade. 1988. *Herb Doctors: Pioneers in Nineteenth Century Botanical Medicine.* East Palestine, Ohio: Buckeye Naturopathic Press.

Bradshaw, William. 1918. "Yungborn, Tangerine, Fla., the Home of Health." *HHN* 23:884-890.

Brauchle, Alfred. 1933. *Handbuch der Naturheilkunde (Handbook of Nature Cure).* Leipzig: Reclam.

Brauchle, Alfred. 1935. "Ärztetagung im Rudolf-Hess-Krankenhaus in Dresden (Physicians' Conference at the Rudolf Hess-Hospital in Dresden)." *Der Naturarzt* 63: 21-22.

Brauchle, Alfred. 1937. *Naturheilkunde in Lebensbildern (Nature Cure in Biographies).* Leipzig: Reclam.

Brauchle, Alfred & Louis R. Grote. 1938-1940. *Ergebnisse aus der Gemeinschaftsarbeit von Naturheilkunde und Schulmedizin (Results of the Cooperation between Nature Cure and Orthodox Medicine).* Leipzig: Reclam.

Brauchle, Alfred. 1951. *Die Geschichte der Naturheilkunde in Lebensbildern (The History of Nature Cure in Biographies).* Stuttgart: Reclam.

Brauchle, Alfred. 1957. *Das grosse Buch der Naturheilkunde (The Great Book of Nature Cure).* Gütersloh: Bertelsmann.

Brauchle, Alfred & Walter Groh. 1971. *Zur Geschichte der Physiotherapie (About the History of Physiotherapy).* Heidelberg, Haug.

Brockmann, J. G. 1895. "Enthüllungen über die Kuhne-Cur! (Disclosures about the Kuhne Cure!)." *Zeitschrift für Erziehung und Unterricht* 9: 79-88.

Brüggemann, Wolfgang 1971. "What is the Kneipp System? Indications, Possibilities, Limitations and Place in Modern Medicine." Translated reprint from *Die Medizinische Welt* No. 48 (27. Nov.) on the occasion of the 150th anniversary of the birth of Sebastian Kneipp.

Brown, P.S. 1988. "Nineteenth-Century American Health Reformers and the Early Nature Cure Movement in Britain." *Medical History* 32:174-194.

———. 1980. (Ed.). *Kneipptherapie: Ein Lehrbuch (Kneipptherapy: A Textbook).* Berlin: Springer.

———. 1982. *Kneipp Vademecum Pro Medico: Principles, Techniques, Indications and Limitations of Kneipp Therapy.* Würzburg: Sebastian Kneipp Publications.

Burghardt, Lothar. 1982. *Bad Wörishofen '82.* Two-page prospectus.

Burghardt, Ludwig. 1988. *Sebastian Kneipp: Helfer der Menschheit (Sebastian Kneipp: Helper of Mankind).* Bad Wörishofen: Kneipp Verlag.

———. 1989. Personal communication. 21. 06.1989 & 11. 08. 1989.

Campanella, M. 1952. "Editorial." *Journal of Naturopathic Medicine* March:3-4.

Campbell, Andy. 1993. "Legislative News." *OANP (Oregon Association of Naturopathic Physicians) News* 84 (4):4.

Carroll, Otis G. 1925. "Letter." *N* 30:170.

———. 1925. "Correspondence." *N* 30: 272-275.

———. 1951. "2nd Vice President's Message." *Journal of American Naturopathic Association* 4(3):5.

———. 1962. Obituary. *Spokane Spokesman-Review.* 26 Feb.

Carroll, Robert V. 1948. "Unity and Progress." *Journal of the American Naturopathic Association* 1(4):3.

Carroll, William 1989. Personal communication. 8 April.

———. 1991. Personal communication. 4 Jan.

Cayleff, Susan E. 1987.*Wash and Be Healed: The Water Cure Movement and Women's Health.* Philadelphia: Temple University Press.

———. 1993. "Keeping to the path: A history of naturopathic healing and professionalism in 20th century America." *Journal of Naturopathic Medicine* 4 (1): 26-27.

Chaitow, Leon. 1987. *Soft-Tissue Manipulation.* Wellingborough, U.K.: Thorons, 1987.

———. 1991. *Palpatory Literacy.* Wellingborough, U.K.: Thorsons.

Chance, Hugh E. 1957. "Naturopathic Scandals Threaten Chiropractic!" *International Review of Chiropractic* 11 (11):6-12.

Claunch, Stanford Kingsley. 1945. *A Brief Outline of Two Advanced Courses of Personal Instruction in Health Building, Scientific Eating, Correct Breathing, Physical Culture, Character Analysis, Vocational Training, Psychology, Psychoanalysis, Scientific Metaphysics: A Complete Philosophy of Life in Two Sections.* Pacific Grove, Calif.: Published by the author.

———. 1981. *The Polarity System.* Vancouver, B.C.: Boucher.

Claridge, R. T. 1843. *The Cold Water Cure.* London: Strange and Smith.

Cody, George. 1985. "History of Naturopathic Medicine." In Joseph E. Pizzorno & Michael T. Murray (Ed.). *Textbook of Natural Medicine.* Seattle: John Bastyr College Publications.

Cole, Ernest I. 1921. "Mark Twain, a Friend of Naturopathy." *HHN* 26:16.

Collins, F.W. 1916. "Dr. Benedict Lust Lectures at 'Mecca of Chiropractic.'" *HHN* 21:21.

———. 1919. (Ed.). *Disease Diagnosed by Obervation of the Eyes.* Newark, N.J.: Published by the author.

———. 1920. "Nomination of Dr. F. W. Collins for President of the U.S.: Announcement by F.W.—Himself." *HHN* 219-220.

———. 1924. "Report of Business Meeting of N.Y.S.S. of Naturopaths." *N* 9:659-665. 1558.

Cordingley, E. W. 1938. "Bilz's Naturopathy of the Nineteenth Century." *NHH* 43:291, 308-309.

Cornaro, Luigi. 1916. *How to Live Long (Discorsi della Vita Sobria).* New York: The Health Culture Co.

Crissinger, K. D. et al. 1990. "Pathophysiology of Gastrointestinal Mucosal Permeability." *Journal of Internal Medicine Supplement (England)* 732:145-154.

Coulter, Harris L.1973-1977. *Divided Legacy: A History of the Schism in Medical Thought.* 3 volumes. Washington, D.C.: Wehawken Book Co.

Davidson, W. McKay. 1923. "Lindlahr's—The Home of Scientific Nature Cure." *N* 28:450-459.

———. 1924. "Henry Lindlahr, M.D." *N 29:1010-1014.*

Day, Harvey. 1979. *Encyclopaedia of Natural Health and Healing.* Santa Barbara: Woodbridge Press.

Debs, Eugene V. 1948. *Writings and Speeches of Eugene V. Debs. Introduction by Arthur M. Schlesinger, Jr.* New York: Hermitage Press.

Detmar, Bernhard. 1951. *Live Wisely—Live Well!* London: Thorsons.

De Terre-Gerard, Anne. 1900. "How Father Kneipp Looked." *KWCM* 1:26-27.

De Vierville, Jonathan Paul. 1991. "Hydrotherapy: Washes, Wraps, Packs and Herbs: Father Sebastian Kneipp and a Hundred Year Health Care Tradition." *Massage Therapy Journal* 30:68-76.

Dextreit, Raymond. 1974. *Our Earth Our Cure.* Brooklyn, N.Y.: Swan House Publishing Co.

Dick, Harold. 1983. Hydrotherapy lecture. NCNM. 9 April. Audiotape.

Directory of the International Society of Naturopathic Physicians. 1955. Graham, Fl.: International Society of Naturopathic Physicians. (Earlier editions:1945 & 1952).

Dixon, Barbara. 1992. Personal communication with Jean Edwards concerning Stanley Lief. 13. 05.

Dodds, Susanna Way. 1915. *Drugless Medicine: Hygeiotherapy.* New York: The Health Culture Co.

Donogan, Jane B. 1986. *Hydropathic Pathway to Health:"Women and Water Cure in Antebellum America.* New York: Greenwood Press.

Dorland's Illustrated Medical Dictionary. 1974. 25th ed. Philadephia: Saunders.

"Drugless Directory of the American Naturopathic Association." 1922. *HHN* 27: 411-413.

Dubos, René. 1959. *Mirage of Health.* Garten City, N.Y.: Anchor Books.

Ebert, Klara. 1905. "Heinrich Lahmann." *Vegetarische Warte* No.12 (23 June):301-305.

Edwards, Jean. 1992. Personal communication about Stanley Lief. 19. 03.

Ehret, Arnold. 1970. *Mucusless Diet Healing System: A Scientific Method of Eating Your Way to Health.* New York: Lust.

———. 1980. *The Story of My Life.* New York: Lust.

Failor, Ralph M. 1955. "History and Present Status of Western States College." *Journal of the AANP* 8(8)6-8.

Farnsworth, G. R. 1990. "A Tribute to Dr. Joseph A. Boucher." *Amercian Association of Naturopathic Physicians Quarterly Newsletter* 5(3):49.

Faulkner, James. 1934. "Speaking of Naturopaths." *NHH* 33:102-103.

Fenn, Axel. 1982. *Welche Kur ist für mich richtig? (What Cure Is Right For Me?).* München: Humboldt-Taschenbuchverlag.

Fenton, Peter. 1992. *Charles Leslie Thomson, B.Sc. (1914-1992).* Mimeographed. Leeds, West Yorkshire: Fenton.

Fey, Christian and Sebastian Kneipp. 1955. *Mein Testament and Codizil (My Will and Codicil).* Munich: Ehrenwirth.

Fey, Christian and Heinrich Lampert. 1978. *Hydrotherapie unter besonderer Berücksichtigung der Kneippschen Wasserbehandlung (Hydrotherapy with Special Consideration of Kneipp's Water Treament).* 3rd. ed. Heidelberg: Verlag für Medizin Fischer.

Findeison, Harry F. 1926. "American Naturopathic Association, Annual Convention, Minutes of the Executive Session, December 17, 1925." *N* 31:43-44.

Finger, M. 1927. "Felkes Stellung zum Vegetarismus" (Felke's Position Towards Vegetarianism) & "Emanuel Felke als Mensch" (Emanuel Felke as a Person). *Vegetarische Presse* No. 2:17-19.

Fishbein, Morris. 1932. *Fads and Quackery in Healing.* New York: Blue Ribbon Books.

Floden, George. 1964. "The Registry and Its Purpose." *Naturopathic Magazette* 16:2.

Franklin, Stanley. 1963. "Stanley Lief: More Personal Tributes." *Health for All* 37-671.

Fraser, Bertram T. 1961. "Herbalism and Nature Cure. *The Kingston Chronicle* 23 (July):1-15.

Freibott, George A. 1990. *The History of Naturopathy or "Pseudomedicalism": Naturopathy's Demise?* (Report submitted to the U.S. Department of Education). Priest River, Idaho: Published by the author.

Fulder, Stephan. 1988. *The Handbook of Complementary Medicine.* Oxford: Oxford University Press.

Gandhi, M. K. 1954. *Nature Cure.* Ahmedabad, India: Navajivan Publishing House, 1954.

Gatterman, Meridel I. 1982. "W.A. Budden: The Transition Through Proprietary Education." *Chiropractic History* 2:21-25.

Gehmann, Jesse Mercer. 1947. (Ed.). *A Commemorative and Descriptive Book on the Light of Naturopathy.* Paterson, N.J.: The Benedict Lust Permanent Memorial Association.

Gehrkes, Clemens. 1881. *John Schroth's Natural Medical Science: Diseases and Ailments of Children.* St. Louis.

Gesser, Charles H. 1966. *The Principles of Natural Living and Natural Healing.* Tampa, Fla.: Published by the author.

Gevitz, Norman. 1982. *The DO's: Osteopathic Medicine in America.* Baltimore: The Johns Hopkins University Press.

———. 1988. (Ed.) *Other Healers: Unorthodox Medicine in America.* Baltimore: The Johns Hopkins Press.

Gibbons, Russell W. 1989. "Fred Collins and his New Jersey 'Mecca.'" *Chiropractic History* 9:41.

Ginger, Ray. 1949. *The Bending Cross: A Biography of Eugene Victor Debs.* New Brunswick: Rutgers University Press.

Gleich, Lorenz. 1860. *Physiatrische Schriften (Physiatric Writings).* München.

Gorst, Elliot. 1963. "Stanley Lief: More Personal Tributes." *Health for All* 37:670.

Gray, John. 1904. "The Schroth Cure." *N* 5:184-185.

Griebel, Karl. 1886. "Der Reichskanzler und seine Krankheit (The Chancellor and His Illness)." *Der Naturarzt* 25 (No.4):54-56.

Griggs, Barbara.1981.*Green Pharmacy: A History of Herbal Medicine.* New York: Viking.

———.1986. *The Food Factor.* New York: Viking.

Groh, Ludwig.1968. *Naturgemässe Lebens-und Heilweise (Natural Method of Living and Healing).* Bietigheim: Turm-Verlag.

Grote, Louis R. & Alfred Brauchle. 1935. *Gespräche über Schulmedizin und Naturheilkunde (Conversations about Orthodox Medicine and Nature Cure).* Leipzig: Reclam.

Haberling, W. et al. 1932. *Biographisches Lexikon der hervorragenden Arzte aller Zeiten und Völker (Biographical Cyclopedia of the Eminent Physicians of All Times and Nations).* 2nd ed. Vol. 4. Berlin: Urban & Schwarzenberg, 1932.

Hahn, Johann Sigmund. 1833. *Unterricht von der wunderbaren Heilkraft des frischen Wassers (Lectures about the Wonderful Healing Power of Fresh Water).* 5th edition, improved and expanded by Prof. Oertel. Ilmenau: Voigt.

Hahn, Peter. 1992. "Dresden, betrachtet vom Dresdner Balkon (Dresden, Viewed from the Dresden Balcony)." *Frankfurter Allgemeine Zeitung* No.13 (16th January)" R 11.

Hahn, Theodor. 1979. *Das Paradies der Gesundheit, das Verlorene und Wiedergewonnene (The Paradise of Health*—Lost and Regained). Cöthen: Schettler.

———.1865. *Praktisches Handbuch der naturgemässen Heilweise (Practical Handbook of Natural Healing).* Leipzig: Grieben.

Hale, Annie Riley. 1926. *These Cults.* New York: National Health Foundation.

Halperson, Maurice. 1925. "To the Memory of Louisa Lust." *N* 30:1017-1021.

Harrison, H. Leslie. 1969. *Getting to Know the Incorporated Society of Registered Naturopaths.* Kingston, Edinburgh: Incorporated Society of Registered Naturopaths.

Hazzard, Linda Burfield. 1927. *Scientific Fasting.* New York: Grant.

———. and Benedict Lust. 1925. "Financial Help Needed for Dr. Hazzard." *N* 30:472-475.

Hentschel, H. D. 1988. "Heublumen-Anwendungen bei rheumatischen Schmerzsyndromen (Hayflower Applications for Rheumatic Pain Syndromes)." *Physikalische Therapie in Theorie und Praxis* 9:69-77.

———. 1989. Personal communication 02. 08. 1989.

Hering, E. 1901. "Louis Kuhne."*Vegetarische Warte.* 23. April: 176-179.

Hewlett-Parson, James. 1968. *Naturopathic Practice: A Valuable Guide to Students and Others in the Principles and Practice of Nature Cure.* New York: Arco Publishing Co.

Hildebrand, Gerhard. 1936. "Adolf Just, ein Kämpfer für naturnahes Leben (Adolf Just, a Fighter for a Natural Life)." *Der Naturarzt* 64:73-75.

Hirsch, Fred. 1923. "Arnold Ehret." *N* 28:11-12.

Hirschel, B. 1840. *Hydriatica oder Begründung der Wasserheilkunde auf wissenschaftliche Prinzipien: Geschichte und Literatur (Hydriatica or the Founding of Water Cure upon Scientific Principles: History and Literature).* Leipzig.

Hoffman. 1986. "The Father of Holistic Medicine." *East West Journal* April 1986:26-29.

Houghton, Roland S. 1851. *Bulwer and Forbes on the Water Treatment.* New York: Fowlers and Wells.

Hudson, Tori. 1992. *Gynecology and Naturopathic Medicine: A Treatment Manual.* Beaverton, Or.: TK Publications.

Hufeland, Christoph Wilhelm. 1870. *Art of Prolonging Life.* Edited by Erasmus Wilson. Philadelphia: Lindsay & Blakiston.

Humphreys, Rob. 1991. *The Real Guide: Czechoslovakia.* New York: Prentice Hall.

Issel, Christine. 1990. *Refexology: Art, Science and History.* Sacramento: New Frontier Publishers.

Jackson, Carlton. 1974. *J. I. Rodale: Apostle of Nonconformity.* New York: Pyramid Books.

Jackson, James C. 1874. *How to Treat the Sick without Medicine.* Dansville, N.Y.: Austin, Jackson & Co.

Jacobs, Michael. 1992. *Blue Guide Czechoslovakia.* London: Black; New York: Norton.

Jayne, Christopher H. 1990. *History of Naturopathic Medicine (1927-1990) in the Northwest.* Student paper based on talks with Dr. William A. Turska and Dr. Jared Zeff. Portland, Or.: National College of Naturopathic Medicine.

Jensen, Bernard. 1952. *The Science and Practice of Iridology.* Provo, Utah: BiWorld Publishers.

———. 1982. *Iridology: Science and Practice in the Healing Arts.* Volume 2. Escondido, Calif.: Published by the author.

"Joseph A. Boucher, N.D., D.C. (1916-1987)." 1987. *Update* (National College of Naturopathic Medicine Alumni Newsletter) Spring, 3-4.

Juettner, Otto. 1916. *A Treatise on Naturopathic Practice.* New York: Lust.

Jungborn-Blätter 1934. Special issue No. 3 (July): *Zu Adolf Justs 75. Geburtag am 8 August 1934 (In Honor of Adolf Just's 75th Birthday on August 8, 1934).* Edited by Rudolf Just.

Just, Adolf. 1903. *Return to Nature!: The True Natural Method of Healing and Living and the True Salvation of the Soul: Paradise Regained . . .* Authorized translation from the 4th enlarged German edition by Benedict Lust. New York: Lust.

———. 1910. "The New Paradise of Health." *NHH* 15:641-650, 712-721.

———. 1912. *Return to Nature!* Authorized translation of "Kehrt zur Natur zurück! by H. A. Nesbitt. London: Routledge.

Just, Rudolf. 1934. (Ed.) "Zu Adolf Just's 75. Geburtstag (In Honor of Adolf Just's 75th Birthday)." *Jungborn-Blätter* 9:65-112 (Special issue).

Kaiser, Joseph H. *Von der originalen Kur Sebastian Kneipp's zur umfassenden Kneipp-Physiotherapie von heute (From Sebastian Kneipp's Original Cure to Today's Comprehensive Kneipp-Physiotherapy).* Undated reprint. Aachen: Published by the author.

———. 1975. (Ed.). *Das grosse Kneippbuch: Handbuch der naturgemässen Lebens-und Heilweise (The Great Kneipp Book: Handbook of Natural Living and Healing).* München: Ehrenwirth.

Kapp, Ernst. 1850. *J. H. Rausse, der Reformator der Wasserheilkunde oder Naturheilkunde (J. H. Rausse: The Reformer of Water Cure or Nature Cure).* New ed. Leipzig: Winkler.

Katz, Dean. 1985. "Naturopathy." *Seattle Times* 14 April: K3.

Kaufman, Martin. 1971. *Homeopathy in America: The Rise and Fall of a Medical Heresy.* Baltimore: The Johns Hopkins Press.

Keating, Joseph C. et al. 1994. "Origins of the LACC (Los Angeles College of Chiropractic), 1901-1922. *Journal of Manipulative and Physiological Therapeutics* 17:93-106.

Keller-Jakob, A. 1950. "Die atmosphärische Kur des Arnold Rikli genannt Sonnendoktor (The Atmospheric Cure of Arnold Rikli called the Sun Doctor)" in C. Fauser, Ed. *Bewährte Naturheilkuren (Proven Nature Cures).* Zurich: Schweizerischer Verein für Volksgesundheit.

Kellogg, John Harvey. 1903. *Rational Hydrotherapy.* 2nd ed. Philadelphia: Davis.

———. 1921. *The New Dietetics.* Battle Creek, Mich.: The Modern Medicine Publishing Co.

Kenny, Elizabeth. 1937. *Infantile Paralysis and Cerebral Diplegia: Methods Used for the Restoration of Function.* Sydney: Angus & Robertson.

———. and Martha Ostenso. 1943. *And They Shall Walk: The Life Story of Sister Elizabeth Kenny.* New York: Dodd, Mead & Co.

Kern, John Hewins. 1925. "Dr. Louisa Lust, An Appreciation." *N* 30:709-710.

Kipnis, Walter Seth. 1926. "State News." *N* 31: 407-409.

Kleinschrod, Franz. 1914. "Sebastian Kneipp." *N* 19:563-561.

"Kneipp Institutes in America." 1898. *AKB* 3:227-228.

Kneipp, Sebastian. 1889. *Thus Shalt Thou Live.* Kempten, Bavaria: Kösel.

———. 1893. *My Water Cure.* Translation & preface by A. de F. Wellingborough, U.K.: Thorsons, 1979 (Reprint of the 1893 ed.).

———. 1894. *My Will.* Kempten, Bavaria: Kösel.

———. 1896. *My Water Cure.* 4th ed. translated from the 36th German ed. Kempten (Bavaria): Kösel.

———. 1897. *The Codicil to My Will.* Kempten, Bavaria: Kösel.

———. and Bonifaz Reile. 1903. *Das grosse Kneippbuch (The Great Kneipp Book).* Wörishofen: Kösel.

———. 1979. *Aus meinem Leben: Selbstbiographie (About My Life: Autobiography).* Bad Wörishofen: Stamm-Kneippverein (Reprint of the 1891 edition).

Kneipp-Bund e. V. 1981. *Die Kneipp-Bewegung: Ihre Entwicklung im In und Ausland (The Kneipp Movement: Its Development Here and Abroad).* Bad Wörishofen: Kneipp-Verlag.

Koegler, Arno R. 1951. "Simplified Homeopathy." *Journal of Naturopathic Medicine.* April: 20-21.

———. 1959. "Greetings to All Naturopathic Physicians." *Journal of Naturopathic Medicine.* August: D-E.

———. 1959. "Can Naturopathic Medicine Take the Place of Antibiotics?" *Journal of Naturopathic Medicine* August: 11-13.

———. 1961. "Some Comments and Observations on Iris Photography." *Journal of Naturopathic Medicine.* October-November:18-19.

Kötschau, Karl. 1960. *Medizin am Schweideweg (Medicine at the Crossroad).* Ulm: Haug.

Krammer, Hans. n.d. *Gesundheit, Lebensfreude, Erfolg durch Kneipp (Health, Joy of Life and Success through Kneipp).* Bad Wörishofen: International Confederation of the Kneipp Movement. (Pamphlet).

Kuhne, Louis. n.d. *The New Science of Healing or The Doctrine of the Unity of Diseases.* Leipzig: Kuhne.

———. 1917. *Neo-Naturopathy: The New Science of Healing or The Doctrine of the Unity of Diseases.* Butler, N.J.: Lust.

———. 1902 & 1917. *The Science of Facial Expression: The New System of Diagnosis, based on Original Researches and Discoveries.* Leipzig: Kuhne & Butler, N.J.: Lust.

Kuts-Cheraux, A. W. 1953. (Ed.). *Naturae Medicina and Naturopathic Dispensatory.* Des Moines, Iowa: American Naturopathic Physicians and Surgeons Associations.

Lahmann, Heinrich. 1885. "Antworten aus dem homöopathischen Lager (Replies from the Homeopathic Camp)." 24 (no.7): 130-133.

———. 1886. "Wie stellt sich die Naturheilkunde zu dem Jaeger'schen System (What ist Nature Cure's Positions toward Jaeger's System)." *Der Volksarzt* 25: 97-99.

———. 1886. "Etwas von meiner Studienreise (Something about My Study Tour)." *Der Volksarzt* 25: 117-120, 148-166.

———. 1890. *Koch und die Kochianer: Eine Kritik der Koch'schen Entdeckung und der Koch'schen Richtung in der Heilkunde (Koch and the Kochians: A Critic of Koch's Discoveries and School of Thought in Medicine).* Stuttgart: Zimmer.

———. 1892. *Die diätetische Blutentmischung (Dysämie) als Grundursache aller Krankheiten (The Dietetic Dysemia as Fundamental Cause of All Diseases).* Leipzig: Spamer.

———. 1893. *Sind gynäkologische Opeationen vermeidbar? (Can Gynecologic Operations Be Avoided?).* Stuttgart: Zimmer.

———. 1894. *Die wichtigsten Kapitel der natürlichen (physikalisch-diätetischen) Heilweise (The Most Important Chapters of the Natural (Physical-Dietetic) Healing Method).* 2nd ed. Stuttgart: Zimmer.

———. 1898. *Das Luftbad als Heil und Abhärtungsmittel (The Air Bath as a Cure and Hardening Method).* Stuttgart: Zimmer.

———. 1901. *Natural Hygiene or Healthy Blood* (English translation of *Dietetic Dysemia*). 2nd ed. London: Sonnenschein.

———. 1905. *Der krankmachende Einfluss atmosphärischer Luftdruck-Schwankungen (The Disease-Producing Influence of Changes in Atmospheric Pressure).*

———. 1921/22. *Dr. Lahmann's Sanatorium Weisser Hirsch: Prospektus und Jahresbericht (Prospectus and Annual Report).* 36th ed.

Lane, Henry Edward. 1904. *Diagnosis from the Eye.* Chicago: Kosmos Publishing Co.

Lang, Walter. N.D. *Investigating the Practical Results of Natural Healing at the Kingston Clinic* (Pamphlet). Edinburgh: Thomson-Kingston Publications.

Leppmann, Wolfgang. 1984. *Rilke: A Life.* New York: Fromm.

Levental, Zdenko.1977. "Der 'Sonnendoktor' Arnold Rikli (The 'Sun Doctor' Arnold Rikli)." *Gesnerus* 34:394-403.

Leviton, Richard. 1990. "How the Swamis Came to the States." *Yoga Journal* No. 91 (March/April):42-45, 119-128.

Licht, Sidney. 1967. (Ed.) *Therapeutic Electricity and Ultraviolet Radiation.* 2nd. edition. New Haven: Licht

Lief, Stanley. 1930. "Our Third Birthday." *Health for All* 4:5.

———. 1930. "Simple Rules Regarding Food." *Health for All* 4:85.

———. 1930. "Fasting is a True Science." *Health for All* 4:125.

———. 1930. "Disease versus Common Sense." *Health for All* 4:141.

———. 1930. "How I Keep Fit." *Health for All* 4:165.

———. 1930. "While There's Life There's Hope." *Health for All* 4:205.

———. 1930. "The Real Cure for Rheumatism." *Health for All* 4:219,

———. 1930. "How Soon Can I Be Cured?" *Health for All* 4:249.

———. 1931. "The True Treatment for Colds." *Health for All* 5:342-343.

———. 1931. "Nature Cure Explained." *The Health and Nature Cure Handbook.* 1:18-20. London: The Nature Cure Educational Association.

———. 1931. "Curative Fasting." *Health and Nature Cure Handbook* 2:67-71. London: The Nature Cure Educational Association.

———. 1962. "Diet Does Not Cure." *Health for All* 36:271.

———. 1962. "Disease is Beneficial." *Health for All* 36:407.

Lief, Stella. 1963. "Stanley Lief: More Personal Tributes." *Health for All* 37:670.

Liek, Erwin. 1930. *The Doctor's Mission.* London: Murray.

Lindlahr, Anna. 1910. "The Vegetarian Kitchen." *Naturopath* 15:239.

Lindlahr, Henry. 1910. "We Can Take Care of Our Enemies, But God Save Us From Our Friends." *N* 15:289-291.

———. 1910. "The New Psychology." *N* 15:458-461.

———. 1910. "The Most Valuable Asset of a Nation is the Health of Its Citizens." *N* 15:608-611.

———. 1913. *Nature Cure: Philosophy & Practice Based on the Unity of Disease & Cure.* Chicago: The Nature Cure Publishing Co. (The Nature Cure Series, vol.1).

———. 1913. "Venereal Diseases." *N* 18:11-16.

———. 1914. "Brief 6, Nature Cure." *N* 19:251-253.

———. 1918. "How I Became Acquainted with Nature Cure." *HHN* 23:122-130.

———. 1922. *Nature Cure.* 20th ed. Chicago: The Nature Cure Publishing Co.

———. 1923. "Henry Lindlahr, M.D., The Father of Scientific Natural Therapeutics" (Reprint of his "How I Found Nature Cure"). *N* 28:438-441.

———. 1923. "The New Blood Wash Treatment." *N* 28:527-530.

———. 1924. "The Marathon Bath—Also Known as BioBath or the Blood Wash Treatment." *N* 29:420-427.

———. 1981. *Natural Therapeutics. Volume II: Practice.* Reprint of the 1919 edition, edited and revised by Jocelyn C. P. Proby. Saffron Walden, U.K.: Daniel.

Lindlahr, Victor H. 1924. "In Memoriam Henry Lindlahr, M.D." *N* 19:1009-1010.

———. 1973. *The Natural Way to Health.* Hollywood, Calif.: Newcastle Publishing Co.

Lucas, William R. 1938. *The Growth and Development of the Naturopathic Movement in Great Britain. NHH* 43:4, 15, 21, 23

Lust, Benedict. 1900. "A Brief History of Natural Healing." *KWCM* 1:2-5.

———. 1900. "Father Kneipp—His Life and His Works." *KWCM* 1:34-36, 51-52, 67-68.

———. 1901. "The Kneipp Cure." *KWCM* 2:211-213.

———. 1902. "A Happy New Year." *NHH* 3:13-14.

———. 1902. "Editorial Drift." *NHH* 3:32-33.

———. 1902. "Editorial Drift." *NHH* 3:168-171.

———. 1902. "New Year Expectations." *NHH* 3:483-485.

———. 1902. "Introducing the New Editor." *NHH* 3:522-523.

———. 1903. "The Origin of the Naturopathic Society." *NNH* 4:36-37.

———. 1903. "Health Incarnate." *NHH* 4:164-167.

———. 1903. "Naturopathy: What Hinders the Propagation of Naturopathy?" *NHH* 4:194-195.

———. 1904. "Naturopathic Progress." *NHH* 5:110-112.

———. 1904. "Father Kneipp and His Methods." *NHH*: 5:145-149.

———. 1905. "Naturopathy: What It Was, What It Is and What It Will Be." *NHH* 6:92-94.

———. 1905. "Health Incarnate: A Naturopathic Silhouette." *NHH* 318-320.

———. 1908. "The Science of Nature Cure." *NHH* 9:1-3.

———. 1908. "Correspondence." *NHH* 9:94-95.

———. 1908. "The Chinese Ambassador, Wu Ting Fang, at the Yungborn." *NHH* 9:288-289.

———. 1908. "Naturopathic News." *NHH* 9:329-330.

———. 1909. "A Family Chat Conerning Our Growth." *NHH* 14:1-4.

———. 1909. "Our New Naturopathic Hospital." *NHH* 14:87-89.

———. 1912. "The Editor's Lecture Tour." *NHH* 17:319-321.

———. 1913. "Naturopathic News." *NHH* 18:240.

———. 1915. "Naturopathic News." *HHN* 20:54-57.

———. 1915. "Letter to Ladies Home Journal by the American Naturopathic Association." *HHN* 20:385.

———. 1916. "Naturopathic News." *HHN* 21:157-158.

———. 1918. "Priessnitz, Introductor of Hydropathy." *HHN* 23:223-224.

———. 1918. "The Principles, Aim and Program of the Nature Cure System." *HHN* 23:423-429.

———. 1918. "Great Pioneers." *HHN* 23:446-447.

———. 1918 "Naturopathic News." *HHN* 23:580-581.

———. (Ed.) 1918. *Universal Naturopathic Encyclopedia, Directory and Buyers' Guide: Yearbook of Drugless Therapy for 1918-19.* Butler, N.J.: Published by the author.

———. 1919. "Intolerance of Official Medicine." *HHN* 24:438-440.

———. 1920. "Proclamation for the 24th Annual Convention of the ANA." *HHN* 25:368-371.

———. 1921. "History of the Naturopathic Movement." *HHN* 26:479-480.

———. 1922. "Naturopathic News." *HHN* 27:499-506, 557-559.

———. 1923. *The Fountain of Youth or Curing by Water.* New York: Macfadden.

———. 1923. "Naturopathic News." *N* 28:37-38.

———. 1924. "Naturopathic News." *N* 29:359-360.

———. 1924. "Naturopathic News." *N* 29:567-569.

———. 1925. "Naturopathic News." *N* 30:363-380.

———. 1925. "To Members of the ANA and Progressive Doctors of Every Kind." *N* 30:673.

———. 1925. "Naturopathic News." *N* 30:759.

———. 1926. "We are on the Brink of a New Era." *N* 31:5-9.

———. 1926. "Report of Dr. Benedict Lust's Trip West." *N* 31:396-402.

———. 1926. "Our Trip to the Fatherland." *N* 31:580-585.

———. 1927. "Our Trip to the Fatherland."*N* 32:7-14, 59-66, 111-118, 165-172, 270-276.

———. 1927. "Naturopathic News." *N* 32:143-144.

———. 1928. "The Centenary of the Triumph of Genius: Vincent Priessnitz of Grafenberg." *NP* 33:12-13, 26.

———. 1928. "The Great Emanuel Felke Passes Away." *NP* 33:44, 69.

———. 1928. *Zone Therapy: Relieving Pain and Sickness by Nerve Pressure.* NewYork: Benedict Lust Publicatins. (Reprinted in 1980).

———. 1932. "On Air School of Naturopathy." *NP* 37:325.

———. 1934. "Dr. Lust Reports . . ." *NHH* 33:36-37.

———. 1934. "Medical Liberty versus Unconstitutional Health Laws . . ."*NHH* 33:296-298, 316.

———. 1935. "Dr. Lust Speaking." *NHH* 40:226-227, back cover.

———. 1935. "Address of Welcome." *NHH* 40:248-252.

———. 1936. "Adolf Just." *NHH* 41:69.

———. 1936. "Allopathy and Naturopathy Reconciled." *NHH* 41:99-100, 114.

———. 1937. "Dr. Lust Speaking." *NHH* 42:162-163, 175; 290-291, 303.

———. 1938 "Proclamation to the People of the United States . . ." *NHH* 43:265-266, 282.

———. 1940. "Forty-fourth Annual Congress of the American Naturopathic Association." *N* 45:186.

———. 1942. "The American Naturopathic Association, Its Purposes and Objectives." *NHH* 47:198-200.

———. 1944. *What is Naturopathy?* American Naturopathic Association.48th Annual Congress, October 19-21. Philadelphia (Program brochure).

———. 1961. *About Herbs.* Wellingborough, U.K. : Thorsons.

Lust, Louisa. 1907. *The Practical Naturopathic-Vegetarian Cook Book.* New York: Lust.

———. 1911. "How to Avoid Pain and Sickness." *N* 16:99.

———. 1911. "Water Cure, Water Applications." *N* 16:231, 233.

———. 1923. "The Curative Agency of Water and Herbs for Treatment of Fever." *N* 28:437.

———. 1924. "Vegetarian Regime Important in Health and Disease." *N* 29:812.

Lust, John B. 1953. *Lust for Living: How to Live and Grow Younger, Healthier and Happier.* New York: Lust.

———. 1974, *The Herb Book.* New York: Benedict Lust Publications, 1974.

Macfadden, Bernarr. 1914. *Macfadden's Encylopedia of Physical Culture.* 5 volumes. New York: Physical Culture Publishing Co.

Macfadden, Mary & Emile Gauvreau. 1953. *Dumbbells and Carrot Strips: The Story of Bernarr Macfadden.* New York.

Madaus, Udo. 1991. Personal communication. 09.24.1991.

Mader, Max. 1926 &1927. "The Schroth Cure."*N* 31:529-533; 32:15-17.

Maimonides, Moses ben. 1958.*The Preservation of Youth: Essays on Health.* New York: Philosophical Library.

Mariafai, Judith M. N.D. *Kneipp and the Kneipp Cure.* Bad Wörishofen (Pamphlet).

———. 1974. *Bibliographie des Kneippschrifttums (Bibliography of Kneippliterature).* Bad Wörishofen: Kneipp-Bund.

———. 1982. *Das Leben des Sanitätsrat Dr. med. Franz Kleinschrod (The Life of Honorable Franz Kleinschrod, M.D.).* Bad Wörishofen: Kneipp-Verlag.

Matsen, Jonn. 1887. *Eating Alive: Prevention through Good Digestion.* North Vancouver, B. C.: Crompton Books.

McReynolds, Margery E. 1991. Personal communication. 8 Dec.

Melville, Herman. 1967. *The Confidence-Man.* New York: Bobbs-Merrill.

Menschel, Thea. 1975. "Felkes Persönlichkeit" (Felke's Personality) in *Die Felke-Kur* (The Felke Cure), edited by H. Dhonau et al. Frankfurt/Main: Kramer.

Metcalfe, Richard. 1898. *The Life of Vincent Priessnitz, Founder of Hydrotherapy.* Richmond Hill, Surrey: Metcalfe's London Hydro., Ltd.

Meyer-Camberg, Ernst. 1977. *Das praktische Lexikon der Naturheilkunde (The Practical Encyclopedia of Nature Cure).* München: Mosaik Verlag.

Milne, Alec. N.D. *Rheumatism* (Pamphlet). Edinburgh: Thomson-Kingston Publications.

Mock, Byrd. 1923. "Echoes of the Naturopathic Convention in the Nation's Capital." *N* 28:442-443.

Moore, J. Stuart. 1993. *Chiropractic in America: The History of a Medical Alternative.* Baltimore: The Johns Hopkins University Press.

Moule, Tom W.1963. "A Great Pioneer—A Great Healer." *Health for All* 37:599.

Moyle, Alan. 1950. *Nature Cure Explained.* London: Health for All Publishing Co.

Müller, Andres. 1904. *Pastor Felke und seine Heilmethoden* (Pastor Felke and His Healing Methods). 3rd rev. ed.. Homberg/Rhine: Hadstein.

Muller, John. 1917. "Six Months with Msgr. Kneipp."*HHN* 22:139-145.

Murray, Michael T., and Joseph E. Pizzorno. 1990. *An Encyclopedia of Natural Medicine.* Rocklin, Calif.: Prima Publishing.

Mundhenk, Michael. 1991. "Visons of the Pioneers: Paavo Airola—Doctor Common Sense." *Alive: Canadian Journal of Health and Nutrition* No.111 (July/August): 12.

Neuburger, Max. 1932. "The Doctrine of the Healing Power of Nature throughout the Course of Time." Translation by Linn J. Boyd. *The Journal of the American Institute of Homeopathy* 25:861-884, 1011-1465.

O'Brien, James G. 1978. *Benedict Lust and Naturopathy.* Stockholm, N.J.: Unpublished manuscript.

Oswald, Jean A. 1989. *Yours for Health: The Life and Times of Herbert M. Shelton.* Franklin, Wis.: Franklin Books.

Overton, Helen. 1989. Personal interview by Alma Howard. JBCNM. 31 March. Audiotape.

Pachter, Henry M. 1951. *Magic into Science: The Story of Paracelsus.* New York: Schuman.

Page, Charles E. 1904. "The Healing Art." *NHH* 5:201.

Paracelsus. 1958. *Selected Writings.* Edited by Jolande Jacobi. 2nd ed. New York: Pantheon (Bollingen Series, vol. 28).

Parasco, Christos & Benedict Lust. 1923. *The Apocalypsis of Physicial Immortality: Essentials of the Biological Blood-Washing Method.* Lesson 1. New York: Lust.

Pattreiouex, J. Allen. 1917. "The Present Position of Naturopathy and Allied Therapeutic Measures in the British Isles." *HHN* 22:217-223.

Pizzorno, Joseph E. 1989. Personal interview by Alma Howard. JBCNM. 30 March. Audiotape.

Pizzorno, Joseph E., and Michael T. Murray. 1985. (Ed.) *Textbook of Natural Medicine.* Seattle: John Bastyr College Publications.

Podszus, W. 1992. "Rückblick auf die Abteilung für natürliche Heilweise im Krankenhaus am Kreuzberg in Berlin: Zur Erinnerung and Dr. Strassburg (Looking Back to the Department for Natural Healing Methods at the Hospital on the Kreuzberg in Berlin: In Memory of Dr. Strassburg). *Ärztezeitschrift für Naturheilverfahren* 33: 863-868.

Pohl, John F. and Sister Elizabeth Kenny. 1943. *The Kenny Concept of Infantile Paralysis and Its Treatment.* Minneapolis: Bruce.

Posner. 1925. "In Memoriam to the Mother of Naturopathy." *N* 30:707-708.

Powell, Milton. 1963. "Stanley Lief: Some Personal Tributes." *Health for All* 37:602.

Price, Weston A. 1945. *Nutrition and Physical Degeneration.* Redlands, Calif.: Price.

Proctor, Lauren Lust. 1991. Personal Communication.

Purinton, Edward Earle. 1903. "The Bible of the Body." *NHH* 4:351-353.

———. 1905. "Most Important: To Students of Naturopathy." *NHH* 6:252-254.

———. 1914. "Where to Find Health." *NHH* 19:275-286.

Rauch, Erich. 1991. *Naturbehandlung der Erkältungs und Infektionskrankheiten (Naturopathic Treatment of Colds and Infectious Diseases).* 15th. ed. Heidelberg: Haug.

Rausse, J. H. (pseud. for Heinrich F. Francke). 1838. *Der Geist der Gräfenberger Wasserkur (The Spirit of the Graefenberg Water Cure).* Zeitz: Schieferdecker.

———. 1848. *Miscellanies to the Graefenberg Water Cure.* Translated by C. H. Meeker. New York: Fowlers and Wells.

———. 1851. *Errors of Physicians and Others in the Practice of the Water Cure as a Remedial Agent in the Prevention and Cure of Diseases.* Translated by C. H. Meeker. New York: Fowlers and Wells (Water-Cure Library, vol. 6).

———. 1852. *Anleitung zur Ausübung der Wasserheilkunde für Jedermann der zu lesen versteht (Instructions in the Application of the Water Cure for Everyone Who Knows to Read).* Edited by Theodor Hahn. Leipzig: Keil.

———. 1858. *The Water Cure Applied to Every Known Disease.* New York: Fowlers and Wells.

———. 1893. *Health and the Various Methods of Cure.* Bitterfeld, Germany & Vineland, N.J.: Baumann.

Renaud, S., and M. de Lorgeril. 1992. "Wine, alcohol, platelets, and the French paradox for coronary heart disease." *Lancet* 339:1523-1526.

Riedel, Gerhard. 1985. *. . . meinte Pfarrrer Kneipp: Ernstes und Heiteres vom Wassdoktor (. . . said Father Kneipp: Serious and Humorous Statements from the Water Doctor).* Bad Wörishofen: Kneipp-Verlag.

Rikli, Arnold. 1861. "Rikli's Bett-Dampfbad (Rikli's Bed-Steambath)."*Der Wasserfreund.* Supplement to No. 6:87-90.

———. 1868. "Auflösung, Aufsaugung, Ausscheidung—die letzten Wirkungen aller Richtungen des Naturheilverfahrens (Dissolution, Absorption, Elimination as the Final Ends of All Nature Cure Methods)." *Der Naturarzt* 7(4):25-31.

———. 1869. *Die Thermodiätetik oder das tägliche thermoelectrische Licht und Luftbad in Verbindung mit naturgemässer Diät als zukünftige Heilmethode (The Thermodietetics or the Daily Thermoelectric Light and Airbath in Combination with Natural Diet as the Future Healing Method).* Vienna (Austria): Braumüller.

———. 1879. "Meine Erfahrungen, Beobachtungen und Schlüsse über Vegetabildiät nach achtzehnjähriger Praxis (My Experiences, Observations and Conclusions about Vegetarian Diet after Eighteen Years of Practice)."*Der Naturarzt* 18(5):72-75, 86-88.

———. 1896. "Die Sonne—der Urquell alles Lebens (The Sun—Primary Source of All Life)." *Zeitschrift für Erziehung und Unterricht* 10:171-178.

———. 1903. "Abschiedsworte an meine verehrten Kollegen und Gesinnungsgenossen (Words of Farewell to My Esteemed Colleagues and Followers)." *Zeitschrift für Geschichte und Unterricht* 17:205-212.

———. 1911. *Die Grundlehren der Naturheilkunde einschliesslich "Die atmosphärische Kure," "Es werde Licht" und "Abschiedsworte"* (The Fundamental Doctrines of Nature Cure including "The Atmospheric Cure," "Let There Be Light," and "Words of Farewell"). 9th revised edition. Wolfsberg, G. Rikli.

Riley, Joe Shelby. 1921. "Benedict Lust: A Tribute to the Leader of the Drugless World." (Poem). *HHN* 26:525.

———. 1924. *Conquering Units, or the Mastery of Disease.* Washington, D.C.: Published by the author.

———. 1942. *Zone Reflex: All Its Applications Made Plain and Simple for Use by Anyone.* Brooklyn, N.Y.: Wendel.

Roeder, Giselle. 1992. "Father Sebastian Kneipp: The Water Doctor." *Alive: Canadian Journal of Health and Nutrition.* No.124 (Nov.):12-13.

Roethke, Theodore. 1975. *The Collected Poems of Theodore Roethke.* Anchor Books. Garden City, NY

Rollier, A. 1923. *Heliotherapy.* London: Frowde and Hodder & Stoughton.

Rosendorff, Alexander. 1964. *Neue Erkenntnisse in der Naturbehandlung (New Knowledge in Nature Cure Treatments).* Bietigheim: Turm-Verlag.

Roth, Julius. 1976. *Health Purifiers and Their Enemies: A Study of the Natural Health Movement in the United States with a Comparison to Its Counterpart in Germany.* New York: Prodist.

Rothschuh, Karl E. 1983. *Naturheilbewegung, Reformbewegung, Alternativbewegung (Nature Cure Movement, Reform Movement, Alternative Movement).* Stuttgart: Hippokrates.

Rousseau, Jean-Jacques.1979. *Emil or Education.* Translation & Notes by Allan Bloom. New York: Basic Books.

Rumfitt, Albert. 1963. "Stanley Lief: Some Personal Tributes." *Health for All* 37:601.

Saine, André. 1982. Hydrotherapy lecture. NCNM. 8 Dec. Audiotape.

———. 1983. "Constitutional Food Intolerance." NCNM. Audiotape.

———. 1983. Hydrotherapy lecture. NCNM. 29 Aug. Audiotape.

———. 1985. Hydrotherapy lecture. NCNM. 5 May. Audiotape.

Schaefer, H. 1982. "So sollt ihr leben!: Kneipp und die moderne Medicine (Thus Shalt Thou Live!: Kneipp and Modern Medicine)." *Ärztezeitschrift für Naturheilverfahren* 23:677-684.

Schicke, Harald. 1985. "Heilen ist Reinigen: Die Ganzheitstherapie nach Pastor Felke (Healing is Cleansing: The Wholistic Therapy according to Pastor Felke)." *Heilpraxis Magazin* 3:4-13.

Schieferdecker, Charles. 1844. *Vincent Priessnitz.* Philadephia: Schieferdecker.

Schimmel, Klaus. 1983. "Zur Geschichte des Zentralverbandes der Ärzte für Naturheilverfahren (About the History of the Union of Physicians for Nature Cure Methods)." *Ärztezeitschrift für Naturheilverfahhren.* 24:463-471.

Schlau, Günter. 1963. *Die Felke-Jungbornkur* (The Felke-Jungborn Cure). Gelnhausen: Schwab.

Schmid, Ronald. 1978. *Dr. John Bastyr on Botanical Medicine and the Heart.* Notes from OANP lecture. 23 June.

Schmidtbauer, Matthäus. 1890. "Mediciner-Zunfthunger (Medical Monopoly)." *Zeitschrift für Eziehung und Unterricht (A Hygienic School and Family Magazine*—Austria) 4:72-74.

———. 1892. "Meine diesjährige Ferienreise (My Vacation Trip in This Year)." *Zeitschrift für Erziehung und Unterricht* 6:227-230.

———. 1897. "Kuhne in Leipzig und die Seinen (Kuhne in Leipzig and His Cronies)." *Zeitschrift für Erziehung und Unterricht* 11:41-50.

———. 1902. "Arnold Rikli (In Honor of His 80th Birthday)."*Zeitschrift für Erziehung und Unterricht* 16:65-67.

———. 1903. "Veldes und Riklis Heilanstalt (Veldes and Rikli's Nature Cure Establishment)." *Zeitschrift für Erziehung und Unterricht* 17:122-123.

———. 1905. "Dr. Lahmann ist tot (Dr. Lahmann Died)." *Zeitschrift für Erziehung und Unterricht* 19:125-126.

———. 1906. "Arnold Rikli" (obituary). *Zeitschrift für Erziehung und Unterricht* 20:126-130.

Scholz, Hugo. 1976. *Zuflucht bei Johann Schroth: Die grosse Heilung (Refuge at Johann Schroth: The Great Cure).* Kempten: Allgäuer Zeitungsverlag.

———. 1978. *Heilendes Wasser: Lebensroman des "Wasserdoktors" Vinzenz Priessnitz (Healing Water: Biographical Novel about the "Water Doctor" Vincent Priessnitz).* Graz/Stuttgart: Stocker.

Schomburg, Eberhard. 1981. *Sebastian Kneipp.* 4th ed. Bad Wörishofen: Kneipp-Verlag.

Schönenberger, Franz. 1906. *Lebenskunst—Heilkunst (Art of Living—Art of Healing).* Zwickau Sa.: Förster & Borries. (Later edition under the title *Der Naturarzt (The Nature Doctor).*

———. 1924. "Ernst Schweninger."*Der Naturarzt* 52 (no.3/4): 13-16.

———. 1930. "Neuherausgabe von Prof. Schönenbergers 'Der Naturarzt' (New Edition of Prof. Schönenberger's 'The Nature Doctor')." *Der Naturarzt* 58 (8):205-207.

———. 1931. "Worte von Vincent Priessnitz (Words of Vincent Priessnitz)."*Der Naturarzt* 59:3-4, 46-48.

———. 1931. "Priessnitz und das Luftbad" (Priessnitz and the Air Bath)." *Der Naturarzt* 59:136-138.

———. 1931. "Priessnitz und Kneipp (Priessnitz and Kneipp)." *Der Naturarzt* 59:172-173, 260-261.

"Schools of Chiropractic and of Naturopathy in the United States: Report of Inspections." 1928. *JAMA* 90:1733-1738.

Schweninger, Ernst. 1893. "Badekuren (Spa Cures)." Der Naturarzt 21 (6): 211-218.

———. 1926. *Der Arzt (The Physician).* 2nd ed. Radeburg/Dresden: Madaus (1st ed. Frankfurt/Main: Rütten & Loening, 1906).

Scott, Leo. 1989. Personal communication. 27 Aug.

———. 1992. Personal communication. 15 July.

Selige, Adolphe. 1919. "Some Day." *HHN* 24:476.

Sensenig, James S. 1991. Speech before the North American Convention of Naturopathic Physicians on September 4, Whistler, B.C.

Shaw, J. Austin. 1911. "Austin Shaw Explains Yungborn Nature Cure." *NHH* 16:145-155.

Shelton, Herbert W. 1949. "Keeping Naturopathy's Record Straight." *Dr. Shelton's Hygienic Review* 11:88-91.

———. 1968. *Natural Hygiene: Man's Pristine Way of Life.* San Antonio: Dr. Shelton's Health School, 1968.

Shew, Joel. 1849. *The Water Cure Manual.* New York: Fowlers and Wells.

———. 1850. *Hydropathy.* New York: Fowlers and Wells.

Smethurst, Thomas. 1843. *Hydrotherapia or The Water Cure . . . Founded on Observations and Experiences Made at Grafenberg . . . and the System There, as Practised by Vincent Priessnitz.* London: Snow.

Shmid L. 1952. "Does Fasting Cure Peptic Ulcer?" *Journal of the American Naturopathic Physicians and Surgeons Association* 5(9):9, 17-18.

Sommer, W. 1925. "Die Naturheilkunde in Amerika (Nature Cure in America)." *Der Naturarzt* 53:316-317.

Spaulding, Frank G. 1956. "New College Organized." *Journal of the AANP* 9(3):6.

Spencer, Charles. 1992. Personal communication with Jean Edwards concerning Stanley Lief. 18. 05.

Spitler, Harry Riley. 1948. (Ed.). *Basic Naturopathy.* Des Moines: American Naturopathic Association.

Strassburg, Lothar. 1979. "Geschichte der Naturheillkunde im Selbsterlebnis (History of Nature Cure Experienced by Myself)."*Der Naturarzt* 101 (7) 4-5 & 101 (8) 4-5.

Stroebele, Louisa. 1899. "Mountain Air Resort 'Bellevue' Butler, N.J." *AKB* 4:141.

Theegarten, Werner. 1986. "Pastor Felke und die Augendiagnose" (Pastor Felke and the Eye Diagnosis). *Heilpraxis Magazin* 4:14-17.

Thomson, C. Leslie. N.D. *But is it Nature Cure?* (Pamphlet). Edinburgh: Kingston Clinic.

———. *Kingston—the Place.* Pamphlet. Edinburgh: Kingston Clinic.

———. *The Naturopathic Approach.* Pamphlet. Edinburgh: Kingston Clinic.

———. 1965. *The Healing Crisis.* Revised ed. Edinburgh: Thomson-Kingston Publications.

———. 1967. "45 Years of the E. S. N. T. (Edinburgh School of Natural Therapeutics)." *Kingston Chronicle* July/August:9-15.

———. 1970. *Water and Nature Cure.* Revised ed. Edinburgh: Thomson-Kingston Publications.

———. 1987. *James C. Thomson: Pioneer Naturopath 1887-1960.* Edinburgh: Thomson-Kingston Publications (Reprinted from the *Kingston Chronicle,* May 1960).

Thomson, James C. 1938. *A New Approach to Cancer.* London: Thorsons.

———. 1939. *The Heart: The Prevention and Cure of Cardiac Conditions.* London: Thorsons.

———. 1950. *The Belfast Lecture: The Way to High Level Health.* Edinburgh: Thomson-Kingston Publications.

———. 1953. *Nature Cure from the Inside.* Edinburgh: Kingston Clinic.

———. 1954. *Two Health Problems: Constipation and Civilisation.* London: Thorsons.

———. 1960. *Toward High Level Health.* Edinburgh: Kingston Clinic.

———. and C. Leslie Thomson. 1970. *A Revised Introduction to Nature Cure.* Edinburgh: Thomson-Kingston Publications.

Thomson, Jessie R. 1952. *Healthy Childhood.* London: Thorsons.

Traub, Michael. 1993. "Wade Francis Boyle, ND: In Memoriam." *The Naturopathic Physician* 8(4):23.

Turner, E. S. 1967. *Taking the Cure.* London: Michael Joseph.

Turner, Roger Newman. 1984. *Naturopathic Medicine: Treating the Whole Person.* Wellingborough, U.K.: Thorsons.

Turska, William A. 1976. "Drugless Physician—A Misnomer?" *Naturopathic Student News* 2:5.

———. 1984. *Thumb-Nail Review of Naturopathic Medicine.* Portland: National College of Naturopathic Medicine.

University of Utah. 1958. The Bureau of Economic and Business Research. *Survey of Naturopathic Schools: Prepared for the Utah State Medical Association.*

Utah Legislative Council Staff. 1958. *A Study of the Healing Arts with Particular Emphasis upon Naturopathy: A Report to the Utah Legislative Council.*

Verus, Justus. 1897. *Vater Kneipp: Sein Leben und sein Wirken (Father Kneipp: His Life and His Work).* Kempten: Kösel.

Vom Walde, Philo. 1898. *Vincent Priessnitz: Sein Leben und Wirken—Zur Gedenkfeier seines hundertsten Geburtstages (Vincent Priessnitz: His Life and Work—at the Occasion of his Hundredth Birthday).* Berlin: Möller.

Wardrip, Diane. 1989. Personal interview by Alma Howard. JBCNM. 3 April.

Wardwell, Walter I. 1992. *Chiropractic: History and Evolution of a New Profession.* St. Louis: Mosby-Year Book.

Weil, Andrew. 1988. *Health and Healing.* Revised and Updated. New York: Houghton Mifflin.

———. 1990. *Natural Health, Natural Medicine: A Comprehensive Manual for Wellness and Self-Care.* Boston: Houghton Mifflin.

Weiss, Harry B. & Howard R. Kemble. 1967. *The Great American Water Cure Craze: A History of Hydropathy in the United States.* Trenton, N.J.: The Past Time Press.

Weiss, J. 1849. *Handbook of Hydrotherapy.* Philadephia

Weiss, Rudolf Fritz. 1988. *Herbal Medicine.* Beaconsfield: Beaconsfield Publishers.

Wendel, Paul. 1947. *Father Kneipp's Health Teachings.* Brooklyn: Published by the author.

———. 1951. *Standardized Naturopathy.* Brooklyn: Published by the author.

Werbach, Melvyn R. 1986. *Third Line Medicine.* New York: Arkana.

White, Arthur. 1992. *Lief, Stanley 1892-1963.* Personal communication with Jean Edwards 11.05.

Whorton, James C. 1982.*Crusaders for Fitness: The History of American Health Reformers.* Princeton, N.J. : Princeton University Press.

———. 1984. *The Hippocrates Diet and Health Program.* Wayne: N.J.: Avery.

Winsch, Wilhelm. 1940. *Über Wärmekultur (About Heat Culture).* 7th edition. Berlin: Verlag Lebenskunst-Heilkunst.

Winternitz, L. 1909. "Is Kneipp's Hydrotherapeutic Treatment Unscientific?" *N* 32:59-66.

Wolf, Friedrich. 1929. *Die Natur als Arzt und Helfer: Das neue naturärztlihe Hausbuch (Nature as Doctor and Helper: The New Nature Cure Book for the Home).* Stuttgart: Deutsche Verlagsanstalt.

Wolf, Josef, and Ludwig Burghardt. 1965. *Ein Bauerndorf wird Weltbad: Sebastian Kneipp und sein Wörishofen (A Village Becomes World Spa: Sebastian Kneipp and His Wörishofen).* Bad Wörishofen: Geyer.

Wood, John H. G. 1963. "In Memoriam: Stanley Lief 1892-1963." *Health for All* 37:600-602.

Wood, Matthew. 1992. *The Magical Staff: The Vitalist Tradition in Western Medicine.* Berkeley, Calif.: North Atlantic Books.

Wright, Jonathan V. 1987. *Return to the Memory: What is a Naturopathic Physician? Compiled Thoughts of 48 Clinicians.* Kent, Wash.: Meridian Valley Clinical Laboratory, 1987.

Yearbook of the International Society of Naturopathic Physicians and of Emerson University Research Council. 1945. Los Angeles: Schramm.

Useful Contacts

The American Association of Naturopathic Physicians
3201 New Mexico Ave., NW Suite 350
Washington, DC 20016
USA
866-538-2267
www.naturopathic.org

National College of Naturopathic Medicine
049 SW Porter Street
Portland, OR 97201
USA
503-552-1555
www.ncnm.edu

Bastyr University
14500 Juanita Dr., NE
Kenmore, WA 98028
USA
425-823-1300
www.bastyr.edu

Southwest College of Naturopathic Medicine
2140 East Broadway Rd.
Tempe, AZ 85282
USA
480-858-9100
www.scnm.edu

University of Bridgeport
College of Naturopathic Medicine
60 Lafayette Street
Bridgeport, CT 06604
USA
203-576-4108
www.bridgeport.edu/pages/3240.asp

Canadian College of Naturopathic Medicine
1255 Sheppard Ave. E
Toronto, ON M2K 1E2
Canada
866-241-2266
www.ccnm.edu

Index

I

O

P

T

U

V

W

Y

Z

ABOUT THE AUTHORS

Wade Boyle, N.D. graduated from the National College of Naturopathic Medicine in Portland, Oregon. He taught at National College and at the Canadian College of Naturopathic Medicine in Toronto, and was a continuing education instructor for the American Association of Naturopathic Physicians (AANP). He authored two books on the history of botanical medicine, *Herb Doctors* and *Official Herbs*, and co-authored *Lectures in Naturopathic Hydrotherapy*. He maintained a private practice in Evans City, Pennsylvania and East Palestine, Ohio until his death in 1993.

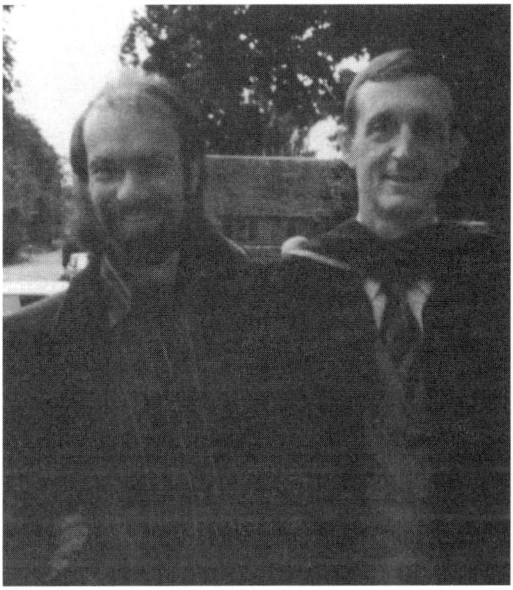

Friedhelm Kirchfeld and Wade Boyle at Boyle's graduation from National College of Naturopathic Medicine

Friedhelm Kirchfeld, M. L. S. is a graduate of the University of Denver. He was hired as a librarian by the National College of Naturopathic Medicine in Portland in 1978 to develop this country's first naturopathic college library. As a native of Germany he also had access to the German sources used in Nature Doctors.

Ronald L. Johnson is a Portland editor and writer who was educated at University of California, Santa Cruz, and University of Oregon.

Howard Asinoff, N.D. is a 1992 graduate of the National College of Naturopathic Medicine who received his premedical training in New York.